Nursing Diagnosis and Process

in Psychiatric Mental Health Nursing

Nursing Diagnoses and Process
in Psychiatric Mental Health Nursing

Third Edition

Gertrude K. McFarland, RN, DNSc, FAAN

Health Scientist Administrator
Nursing Research Study Section
Division of Research Grants
National Institutes of Health
U.S. Department of Health and Human Services
Bethesda, Maryland

Evelyn Wasli, RN, DNSc

Chief Nurse
Emergency Psychiatric Response Division
Community Mental Health Services
D.C. Commission of Mental Health Services
Washington, DC

Elizabeth Kelchner Gerety, MS, RN, CS, FAAN

Clinical Nurse Specialist, Psychiatry
Psychiatry Consultation Service
Portland Veterans Affairs Medical Center
Instructor, Department of Mental Health Nursing
School of Nursing
Oregon Health Sciences University
Portland, Oregon

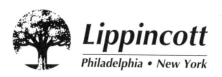

Lippincott

Philadelphia • New York

Acquisitions Editor: Margaret Zuccarini　　*Production Coordinator: Nannette Winski*
Sponsoring Editor: Emily Cotlier　　　　　*Design Coordinator: Melissa Olson*
Project Editor: Tom Gibbons　　　　　　　*Indexer: Lynne Mahan*
Production Manager: Helen Ewan

Third Edition

Library of Congress Cataloging in Publications Data

McFarland, Gertrude K., 1941–
　　Nursing diagnoses and process in psychiatric mental health nursing
　/ by Gertrude K. McFarland, Evelyn Wasli, Elizabeth Kelchner Gerety.
　—3rd ed.
　　　p.　cm.
　　Includes bibliographical references and index.
　　ISBN 0-397-55317-X (alk. paper)
　　1. Psychiatric nursing.　2. Nursing diagnosis.　I. Wasli, Evelyn L.
II. Gerety, Elizabeth Kelchner.　III. Title.
　　[DNLM:　1. Psychiatric Nursing—methods—outlines.　2. Mental
Disorders—nursing—outlines.　3. Nursing Process—outlines.
WY 18.2 M4777n　1997]
RC440.M32　1997
616.89′075—dc20
DNLM/DLC
for Library of Congress　　　　　　　　　　　　　96-41727
　　　　　　　　　　　　　　　　　　　　　　　　　CIP

Care has been taken to confirm the accuracy of the information presented and to describe generally accepted practices. However, the authors, editors, and publisher are not responsible for errors or omissions or for any consequences from application of the information in this book and make no warranty, express or implied, with respect to the contents of the publication.

The authors, editors and publisher have exerted every effort to ensure that drug selection and dosage set forth in this text are in accordance with current recommendations and practice at the time of publication. However, in view of ongoing research, changes in government regulations, and the constant flow of information relating to drug therapy and drug reactions, the reader is urged to check the package insert for each drug for any change in indications and dosage and for added warnings and precautions. This is particularly important when the recommended agent is a new or infrequently employed drug.

Some drugs and medical devices presented in this publication have Food and Drug Administration (FDA) clearance for limited use in restricted research settings. It is the responsibility of the health care provider to ascertain the FDA status of each drug or device planned for use in their clinical practice.

The opinions expressed herein are those of the authors and do not necessarily reflect those of the U.S. Department of Health and Human Services, the National Institutes of Health, or the Department of Veterans Affairs.

9 8 7 6 5 4 3 2 1

CONTRIBUTORS AND CONSULTANTS

Suzanne Beverlee Millar, PharmD
Clinical Pharmacist Specialist
Portland Veterans Affairs Medical Center
Portland, Oregon

Assistant Professor of Clinical Pharmacology
Oregon State University, College of Pharmacy
Corvallis, Oregon

David Morrison Smith, MD
Psychiatrist
Mental Health Division
Portland Veterans Affairs Medical Center
Portland, Oregon

PREFACE

While practicing in an era of health care reform and cost containment, every nurse has the goal of providing the highest quality nursing care possible. *Nursing Diagnoses and Process in Psychiatric Mental Health Nursing* 3/E contains the concepts and principles essential to providing the highest quality nursing care for clients who have behavioral problems. Easy-to-access content is presented in a handy pocket-sized format, so that nurses can be guided in caring for the client who is experiencing behavioral or mental health problems, wherever care is being given.

The third edition is organized into two major parts. Part One presents an overview of mental health care and psychiatric nursing. The authors have thoroughly updated the five chapters in this part. They have expertly summarized necessary information to support the basic understanding of mental health and mental illness. They have summarized and presented the necessary information to support the provision of quality psychiatric mental health nursing care.

This includes:

- the major schools of psychiatric thought
- techniques and concepts useful in developing the therapeutic nurse–patient relationship and in facilitating therapeutic communication
- the nursing process
- a systems theory–based conceptual model for the practice of psychiatric nursing
- a biopsychosocial assessment guide
- the components of conducting a mental status examination
- nursing interventions
- psychopharmacology

The chapter on psychopharmacology has been thoroughly updated and expanded to include the latest information on drug therapy for mental disorders. The chapter on major nursing interventions has been fully updated and expanded to include an appropriate range of interventions, including abuse protection, contracting, crisis intervention, decision making, discharge planning, family and client education, group treatment, protective interventions (activity area restriction, observation for suicide, seclusion, restraints, seizure management), social skills training, stress management, and supportive therapy—offering hope.

Part Two presents 15 chapters covering the nursing interventions and process for the major psychiatric disorders.

▌ DSM-IV Organization and Content

Based on input from many of you, the authors have completely reorganized this part of the text to make it easier to access information on the major psychiatric disorders identified in the DSM-IV. Chapters focus on the major psychiatric disorders—Delirium, Dementia, Amnestic, and Other Cognitive Disorders; Mental Disorders Due to a General Medical Condition; Substance-Related Disorders; Schizophrenia and Other Psychotic Disorders; Mood Disorders; Anxiety Disorders; Somatoform Disorders; Factitious Disorders; Dissociative Disorders; Sexual and Gender Identity Disorders; Eating Disorders; Sleep Disorders; Impulse Control Disorders; Adjustment Disorders; and Personality Disorders. Content in each chapter addresses definition/major symptoms; definition/major symptoms of selected major categories; incidence; course; contributing factors; laboratory and physical examination findings; special assessment considerations; and treatment.

▌ Nursing Content

Nursing care is strongly emphasized for each major psychiatric disorder by sections on commonly occurring nursing diagnoses, selective nursing diagnoses, outcome criteria, and nursing interventions with rationale. For each major psychiatric disorder, the authors have selected the most current and relevant North American Nursing Diagnoses Association (NANDA) nursing diagnoses.

▋Features and Benefits

- Easy-to-access information in a pocket-sized book maximizes clinical applicability of psychiatric nursing information.
- DSM-IV organization provides a brief description, laboratory findings, assessment, and medical treatment for frequently encountered psychiatric diagnosis.
- Consistent chapter format, presentation of content, and clear bold headings promote access to information in any setting.
- Commonly occurring nursing diagnoses and related nursing interventions enable students to grasp a complete, current, and accurate picture of nursing management of psychiatric disorders.
- Rationale for nursing interventions enables students to plan and implement sound nursing care.
- Outcome-based care consistent with the desired goals of current health care reimbursement agencies focuses nursing care on achieving a specific outcome, consistent with goals of current health care practice and reimbursement policies.
- Documented content and complete chapter reference lists provided at the end of the book present the reader with current resources for further reading and knowledge development.

The authors envision that as the NANDA and other nursing diagnoses continue to be tested and utilized in clinical practice, additional knowledge will be generated that will provide input to the ongoing development work. In addition, nurses are encouraged to continue to identify and develop major nursing interventions and build upon the present knowledge base.

ACKNOWLEDGEMENT

The authors wish to acknowledge their families—Al McFarland, Emma Ramseier, and the late John Ramseier; Arne Wasli and sons Kevin and Eric; and Dick Gerety, Danica Kelchner, and the late John Kelchner, for their general encouragement in life and/or patience during the preparation of this project. Our appreciation is also extended to all those nurses who are working to identify, develop, clinically utilize, and research nursing diagnoses and nursing interventions.

CONTENTS

CHAPTER **7**

Mental Disorders Due to a General Medical Condition 177

CHAPTER **8**

Substance-Related Disorders 185

CHAPTER **9**

Schizophrenia and Other Psychotic Disorders 217

CHAPTER **13**

Factitious Disorders   305

CHAPTER **14**

Dissociative Disorders   315

CHAPTER **15**
Sexual and Gender Identity Disorders 325

CHAPTER **16**
Eating Disorders 342

CHAPTER **17**
Sleep Disorders 359

CHAPTER **20**

Personality Disorders 401

OVERVIEW OF MENTAL HEALTH CARE AND PSYCHIATRIC NURSING

CHAPTER 1

Contemporary Mental Health/Psychiatric Nursing Practice

■ Major Views of Mental Health and Mental Illness*

Mental health is characterized by the client's ability to modify behavior and engage in a dynamic and successful adaptation process between his or her needs and desires and community and environmental expectations.[53]

Mental health—"A state of being, relative rather than absolute. The best indices of mental health are simultaneous success at working, loving and creating with the capacity for mature and flexible resolution of conflicts between instincts, conscience, important other people, and reality."[69]

Jahoda's six cardinal aspects of mental health—These aspects include a positive attitude toward self, active growth and development toward self-actualization, integration, autonomy and independence from social influences, accurate perception of reality, and environmental mastery.[24]

Roger's process of self-actualization—The person engaging in the process exhibits openness to experience, lack of defensiveness, accuracy in symbolization, congruency, flexibility, unconditional self-regard, creative adaptation, effective reality testing, and harmony with others.[48-51]

*References 1–72

Maslow's view of health—The achievement of self-actualization, including an understanding of self and reality, the expression of emotionality and spontaneity, and the achievement of life goals.[42]

Mental illness—Characterized by maladaptive behavior that is a product of disordered body processes, disordered psychological functions, and/or a disordered social environment.[53]

Mental illness—"An illness with psychologic or behavioral manifestations and/or impairment in functioning due to a social, psychologic, genetic, physical/chemical or biologic disturbance. The disorder is not limited to relations between people and society. The illness is characterized by symptoms and/or impairment in functioning."[61] Some common indicators of mental illness are depression, feelings of anxiety that are not proportionate to a possible cause, physical complaints without medical condition, any sudden change of behavior or mood, unreasonable and unrealistic expectations of self or others, and failure to achieve potential.

▌ Selected Trends and Issues in Psychiatric Mental Health Nursing Practice and Mental Health Services*

Mental Health Needs and Care Are in Transition

- The current "Decade of the Brain" gives psychiatric nurses the opportunity to support a genuine biopsychosocial synthesis and approach to care. "Psychiatric nursing, like psychiatry, has returned to an era where the bio is a focus of investigation in the search for an etiology of mental disorders."[43]

- Deinstitutionalization of state mental hospitals, begun in 1955, was stimulated by such developments as the Community Mental Health Care Centers Act in 1963, Aid to the Disabled/Supplemental Security Income/Social Security Disability Insurance legislation, and change in commitment laws.

- Deinstitutionalization has resulted in an 80% reduction in public mental hospital beds while there has been a

*References 12–13,23,28,33–35,39,40–41,43,46,55–57,60,66

90% increase in mental health admissions due to high recidivism rates, increased use of community emergency services by acutely disturbed persons, and increased admissions to general hospital psychiatric units.

- Growth in the mentally ill homeless population continues. Estimates of the prevalence of illness vary (e.g., 25% to 50% psychosis, 33% to 50% alcoholism); support systems for the mentally ill homeless are often lacking; an adequate shift of expenditures for mental health care services to community-based services from state hospital expenditures has not occurred; adequate retraining and redeployment of personnel from state hospital staffs has not occurred.[41]

- Cost-containment pressures are leading to changes in health care delivery models, e.g., emphasis on managed care with increased focus on ambulatory care and decreased focus on institutional services. Nurses can play an essential role in coordinating care, allocating resources efficiently, documenting outcomes of care, and documenting the cost-effectiveness of nursing care.[35]

- Inpatient facilities are still undergoing downsizing.

- Length of inpatient stay has been reduced.

- Care is now provided to only the most acutely ill psychiatric clients in inpatient facilities.

- Violence and safety can be issues in current work environments.

- "For-profit" psychiatric hospitals are more common.

- Psychiatric nurses may sometimes encounter ideological tensions between professional and ethical values and the market-oriented mental health care system.

- Primary care (clinics—primary care, community health, school health or pediatric offices) is sought more often than mental health care by vulnerable populations, e.g., the young, elderly, homeless, clients with substance abuse problems, and impoverished persons.

- Primary care providers need appropriate training in order to make appropriate mental health referrals.

- New models of mental health care delivery are being sought; nurses advocate for the following mental health care services/benefits: consumer choice; accessibility to a wide range of mental health care services; equality of mental health care benefits with benefits for general health care; cost-effective mental health care, including facility care and continuous biopsychosocial outpatient care; organized not-for-profit models that specialize in the care of the severely mentally ill.[41]

- Hospital case management used for psychiatric diagnoses can reduce fragmentation, promote collaboration, streamline resources and care, and enhance access to services.
- Critical pathways tools can be used to manage care to achieve expected outcomes within appropriate length of stay.
- Psychiatric home care nursing is a cost-effective alternative to inpatient care.
- Psychosocial rehabilitation can be used to facilitate persons with mental health problems to function optimally in the community.
- Health status, risk reduction, and protection objectives are stressed in Healthy People 2000.[12]
- Community mental health (CMH) is care with an emphasis on health promotion/disease prevention, smooth transitions and continuity in care, client and family involvement in care, education of communities about CMH goals, identification of residential alternatives, and enhancement of job-training opportunities.

Primary Mental Health Care Model

- Mental health services are designed to promote optimal mental health, prevent mental illness, maintain mental health, and manage mental health problems prior to or during client's first contacts with the mental health care delivery system.
- Universal preventive interventions are targeted at whole population groups.
- Selective preventive interventions are targeted at subgroups or individuals at risk for mental health problems.
- Treatment or management interventions are designed to identify mental health problems early, reduce the duration of the problem, decrease severity of progression, and prevent relapse.
- Maintenance interventions provide coordinated management of mental health problems faced by clients with chronic mental illness.

- Interventions promote and maintain general physical health.
- Advanced practice psychiatric mental health nurses, e.g., clinical nurse specialists and psychiatric nurse practitioners, play a key role in the Primary Mental Health Care Model by providing home care services; individual, family, and group psychotherapy; counseling and crisis intervention; psychobiological interventions; case management; milieu therapy; and in consultation-liaison roles.

Strategies of Psychiatric Mental Health Nurses in Health Care Debate*

Strategies used by psychiatric mental health nurses to influence policy and to actively participate in the current health care debate and change include the following: proactively managing change effectively; actively participating in committees focusing on issues related to mental health/illness; assuming leadership positions in organizations relevant to mental health care; becoming advocates of quality psychiatric nursing care; identifying ways to document clinical outcomes of quality psychiatric nursing care; facilitating clients to become empowered and to overcome the stigma that may be associated with mental illness; publicly recognizing psychiatric nurses in leadership positions; becoming active politically in order to influence mental health care and services; actively promoting such national efforts at improving mental health care research as The National Plan for Research on Child and Adolescent Mental Disorders launched by the National Institute of Mental Health; actively defining nursing practice and developing models of nursing care that incorporate both physical and psychosocial aspects; incorporating physical assessment skills into clinical practice; and focusing on current issues such as women's health, managed care, case management, and prescriptive authority.

Objectives of the American Academy of Nursing†

Objectives outlined by the American Academy of Nursing that all professional nurses support include the following:[23]

*References 56,57
†Reference 23

   Accessibility of health care services regardless of the
      ability to pay
   Comprehensive health care coverage that takes into
      account changing disease processes; care of the
      elderly, the mentally ill, and other vulnerable popula-
      tions; and delivery of care in the most appropriate and
      cost-effective setting
   Availability of preventive, specialized, and emergency
      care services to rural populations
   Cost management through managed care, planning, pre-
      ventive care, research on clinical outcomes, and
      reduction of unnecessary administrative expenditures
   Use of a cost-effective and efficient mix of providers
   Increased focus on preventive care
   Use of the most appropriate therapy in the best setting
   Reduction in administrative costs

Predictions for the Future[*]

Predictions for the future of psychiatric mental health
nursing include:

   Increasing emphasis on epidemiology and public health
   Increasing focus on case management and mental health
      managed care
   Increasing focus on comprehensive assessment
   Increasing emphasis on health promotion/disease pre-
      vention interventions across settings
   Increasing collaboration and participation with other
      disciplines in an integrated mental health team

Needs to Be Addressed

There remains a need to conduct research in the areas of
mental health promotion/mental illness prevention, psychiatric mental health nursing care and clinical outcomes, and
cost effectiveness of psychiatric and mental health nursing
care.

   There is a need to facilitate undergraduate and graduate
professional nursing curriculum changes to incorporate
new content so that graduates are culturally competent,
can manage change, can engage consumers as active par-

[*]References 56,57

ticipants in care, can negotiate complex systems, are knowledgeable about community-based models of care, possess critical thinking skills, possess management skills, and have competency in psychopharmacology and neuroscience. "In the future, psychiatric nurses will need to know normal neuroanatomy, physiology, psychoneuroendocrinology, and immunology to understand deviations occurring with mental disorders."[43]

▌ Concepts of Mental Health and Mental Illness

Neurobiological Approach*

This approach emphasizes a scientific approach to the study of the nervous system, to explain and treat mental disorders. *Illness* is defined as a disturbance in the neurobiological system.

A. Theoretical basis: genetics.
　　1. Family risk, twin, and adoption studies have found increased risk for relatives of persons with mental illness.
　　2. See also discussion in chapters on major psychiatric disorders.
B. Theoretical basis: neurotransmitters
　　1. Each neuron receives information through its many dendrites from thousands of other axons of neurons. Consequently, each neuron sends messages by its network of axons. The gap between the axon of one neuron and the dendrite of another neuron is the synapse; the transaction occurring is the synaptic transmission.
　　2. Chemical substances called neurotransmitters are active in the synapse. The neurotransmitter is released from the endings of the axon. Other neurons are specifically sensitive to the neurotransmitter and respond via membrane receptors. These receptors are the target of psychoactive drugs.
　　3. The transmitters produce an excitatory or inhibitory effect at the synapse. One neuron has many synapses, with excitatory forces firing the neuron and inhibitory forces decreasing the firing. An imbal-

*References 1–72

ance of these forces may be related to aggressiveness, rage, or lethargy.

4. Thousands of these chemical reactions are occurring at any one time and are the biological basis for thinking and feeling.

5. Characteristics of the neurotransmitter are:
   a. synthesis and storage of substance in neuron;
   b. release of substance upon depolarization of neuron;
   c. neurotransmitter is physiologically active on specialized receptors;
   d. termination of activity by enzymes and uptake process.

6. The cell bodies of neurons containing certain transmitters—norepinephrine, dopamine, serotonin, gamma-aminobutyric acid (GABA), glutamate and others—have been located in brain stem, and their pathways extending to the brain and spinal cord have been identified by histochemical fluorescence method. Further study of the pathways or tracts will explain seemingly unrelated symptoms.

7. Selected neurotransmitters:
   a. *Dopamine.* Tracts are found in the substantia nigra, hypothalamus, neocortex, and limbic system. Overactivity of the dopaminergic system (tracts and receptors at synapses) is associated with Schizophrenia and Mood Disorders.
   b. *Norepinephrine and epinephrine.* Tracts are found mostly in the pons with pathways to the brain stem, limbic system, thalamus, hypothalamus, and spinal cord. Tricyclic antidepressant and monoamine oxidase inhibitor effects have been related to this system.
   c. *Serotonin.* Tracts are found in pons and midbrain with pathways to basal ganglia, limbic system, cerebral cortex, and spinal cord. Decreased concentrations of serotonin in the synapse have been associated with Schizophrenia, Mood Disorders, Anxiety Disorders, and episodes of violence.
   d. *Acetylcholine* (produced at the cholinergic synapse). Tracts are found in nucleus basalis with pathways to the cerebral cortex, limbic system, thalamus, and hypothalamus. Dementia has been

associated with degeneration of these neurons. Disruption in the physiology of the cholinergic system has been associated with movement disorders, e.g., the parkinsonian side effects of antipsychotics.

   e. GABA is the main inhibitory neurotransmitter and GABA receptors are the principal site of action of benzodiazepines, barbiturates, and anticonvulsants.

C. Diagnostic aids and therapy

Diagnostic aids such as computed tomography (CT) scans, electroencephalograms (EEGs), laboratory studies, radiographs, history of present illness, history of familial incidence of disorders, physical examination, and behavioral observations are used to determine the areas of dysfunction. Drugs that effect change in the neurobiological system are prescribed and changes are monitored. Genetic counseling is provided.

Stress–Adaptation Approach*

This method emphasizes the role of stress in the increased incidence of illness. Illness is viewed as a human reaction pattern to stress or maladaptation.

A. Theoretical basis

   1. Examples of risk factors that have been identified by various writers as being associated with the development of mental disorders are prematurity, poor diet, chromosomal disorders, accidents, and racial discrimination.

   2. Life events that are stressors and contribute to development of crises include death of a spouse, divorce, marital separation, and assuming the caregiver role. There remains controversy over how stress mechanisms affect a person. If a person receives adequate support, the risk of illness lessens.

   3. A crisis exists when a person is unable to cope with a threat and experiences an increase in anxiety, then tries other coping mechanisms and the problem is still not resolved. If the problem is not resolved, the anxiety increases and a variety of symptoms can emerge, e.g., suicidal and homicidal thoughts,

*References 1–72

somatic symptoms, confusion, depression, isolation, and nonproductivity. Crises can be divided into three groups: maturational (e.g., transition into retirement), situational (e.g., loss of a job), and adventitious (e.g., earthquake).

4. The competence of a person in adapting to crisis affects the adaptation process.
   a. A person makes a cognitive appraisal of the stressor. For example, a situation can be viewed as a challenge by one individual and as a catastrophe by another.
   b. Many coping behaviors, mechanisms, and strategies exist and are classified in various ways.
   c. Vaillant offers a hierarchy of ego defenses.[67,68]
      (1) Psychotic mechanisms: denial, distortion, delusional projection
      (2) Immature ego defenses: fantasy, projection, passive aggression, hypochondriasis, acting out
      (3) Neurotic ego defenses: intellectualization, repression, displacement, dissociation, reaction formation
      (4) Mature ego defenses: sublimation, altruism, suppression, humor, anticipation
5. The presence of social support assists a person in problem solving and offers sustenance during a crisis period.

B. Therapy
   The focus is on establishment of a working relationship with the client, problem identification and steps in resolution, support of coping strategies, enhancement of self-esteem, anticipatory guidance, and preventive interventions (e.g., assisting a mother in parenting techniques).

Psychodynamic Approach

This approach emphasizes the influences of intrapsychic forces on observable behavior. This approach and theoretical framework is now viewed as less important than 10 years ago: it is viewed as somewhat controversial because some view this theory as difficult to test. *Illness* is defined in terms of behavior disorders that originate in conflicts occurring before 6 years of age among the id, ego, super-ego, and/or environment. Anxiety is then experienced as a result of these conflicts. Excessive use of mental defense mechanisms leads to serious behavioral disturbances.

A. Theoretical basis[8,11,36–38,53]
   1. Freud is recognized as the founder of the psychoana-lytic school of thought.
   2. Psychic activity is influenced by two drives: sexual and aggressive.
   3. The psyche is divided into levels of consciousness:
      a. *Conscious*—The awareness of self and environ-ment that occurs when a person is awake
      b. *Preconscious*—Contains memories and thoughts that are easily recalled
      c. *Unconscious*—Contains memories and thoughts that ordinarily do not enter consciousness
   4. Structural aspects of the psyche are
      a. *Id*—The part containing instinctual drives and impulses. The ego and superego develop from the id.
         (1) *Pleasure principle*—The id seeks immediate release from tension or pleasure and avoids displeasure without regard for consequences.
         (2) *Primary process thinking*—Mental activity of the id is characterized by a collapse of time periods and by images mistaken for reality, occurring naturally in infants, during dreams, and in some mental illnesses.
      b. *Ego*—The part that assists the psyche in relating to the environment through such functions as memory and thinking and in resolving psyche conflicts. One of the more important functions is reality testing (the ego's function in sorting per-ceptions coming from the id and from the envi-ronment). Its primary growth period is 6 months to 3 years of age. It is the "I."
         (1) *Reality principle*—States that the ego tends to delay satisfaction by accommodation to situa-tional factors
         (2) *Secondary process thinking*—Mental activity of the ego characterized by reason, logic and dif-

ferentiating among people, situations, and things

   c. *Superego*—The part that evaluates thought and actions, rewarding the good and punishing the bad

5. *Anxiety*—An automatic response occurring when the psyche is flooded with uncontrollable stimulation

   a. *Signal anxiety or reality anxiety*—Type of anxiety produced by the ego in anticipation of danger, such as loss of a loved one or disapproval of superego

   b. *Moral anxiety*—Type of anxiety from overwhelming feelings of guilt or shame about an act or thought

   c. *Neurotic anxiety*—Type of anxiety in which impulses from the id, such as aggressive or sexual impulses, threaten to overpower the ego

B. Psychosexual stages of development

These stages are crucial because they are periods during which unconscious conflicts among id, ego, and superego develop. Fixation, or the arrest of development, may occur at any stage as a result of excessive gratification or deprivation.

1. *Oral stage* (birth to 1½ years)

   a. The infant obtains relief from biological and psychological tensions through his or her mouth and lips.

2. *Anal stage* (1½ to 3 years)

   a. The infant achieves control over the anal sphincter and then gives up some control as he or she experiences toilet training.

   b. The infant and the parents are involved in issues of control over defecation.

3. *Phallic stage* (3 to 6 years)

   a. Child experiences the genitals, particularly the penis, as the main source of pleasurable sensation and interest.

   b. Oedipus complex—Refers to the emotional attachment of a boy for the mother and ambivalent feelings toward the father.

   c. Electra complex—Describes a girl's wishes for penis of father and hopes to take the place of mother, whom she blames for not having penis.

   4. *Latency stage* (6 to 12 years)
      Child experiences a quiet period during which the sexual drive is dormant.
   5. *Genital stage* (12 years to adulthood)
      The person experiences onset of puberty, renewed interest in sexual activity, and conflicts that were unresolved in past developmental stages.
C. Defense mechanisms
   The following are mental processes used by the ego to reduce anxiety and conflict by modifying, distorting, or rejecting reality. The most frequently used defense mechanisms include:
   1. *Repression*—Response that keeps painful thoughts, feelings, and impulses from consciousness.
   2. *Denial*—Response that does not acknowledge awareness of a painful event.
   3. *Reaction formation*—Response that expresses feelings opposite to those being experienced.
   4. *Projection*—Response that ascribes the unacceptable thoughts and feelings to another person.
   5. *Rationalization*—Response that justifies behavior by an attempt to explain it logically.
   6. *Undoing*—Response that cancels the effect of another response just made.
   7. *Displacement*—Response that is misdirected from original person or object to a safer target.
   8. *Sublimation*—Response that partially substitutes socially acceptable activities for unacceptable impulses.
   9. *Regression*—Response that involves behaving at a level more appropriate to an earlier age.
   10. *Identification*—Response that involves acting and feeling in the same manner as a significant other.
   11. *Introjection*—Response that involves taking an aspect of behavior or thought of another into the ego structure.
   12. *Isolation*—Response that involves blocking the feeling associated with an unpleasant, threatening situation or thought.
   13. *Suppression*—Response that involves consciously and deliberately forcing certain ideas from thought and action.

D. Grouping of defense mechanisms[67,68]
   1. Psychotic mechanisms
      a. Denial of external reality
      b. Distortion of external reality
   2. Immature mechanisms
      a. Autistic fantasy
      b. Projection
      c. Dissociation
      d. Devaluation, idealization, splitting
      e. Passive-aggressive behavior
      f. Acting out
   3. Intermediate defenses
      a. Intellectualization
      b. Repression
      c. Reaction-formation
      d. Displacement
      e. Somatization
   4. Mature mechanisms
      a. Sublimation
      b. Altruism
      c. Suppression
      d. Humor
E. Therapy
   1. *Psychoanalysis* is an intense relationship with a psychoanalyst for a period of time for the purpose of helping the person establish conscious control over affect and behavior.
   2. Through dream analysis, free association, interpretation, analysis of resistance and *transference* (ascribing to the analyst the thoughts and feelings associated with parents or other important people), and neutrality, the analyst assists the patient in reducing the anxiety associated with thought.
   3. Conflicts are brought into awareness and thus resolved.

Interpersonal Approach[*]

This approach emphasizes the importance of interpersonal relationships and communication on behavior. *Behavior disorders* are a result of patterns of avoidance, use of substitutive processes, and experiences with significant adults.

[*]References 63–65

A. Theoretical basis
  1. Sullivan[63–65] is noted for interpersonal theory of psychiatry.
  2. *Satisfaction* is achieved through an interaction to obtain relief from tension from biological drives or needs.
  3. *Security* is achieved when basic needs are satisfied in relationship to a mothering person without the presence of anxiety.
  4. *Self system* develops from the dynamic interplay of the basic needs and the interpersonal process to achieve satisfaction and security and to avoid or decrease anxiety.
     a. Modes of experiencing describe one's perception and thoughts:
        (1) *Prototaxic mode*—Person identifies with the whole world; thoughts and responses are undifferentiated.
        (2) *Parataxic mode*—Person recognizes that things go together, but there is no logic. Things are put together only because one event occurs and is followed by another.
        (3) *Syntaxic mode*—Person is able to use logic in explaining events.
     b. Person appraises self through significant others' reactions and organizes the appraisals in terms of:
        (1) bad me—acts that result in anxiety
        (2) good me—acts that cause no anxiety
        (3) not me—acts that are totally disapproved; severe anxiety is experienced.
B. Stages of growth and development:
   These stages reflect the interpersonal approach.
  1. Infancy—Lasts until the appearance of speech, which enables infant to change environment
  2. Childhood—Lasts until emergence of need for peers
  3. Juvenile—Lasts until need for close relationship
  4. Preadolescence—Lasts until puberty and beginning interest in opposite sex
  5. Early adolescence—Lasts until development of relationships with opposite sex

  6. Late adolescence—Lasts until the establishment of a stable love relationship with another person

C. Anxiety
  1. First develops when infant experiences tension or insecurity of mother.
  2. Later it is experienced whenever a threat of disapproval from a significant person occurs.
  3. Avoidance behaviors develop to deal with anxiety:
   a. Physically avoiding the situation
   b. Changing the interaction in the situation
   c. Using selective inattention, which is the process the person employs to not attend to that which causes anxiety
   d. Using substitutive processes in which the person dissociates certain aspects of interpersonal system. The term *security operations* also is used to describe these processes; these are similar to the defense mechanisms described by Freud.

D. Therapy
  1. The therapist is a participant observer and not a neutral object.
  2. *Elucidation* is a principle that states that a behavior change can occur when one can identify, conceptualize and evaluate behavior.
  3. The focus of the interview is on exploring the avoidance behaviors, anxiety experiences, and the interpersonal context in which the avoidance behaviors and anxiety occur.

Ego Development Approach

This method emphasizes the development of ego identity throughout the life span; it was developed by Erikson.[15-19] *Illness* is characterized by problems with self, relationships, or society that may cause extension of the developmental period. Behavioral disorders result from unresolved conflicts during the stages of the life cycle.

A. Theoretical basis
  1. Human beings progress through a series of eight psychosocial developmental stages.

   2. The growth plan is governed by both social experiences and innate capacities—the epigenetic principle.
   3. In each developmental stage, the potential exists for the person to develop a new task that serves as a building block for subsequent stages. Physical and psychosocial hazards may thwart the person from achieving the task central to a given developmental stage. The lack of achievement of the task has a negative effect on subsequent developmental stages and may lead to maladaptive behavioral patterns.
B. Erikson's eight developmental stages[15–19]
   1. *Infancy* (birth to 18 months)
      a. During this stage, the infant learns to *trust* self and others, provided his or her needs have been met in a consistent and satisfying manner.
      b. Confidence, realistic trust, hope, optimism, and the ability to form relationships in later life stem from such an attitude of trust.
      c. When subject to hazards such as mistreatment, the infant may develop *mistrust* that is later reflected in hostility, suspiciousness, and a general feeling of dissatisfaction.
   2. *Early childhood* (18 months to 3 years)
      a. In this stage, *autonomy* results from reassuring, constructively guided experiences in which the child is allowed to exercise self-control of behavior without being subjected to experiences beyond the child's capabilities.
      b. The socially acceptable behaviors of holding and letting go, on which toilet training focuses during this stage, become generalized to other aspects of living.
      c. The development of autonomy leads to self-control without loss of self-esteem, a sense of pride and good will, the ability to initiate activities yet be cooperative, and appropriate generosity and withholding.
      d. Difficulties, such as external overcontrol, can lead to *shame and doubt* (i.e., feelings of being exposed, lack of a belief in being able to control one's life, and a lack of self-worth).
   3. *Late childhood* (3 to 5 years)

   a. The child develops *initiative,* the ability to under-
      take and plan tasks, the pleasure of being active,
      and the experience of a sense of purpose.
   b. Pleasure in attack and conquest aids in develop-
      ing sexual identity and roles.
   c. Initiative is controlled by a developing conscience.
      The person grows to develop and strives to utilize
      potentials in a socially appropriate manner.
   d. *Guilt,* accompanied by self-restriction and denial,
      can result from an unsuccessful negotiation of this
      stage. The person fails to develop potential.
4. *School age* (6 to 12 years)
   a. The major task is *industry,* characterized by
      involvement in the world, construction and plan-
      ning, development of relationships with peers,
      development of specific skills, and identification
      with admired others.
   b. A sense of competence and the pleasure of dili-
      gence develops.
   c. *Inferiority,* the feeling that one is unworthy and
      inadequate, can result from hindrances.
5. *Adolescence* (12 to 20 years)
   a. The developmental task is *identity,* a confident
      sense of self, commitment to a career, and finding
      one's place in society.
   b. Successful resolution leads to the ability to work
      toward long-term goals, self-esteem, and emo-
      tional stability.
   c. The danger is *role* confusion, characterized by
      feelings of confusion, lack of confidence, indeci-
      sion, alienation, and possibly acting-out behavior.
   d. Unsuccessful resolution may require the adult to
      spend life-long energies attempting to resolve
      remaining conflicts.
6. *Young adulthood* (18 to 25 years)
   a. *Intimacy* is the major developmental task. The per-
      son develops the ability to love, to develop com-
      mitments to other persons, and to enter true
      mutual relationships.
   b. *Isolation* is the danger. The person remains distant
      from others, withdraws, enters into superficial
      relationships, or develops prejudices.

7. *Adulthood* (28 to 65 years)
    a. *Generativity* is the task. The adult becomes responsible for guiding children or for the creation and development of productive and constructive tasks.
    b. Failure leads to *stagnation*, personal impoverishment, and self-indulgence.
8. *Old age* (65 years to death)
    a. The last stage is characterized by feelings of acceptance, importance, and self-worth about the value of one's life—*integrity.*
    b. *Despair,* the negative outcome of this stage, is the sense of loss, a feeling of life's meaninglessness, and the feeling that life's goals have not been achieved and that it is too late to start over.
C. Therapy
    The focus is on establishing trust not obtained early in life and helping patient gain insight into unconscious motivations, thus reducing anxiety.

Behaviorist Approach

This approach emphasizes observable and measurable behavioral processes. *Maladaptive behavior* can be classified as behavior excess, behavioral deficit, distortion of reinforcing stimuli, distortion of discrimination stimuli, and aversive behavior.

A. Theoretical basis[8,11,36–38,53]
    1. Watson, Pavlov, and Skinner have contributed to the development of the behaviorist school of thought.
    2. Two schools of thought have developed.
        a. *Behaviorism*—All behavior follows learning principles; therefore, behavior may become maladaptive but is not considered abnormal.
            (1) *Respondent conditioning*—Concept that states that a specific stimulus elicits a certain response.
            (2) *Operant conditioning*—Concept that states that behavioral responses are influenced by what follows the response.

(3) *Reinforcement*—Concept that states that a behavioral response can be influenced by positive and negative rewards.

b. *Cognitive behaviorism*—Behavior is influenced by cognition, independently of the stimulus.

(1) Important variables determining behavior include: plans, beliefs, expectancies, encodings, and competencies.

(2) Feelings are believed to follow thoughts.

B. Therapy

1. *Functional analysis* is analysis of the manifest behavior.
   a. What behaviors are problematic?
   b. Under what conditions does the behavior occur?
   c. What are the positive reinforcers?
   d. What are the negative reinforcers?
   e. What are the effective behaviors that could be used as substitutes or as reinforcers?

2. Techniques frequently used in behavioral therapy are systematic desensitization, flooding, implosion, positive reinforcement, and programs such as assertiveness training, relaxation exercises, token economy, and sex therapy.

3. Cognitive therapy focuses on changing the internal contingencies, such as expectancies, distortions, self-injunctions, self-reproaches, and sequence of thoughts, to effect a behavior change.

4. Techniques in cognitive therapy include verbal probing, reality testing, thought substitution, role playing, self-monitoring, assignment of tasks, use of humor, and reflection.

Humanistic-Existential Approach

This approach emphasizes the holistic view of man, man's individuality and intrinsic worth, the importance of experiencing the present and the personal meanings of experience. According to Rogers, Maslow, and Frankl, abnormal behavior is a consequence of the following:

Rogers—An incongruence exists between one's self-image and experience.[48–51]

Maslow—Basic needs are not satisfied (air, food, water, safety, love, belonging, self-actualization).[42]

Frankl—Lack of meaning of life may result in illness.[20,21]

A. Theoretical basis: Rogers
1. *Self* is a central concept because one's evaluation of life is related to views of the self: Who am I? What can I do? What am I able to do? What do I want to be? Man strives for self-actualization.
2. Incongruence can develop between the ideal self and the real self and/or reality. This causes dissatisfaction, anxiety, and activation of a self-defense mechanism.
3. Continuous feedback about behavior is given to the child by others. These experiences are integrated, denied, or accepted as truth by the child, thus affecting the self.
4. The importance of accepting one's feelings and not denying them and of recognizing one's own values and beliefs and not generally accepting the values of others is stressed.

B. Therapy
Therapist demonstrates unconditional positive self-regard (genuine acceptance), empathetic understanding (ability to perceive another's world), correctness, and congruence to assist patient in exploring his uniqueness and worth.

Family Approach*

Differing conceptual views of family theory and family therapy exist. There is no accepted typology or diagnostic view of families.

A. Structural framework
1. Minuchin[44,45] views the family as a social system with structure and organization in which the individual lives and responds. Transactional patterns develop that control the interaction and behavior of family members.
2. Maladaption is noted in the transactional patterns (i.e., disengagement with no or minimal contact among the family members and enmeshment with an overinvolvement between and/or among members).

*References 25–27

    3. Therapy is directed toward initiating change in the family structure by clarifying boundaries, rules and expectations.
B. Interactional framework: Satir[54] and Haley[30–32]
    1. The double bind theory offers a way to view the development of dysfunction in a family system. Its characteristics are as follows:
        a. The individual is in an important relationship that necessitates understanding what is being communicated.
        b. The other person in the relationship is communicating two orders of messages and they are contradictory.
        c. The individual is unable to make a comment about either order of the messages and therefore is in a double bind.
    2. Dysfunctional communication is produced by denying, rejecting, or disqualifying the relationship aspect as the message aspects of the communication; by differing punctuation in the interactions between two persons, which results in greater and greater differences; and by having symmetrical or rigid interaction patterns.
    3. Problems are viewed as consequences of using solutions that obviously are not working. Mishandling occurs as
        a. steps are not taken and action is needed;
        b. steps are taken and no action is needed; or
        c. steps are taken at every level of communication.
    4. Therapy is directed toward a change in the individual interaction patterns in the family system (e.g., Satir) and/or change in the structure or transaction pattern (e.g., Haley) by setting goals, giving tasks, symptom prescription, advertising symptoms, reframing behavior, and so on.
C. Bowen system theory*
    The Bowen system presents a conceptualization of the emotional system over several generations. It emphasizes variables of anxiety and level of integration and their influence on the family system. Illness is viewed as an aspect of human adaptation in which a person experiences a level of undifferentiation resulting from the transmission of low levels of differentiation from past generations.

*References 25–27

1. Theoretical basis
   a. *Sibling position*—Personality characteristics are related to sibling position (10 have been identified) and provide predictive data.
   b. *Triangles*—The basic unit of the emotional system (i.e., a twosome and an outsider). When tension is experienced, each person will attempt to obtain the outside position. If the tension increases, one of the persons will triangle another; a larger and larger interlocking system is thus formed.
   c. *Family projection process*—Anxiety is experienced by the mother, who may respond by becoming sensitive to the child and overconcerned. The mother's overattachment to the child is supported by the father. The child becomes anxious, demanding, and unable to function alone. Schizophrenia may develop following several generations of lower levels of differentiation as a result of the family projection process.
   d. *Multigenerational transmission process*—The family projection process involves multiple generations, with one child in each generation becoming less differentiated and less able to function.
   e. *Emotional cut-off*—This concept describes the process of separation from parents as people attempt to resolve their emotional attachments. The more intense the cut-off from parents, the more likely that the person and the person's children will have similar problems in life.
   f. *Differentiation*—This concept is related to a state of being and to the process of becoming more responsible for oneself at emotional and intellectual levels. Profiles are developed for different levels of differentiation.
   g. *Nuclear family emotional system*—Patterns of functioning of mother, father, and children are identified. Major patterns include marital conflict, dysfunction in one spouse, projection of problems to a child, and/or a combination of these patterns.
   h. *Societal regression*—When a society is exposed to chronic anxiety, it responds with emotionality to

relieve the anxiety; thus, functioning regresses. An example of regression response is overuse of drugs in society.

2. Therapy
   a. Therapy focuses on reducing reactivity and increasing one's differentiation.
   b. The expression of feelings is not encouraged or interpreted, but the person is assisted in thinking about processes.
   c. The exploration of family's past history is encouraged.
   d. Reestablishment of contact with family is supported.
   e. Therapist remains out of the interlocking triangles, thereby increasing flexibility and ability to decrease anxiety.

Group Approach: Types of Groups Based on Theoretical Frameworks*

A. Client-centered groups—based on theories of Carl Rogers
   1. *Goals*—increased awareness and acceptance of oneself and others, self-actualization, self-responsibility.
   2. *Role of therapist*—nondirective; shows genuineness, unconditional positive regard and empathy; focuses on being with the individuals in group and on group process.
B. Transactional analysis groups—based on theories of Eric Berne
   1. *Goals*—increased insight; reconstruction of personality structure; assumption of self-responsibility; and autonomy in spontaneity and intimacy.
   2. *Role of therapist*—identifies ego states, transactions, and games used by group members and then facilitates more adaptive behaviors; relates openly and honestly in a manner that is free from personal games; serves as teacher and facilitator.
C. Interpersonal groups—based on theories of Harry S. Sullivan[65]
   1. *Goals*—increased insight and personality reconstruction.

*References 4–5,10,11,37,59,70

    2. *Role of therapist*—serves as participant observer, catalyst, and facilitator; supports enhancement of self-esteem; focuses on link between current problems and prior distorted experiences; encourages consensual validation of behavior in order to correct developmental distortions.

D. Psychoanalytic groups—based on theories of Sigmund Freud
    1. *Goal*—reconstruction of personality structure.
    2. *Role of therapist*—serves as neutral sounding board and authority figure; listens actively; focuses on analyzing individuals in group dealing with transferences, dream content, resistance, past traumatic relationships and link to present behavior; focuses on needs of group by identifying group processes that are operant.

E. Gestalt groups—based on theories of Frederick Perls
    1. *Goals*—assuming responsibility for self; increasing awareness of personal feelings and behavior; increasing awareness of the behavior and feelings of others; completing unfinished business (e.g., by experiencing past experiences in the present)
    2. *Role of therapist*—confronts, supports, and takes an active role in directing structured exercises; works with individual group members on the "hot seat" in the "here and now."

F. Existential groups—based on such theorists as Rollo May
    1. *Goals*—fully experiencing and relating to others; self-actualization.
    2. *Role of therapist*—shares self intimately with group as whole; nondirective but guiding when appropriate.

CHAPTER 2

Therapeutic Relationship and Communication

The One-to-One Nurse–Client Relationship*

A. Definition and characteristics of the one-to-one relationship include:

1. A professional relationship that incorporates theories of human behavior and is based on the purposeful use of "self"; the focus is on the client's emotional, cognitive and behavioral responses and concerns over a specified period of time.

2. Mutually determined, goal directed, nurse–client interactions that incorporate specific interpersonal techniques, to assist the client to explore problem areas, learning, change and personal growth.

3. Interpersonal techniques are used to assist the client to focus on thoughts, feelings and behaviors; to reinforce constructive client behaviors and interaction; and to assist the client to modify or discontinue unhealthy behaviors and patterns of interaction.

4. Scope: ranges from brief interactions and counseling that is provided by a basic level psychiatric mental health nurse to individual psychotherapy provided by a Psychiatric Mental Health Advanced Practice Nurse, e.g., Clinical Nurse Specialist or Nurse Practitioner.

*References 3, 41, 42

B. Phases of the nurse–client relationship (phases are overlapping and interlocking throughout the nurse–client relationship)[3,6,8,9,14–18,20,22,23,25,30,31,34,36,40]
  1. Phase I (beginning or orientation phase)
    a. Common client characteristics and behaviors include:
      (1) experiences a felt (but sometimes poorly understood) need for assistance and seeks assistance for this need;
      (2) experiences tension or anxiety that is not always observable;
      (3) frequently bases preconceptions and expectations of current nurse–client relationship on past experiences;
      (4) hesitates at certain points and states there is nothing more to say;
      (5) often tests parameters of the nurse–client relationship, i.e., unexpected tardiness or absence or other actions that test the extent of the nurse willingness to meet the client's needs;
      (6) often uses cognitive words and phrases to describe situations and events, with minimal focus on identification and description of feelings.
    b. Therapeutic nursing tasks during orientation phase:
      (1) Assess, identify and clarify client's current needs and problems.
      (2) Formulate initial nursing diagnoses and participate in formulating psychiatric diagnoses.
      (3) Begin to identify client's health pattern responses to actual or potential psychiatric health problems.
      (4) Clarify one's own preconceptions and expectations.
      (5) Evaluate need for referral to another mental health professional when client's needs exceed the nurse's expertise; discuss rationale for referral with client to reduce client anxiety; obtain client permission to share information with referred resource.

(6) Establish a mutually agreed upon therapeutic contract for the one-to-one nurse–client relationship. This contract includes:
  (a) explanation of the nurse's role and responsibilities in the relationship;
  (b) description of the overall purpose of the relationship;
  (c) identification of mutually defined cognitive, emotional and behavioral goals;
  (d) agreement on place, time and length of meetings;
  (e) establishment of fee/reimbursement (if applicable);
  (f) statement of actual or tentative length of therapy/nurse–client relationship (preparation for termination phase);
  (g) statement on policy for cancellation of appointments;
  (h) discussion of parameters regarding the role of family/significant others;
  (i) agreement on the client's responsibilities;
  (j) clarification of client's understanding of orientation information, explanations and the therapeutic contract.
(7) Discuss confidentiality of information.
  (a) Inform client that progress in therapy will be shared in general terms with health care team members.
  (b) Inform client whether written progress reports by the nurse will be shared with the client prior to being placed in the client's record.
  (c) Inform client who verbalizes intent to harm self or others that this information will be shared with appropriate professional staff, family or significant others who would need to be informed in case of danger to self or others. Give client rationale for this action.
  (d) Do not promise client to withhold specific client information from other team

members; instead, emphasize that sharing with the interdisciplinary team specific client information, i.e., suicidal or homicidal ideation, alcohol and drug use, is a decision that is based upon the nurse's professional judgment.

(8) Build trusting relationship by maintaining the stipulations of the contract and informing the client of any changes, including unavoidable absences.

2. Phase II (middle or working phase)
    a. Common client characteristics and behaviors:
       (1) responds to offers of help from the nurse;
       (2) identifies and describes specific problems to be explored;
       (3) decreases testing maneuvers that were evident during the orientation phase, i.e., asking personal information about nurse, questioning focus, length and frequency of interviews;
       (4) fluctuates in the need for dependency, independence and interdependency in the nurse–client relationship;
       (5) demonstrates increased ability to discuss problems and to identify, describe and explore feelings;
       (6) imitates or copies behaviors or appearance of the nurse to convey identification with or wishing to be like the nurse;
       (7) demonstrates movement toward therapeutic goals that were formulated during the orientation phase;
       (8) makes full use of the services offered by the nurse and attempts to obtain maximum benefits from the nurse–client relationship.
    b. Therapeutic nursing tasks during the working phase:
       (1) Recognize behavioral manifestations of ambivalence and resistance, i.e., rejection, avoidance, denial, hostility and reaching a plateau in therapy.
       (2) Note the frequency of client's use of affective words and phrases as well as the client's

descriptions of behavioral trends and patterns.

(3) Periodically devote a portion of the nurse–client interaction to a mutual nurse–client review of the progress that has been made in the achievement of the goals that were formulated during the orientation phase. Use the findings from this review to determine the need for re-formulation of therapeutic goals.

(4) Avoid making observations about the client's copying or imitating the nurse's appearance or behaviors.

(5) Facilitate the resolution of emotional conflicts, the reduction in self-defeating behavioral patterns and the attainment of the mutually defined behavioral goals of the client.

　　(a) Identify together the forces that hinder client behavioral change.

　　(b) Facilitate problem-solving strategies to formulate behavioral alternatives.

　　(c) Promote changes in undesirable cognitive and behavioral patterns through the use of assignments between counseling sessions.

　　(d) Capitalize on opportunities that allow the client to test new behaviors and work through associated thoughts and emotions, i.e., anxiety.

(6) Continue preparation for termination by periodically reminding the client of the remaining length of time that the nurse and client will be meeting together.

3. Phase III (termination or resolution phase)

　a. Common client characteristics and behaviors:

　　(1) responds to the actual termination with the nurse according to prior termination experiences, type of treatment, present problems, actual and perceived rationale for termination;

　　(2) reactions to impending loss of the nurse–client relationship can include grief, sadness, depression, displacement of feelings, ambivalence, reaction formation, dependency, regression,

frank hostility, missed appointments, rejection of the nurse;

(3) maximizes learning that has occurred throughout the one-to-one relationship;

(4) participates in evaluation of progress made toward achievement of the goals that were identified during the orientation phase;

(5) demonstrates increased ability to use cognitive words and themes in relation to the ending of the nurse–client relationship and in the formulation of future plans.

b. Therapeutic nursing tasks during the termination phase:

(1) Clearly establish that the therapeutic relationship is ending.

(2) Determine the extent of the client's readiness for termination by evaluating factors such as progress toward resolution of identified problems and attainment of treatment goals and client outcomes.

(3) When possible, mutually determine termination date.

(4) Anticipate one's own reactions to ending of relationship.

(5) Assist client to identify feelings and reactions to impending loss of relationship with nurse.

(6) Help client tolerate the discomfort involved in termination by encouraging client to experience and discuss feelings associated with current and past ending of relationships.

(7) Acknowledge own feelings and reactions in a constructive manner without placing a burden on the client.

(8) Encourage client to review, summarize and evaluate perceptions of experiences throughout the one-to-one relationship; and also to review and evaluate the therapeutic contract.

(9) Encourage and support client's transition to emotional investments in other relationships.

(10) Convey recognition of client's progress during the relationship.

(11) Share recommendations of areas for further growth for client to consider.

(12) Emphasize importance of preventive measures, i.e., recognizing early signs of relapse and use of available community resources for continuation of medications or individual therapy.

▌ Principles and Strategies for Developing and Maintaining a Therapeutic Nurse–Client Relationship

A. Develop effective communication skills.[6,7,10,11,15,19,22,27,28,41]

1. Recognize factors that influence nurse/client communication

   a. Culture, customs, gender differences, education, social background, physical attributes, mental well-being, body image, self-esteem, intellectual ability and past experiences of the nurse and client

   b. Language and words, including slang and jargon, used to transmit messages

   c. Context in which communication occurs

   d. Nature of the relationship between client and nurse

   e. Intentions or goals of client and nurse

   f. Interpersonal competence of nurse

   g. Anxiety or stress level of client or nurse

   h. Sensory impairment or physical disorder that interferes with client's ability to communicate

   i. Disorders interfering with client's cognitive function and/or information processing

2. Use goal-directed verbal and nonverbal communication techniques that are based on a working knowledge of communication theories.[4,6,10,15,21,22,28,32,33,37]

   a. Use short simple sentences that focus on the client's concerns.

   b. Use *questioning* to obtain specific information, to clarify and to offer assistance.

   c. Avoid closed questions that imply an expected answer.

   d. *Encourage description* by using verbal and nonverbal means to assist the client to keep talking, e.g., open-ended statements and questions, such as "Go on," "Tell me more," "When did you . . . ?", "Where were you?", or nodding head.

e. Use *reflection*; repeat the same key words used by the client to indicate to the client that the nurse has heard what the client overtly or covertly has said.

f. Use *restating*; repeat a main thought using similar words to those used by the client in order to encourage expansion.

g. Use *focusing* to help the client stick to important subject matter or themes, for example, "What did you say that you did after you became angry?" or "You were saying that . . . "

h. Use *active listening*; listen to client's communications in order to interpret what is communicated, to respond selectively, and to decrease client resistance level that interferes with development of therapeutic alliance or accomplishment of treatment goals.

i. Share *observations*; verbalize observations about a client's behavior, for example, "You appear to be feeling sad."

j. Use *clarifications* to request feedback and to make certain that the client's communications are accurately understood, for example, "By telling me . . . are you saying that . . . ?" or "To whom are you referring when you say *they*?"

k. Use *silence* to observe, to reflect and to interpret possible meanings of the client's prior verbal and current nonverbal communication. Avoid switching to a superficial topic or introducing a new topic.

l. Use *confrontation*, only after basic trust has been established, to assist client in becoming aware of specific aspects of behavior or problem.

m. Use *humor* in selected situations to decrease anxiety and tension by changing client's perception of an anxiety-producing situation.

n. Seek *consensual validation*; request feedback from the client to check understanding and interpretation of the client's communication and perceptions.

o. Use *summarization*; provide a condensed version of the general content and theme of the conversation to give the client feedback and allow for further clarification and validation.

B. Develop an understanding of the causes of communication breakdown or distortion.[1,4,5,7,10,11,15,19,22,28,30,35,37,40,41]

1. Failure to recognize when nondirective behaviors are appropriate, i.e., listening, encouraging, instead of directive behaviors.
2. Failure to provide privacy for discussion of personal matters
3. Failure to focus on the client's concerns
4. Inattentiveness to client readiness
5. Lack of follow through on agreed-upon interventions
6. Ineffective or inappropriate reassurance
7. Switching topic of conversation to superficial aspects
8. Judgmental, prejudicial or stereotyping attitudes
9. Culturally incongruent verbal or nonverbal behavioral

C. Develop trust.[5,6,15,30,31,37,38,41]

1. Be consistently truthful.
2. Demonstrate genuine interest in and commitment to the client over a period of time.
3. Create an interpersonal relationship in which the client can freely communicate feelings, needs and problems.
4. Don't make promises unless they can be kept.
5. Try to respond to reasonable requests.

D. Be congruent.[5,10,15,30,37]

1. Strive for consistency in expression of feelings, thoughts, verbalization and behavior.
2. Be sincere and nondefensive.
3. Be as natural and spontaneous as possible in the use of interpersonal techniques and therapeutic interventions.

E. Use personal self-disclosure appropriately.[15,26,32,41,44]

1. Avoid self-disclosure to meet nurse's personal needs.
2. Recognize that inappropriate disclosure can be incorporated into the client's delusions or fantasies.

F. Develop and improve self-awareness.[1,3,4,7,11,12,14,15,19,27,30,35,37,41]

1. Develop awareness of one's own verbal and nonverbal communication patterns.
2. Develop awareness of one's own racial, cultural and subcultural values, biases, customs and their influ-

ence on one's own behavior, perception and interpretation of another's behavior.

3. Explore the origins of one's own stereotyping, prejudices and biases, and attempt to work through them.

4. Recognize the influence of one's own motives, feelings, and behavior.

5. Differentiate between one's own feelings and those belonging to the client.

6. Assume the responsibility for acquiring knowledge to increase self-awareness—i.e., institutional inservices, continuing education, formal education.

G. Cultivate use of empathic responses.[6,24,25,29,38, 39,41,43,44]

1. Use empathy as a therapeutic tool to:

   a. Make verbal observations about the client's emotional state that help the client feel understood and soothed;

   b. Help the client discover and communicate hidden emotions and their possible connections to the current situation;

   c. Promote the achievement of mutually determined goals in the nurse–client relationship.

2. Convey recognition of the client's private, inner experiences and feelings by reflecting on client's perception of feelings and using open-ended questions to focus on these feelings.

3. Selectively use self-disclosure, e.g., sharing experiences that model client's expression of feelings to help decrease client's sense of aloneness.

H. Use clinical consultation/supervision in the one-to-one nurse–client relationship to increase self-awareness.[2–4,13,14,27,31,32,36,41]

1. Definition and characteristics of clinical consultation/supervision

   a. *Clinical consultation/supervision*—an interpersonal process between a mental health professional, preferably a certified psychiatric mental health advanced practice nurse and a psychiatric mental health nurse, to facilitate the nurse's clinical competency and problem-solving ability in addressing treatment issues in nurse–client relationships.

   b. The consultation/supervision process is cognitive and didactic, emphasizing the cultivation of the

therapeutic use of self, psychotherapeutic skills and psychotherapeutic interventions.
   c. The focus is on the nurse's behavior and reactions and on their influence on nurse–client relationships.
   d. The consultant/supervisor serves as a mentor guiding the application of theory to the practice of psychotherapeutic nursing interventions.
2. Phases of consultation/supervision:
   a. Preinteraction—the beginning of the developmental process of consultation/supervision; the focus is on nurse's behavior with the nurse experiencing varying degrees of anxiety related to wanting to be accepted by the consultant/supervisor and also fearing rejection.
   b. Beginning/Introductory/Honeymoon—the consultant/supervisor focuses on establishing a learning alliance; the nurse strives to be open to suggestions, learn more about the therapeutic use of the self, and gain knowledge about the nurse–client relationship.
   c. Mid-phase/Working—the nurse may experience feelings of anger and confusion during the process of identifying with the consultant/supervisor's expertise and attempting to incorporate new clinical information. The consultant/supervisor avoids personalization of these feelings and evaluates the nurse's anxiety to determine the extent to which new material can be processed.
   d. Integration phase—the consultant/supervisor facilitates the nurse to move towards becoming an autonomous clinical practitioner. The nurse demonstrates the ability to integrate clinical knowledge and psychotherapeutic interventions that are consistent with the nurse's personality and treatment preferences.
   e. End phase—the consultant/supervisor and the nurse mutually review and evaluate the consultation/supervisory process. Recognition of accomplishments and recommendations for future learning are discussed. Successful termination of the consultation/supervisory relationship is dependent upon the consultant/supervisor and the nurse working through this evaluation process.

CHAPTER **3**

Initial Psychiatric Assessment of the Client

▐ The Nursing Process*

The nursing process is an interactive, systemic, problem-solving process that is used to assist the client to achieve a maximum level of wellness. It should be used throughout the one-to-one nurse–client relationship.

A. Assessment
   Assessment is the systematic and continuous collection of data about the health status of the client. The assessment interview involves interviewing, observing, reviewing interdisciplinary databases and comprehensively assessing the client.

   The comprehensive assessment interview facilitates sound clinical judgment and decision making, enabling the nurse to formulate diagnoses, identify outcomes, and develop an individualized plan of care.[1]

Guidelines for Structuring the Process and Content of the Interview

- Use an assessment guide during the interview to collect data.
- Use open-ended questions.
- Provide for privacy, physical comfort and freedom from interruptions during the interview.

- Conduct the interview with sensitivity so that a positive nurse-client relationship can begin to be established. Use pauses to allow for full disclosure.
- Explain the purpose, nature and length of the interview.
- Inform client that information gained will be used to assist in treatment and will be shared with appropriate clinical staff.
- Ask about the nature of the client's problem and current life situation; show interest and allow client to fully express all concerns.
- Note verbal responses, nonverbal expressions, changes in mood and difficulties in answering any questions.
- Ask questions in a concrete and simple way. Use narrowly focused questions to test hunches.
- Periodically repeat and summarize the client's responses.
- Use a conceptual framework for nursing practice to guide observations, interviewing and assessment.
- Follow health care agency guidelines for documenting observations, assessments and findings.

B. Diagnosis

The diagnosis is formulated from an analysis of client assessment data.

Diagnoses should conform to the classification systems that are accepted and used in clinical practice, e.g., North American Nursing Diagnosis Association (NANDA) and Diagnostic and Statistical Manual of Mental Disorders (DSM-IV).

A nursing diagnosis is a clinical judgment about an individual, a family, or a community's response to actual or potential health problems/life processes.[14,p.7] Nursing diagnoses provide the basis for selection of nursing interventions to achieve outcomes for which the nurse is accountable (Fig. 3-1).[14,p.17]

C. Outcome Identification

Individualized, client-oriented, expected, and measurable outcomes are developed from the diagnosis. Outcomes are developed in collaboration with the client, significant others, and the interdisciplinary team. Outcomes include an estimate of the time for their achievement.

D. Planning

The plan of care is individualized based on the client's need and diagnoses, and it defines priorities of care in order to meet the expected outcomes.

Arrange for input from the client when possible and from significant others and members of the interdisciplinary team as appropriate.

E. Implementation

Intervention strategies are selected to help the client achieve the expected outcomes. A conceptual framework for practice can serve to guide both implementation and outcome identification.

F. Evaluation

Determine the extent to which client outcomes have been met. Data resulting from evaluation are used to plan and redesign intervention strategies to meet, revise or formulate new client outcomes as necessary (Fig. 3-2).

▌ The Mental Status Examination[*]

The mental status review is usually performed by a psychiatrist, advanced practice psychiatric mental health nurse or psychologist. It serves as only one component of the overall assessment of mental health.

A. Objective

The objective is to assess the mental functioning and present emotional state of the client.

B. General appearance

Observe the following about the client:
1. Hygiene, grooming and dress (slovenly, neat, unkempt, overly meticulous, fastidious, disheveled, inappropriate, unusual).
2. Facial expression and mobility (calm, perplexed, stressed, tense, alert, dazed)
3. Physical appearance (noticeable physical deformities, thin, obese, average weight, robust, any idiosyncrasies)
4. Posture (normal, rigid, slouching)
5. Eye contact and movement (eyes closed, eyes open, good contact, avoids contact, stares)
6. Attitude (friendly, cooperative, guarded, suspicious, angry, arrogant, apathetic, tearful, shifting attitude)

C. Motor behavior and activity (observe for unusual bodily movements)

*References 3,6,8,9,12,13,15,16,18–21,23

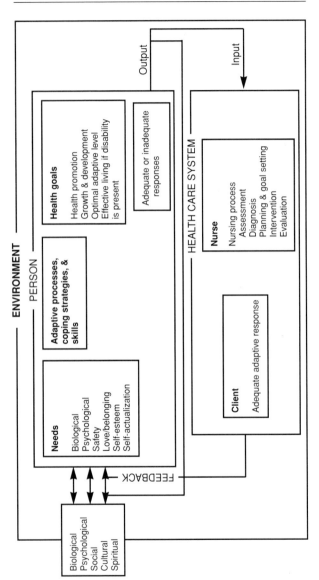

FIGURE 3-1. A conceptual framework for psychiatric nursing practice.

1. Level and pace of motor behavior (appropriate, accelerated, agitated, catatonic excitement, psychomotor retardation, catatonic, catatonic stupor)
2. Movements (goal directed, appropriate, graceful, consistent, excessive, rapid, abrupt, slowed, inconsistent, random)
3. *Impulsiveness*—unpredictable, sudden outbursts of activity
4. *Stereotypy*—repetitive, persistent motor activity or speech
5. *Compulsive*—unwanted repetitive actions
6. *Echopraxia*—repetition of examiner's movements
7. *Waxy flexibility or catalepsy*—posture, imposed by examiner or others, held by client
8. Mannerisms (nail biting, tapping feet, licking lips)
9. Freedom of movement and gait
10. Firmness of handshake
11. Tics, spasms, tremors

D. Speech

Observe for speech activity, normal and unusual patterns, or unusual use of words, such as the following:

1. *Verbigeration*—repetitive, meaningless expression of sentences, phrases, or words.
2. *Rhyming*—interjecting into the conversation regular, recurring, corresponding sounds at the end of phrases or sentences, as in poetry.
3. *Punning*—interjecting into the conversation the clever and humorous use of a word or words.
4. *Mutism*—no expression of words or lack of communication over a period of time.
5. *Aphasia*–partial or total loss of self-expression through language or the ability to understand verbal communication of another person.
6. *Neologisms*—words created by the patient that are not easily understood by others.
7. Unusual rate of speech, volume of voice, intonation, or modulation.

E. Functioning

Assess the patient for the following:

1. Alertness

(text continues on page 49)

GENERAL INFORMATION

Name: _____

Address: _____ Phone: _____

DOB/Age: _____ Sex: _____ Race/ethnic background: _____

Marital status: _____

Name of spouse, relative, or friend: _____

Date _____ Time _____ Mode of admission _____

Patient's statement of current health problem: _____

Allergies: _____

Suicidal thoughts or behavior: _____

Homocidal thoughts or behavior: _____

Use of street drugs or alcohol: _____

Legal problems: Arrests, court dates, prison/jail, probation:

_____

History or current evidence of abuse (e.g., physical, sexual, emotional)

_____

History of mental illness or emotional problems in self or family:

_____

ASSESSMENT OF BIOPHYSICAL FACTORS
(Note alterations, limitations, concerns, strengths)

Current level of growth & development: _____

Vital signs: _____

Height: _____ Weight: _____

Vision: _____ Hearing: _____

Speech (clear, slurred, rapid, pressured): _____

History of physical illness: _____

Current physical problem (frequency & type of complaints): _____

_____

Current treatments & medications: _____

Neurological status: _____

  Level of consciousness: _____

(continues)

FIGURE 3-2. Initial psychiatric nursing assessment. (This is a guideline for assessment, and information can be formatted into check lists for easy computer entry.) (See references 2, 4, 5, 7, 10, 11, 17, 22, and 24.)

Arousal level: _____

Memory impairment: _____

Orientation to time, place, person: _____

History of fainting spells or dizziness: _____

History of seizures: _____

History of blackouts: _____

Tingling or numbness: _____

Presence of tardive dyskinesia: _____

Presence of pain & how relieved: _____

Skin condition: _____

General nutrition: _____

Dentures or dental problems: _____

Elimination: _____

Respiratory (dyspnea, cough, smoking history): _____

Muscular skeletal: _____

Cardiovascular: _____

Reproductive factors: _____

Sexual orientation (heterosexual, homosexual, bisexual): _____

Exposure to sexually transmitted disease (sexual orientation, number of sexual partners, use of protective device, IV drug use, history of blood transfusions, HIV positive): _____
_____

Exposure to infectious disease: _____

ASSESSMENT OF SELF CARE FACTORS

General appearance: _____

General level of functioning: _____

Grooming and dressing: _____

Hygiene and bathing: _____

Eating patterns (usual diet): _____

Elimination patterns: _____

Level of energy: _____

Sleep/rest pattern: _____

Activity pattern: _____

(continues)

FIGURE 3-2. (Continued)

Client's awareness of other's concerns about physical appearance: _____

_____

Activities/habits detrimental to general well being & health: _____

_____

ASSESSMENT OF PSYCHOSOCIAL FACTORS

Problems prior to admission to treatment facility: _____

Current problems/stressors: _____

Use of defense mechanisms: _____ Other coping skills used: _____

Behavior: suicide potential _____

  pre-admission factors _____

    developmental stressors: _____

    situational stressors: _____

    family dynamics: _____

    biological factors: _____

    severity of current illness: _____

  Interaction with staff & significant others _____

    therapeutic interventions: _____

    contacts with significant others: _____

  Previous attempts: _____

  Current thought or plan: _____

  Biological therapies (use & effectiveness): _____

  Environmental safety factors: _____

  External resources (family, significant others, employment

  spiritual/religious): _____

Behavior: potential for violence towards others: _____

Behavior: communications

  Communication skills: _____

    With interviewer: _____

    With spouse: _____

    With children: _____

    With others (specify): _____

(continues)

FIGURE 3-2. (Continued)

Behavior: interpersonal interactions

    Degree and style of social interaction: _____

    Current social network & support system: _____

    Early family relationships: _____

    Current family dynamics: _____

    Relationship with spouse &/or significant other(s): _____

    Consistency of client's behavior: _____

    Spouse &/or significant others' response to patient's illness: _____

    _____

    Expression of needs/goals: _____

    Abuse (current/past): _____

Behavior: sexuality

      High risk sexual behaviors: _____

      Sexual concerns: _____

Behavior: recreational activities _____

      Recreational activities & hobbies: _____

      Use of leisure time: _____

      Pets: _____

Thought/Cognition/Affect _____

      Thought form (disorganized, disoriented, distracted): _____

      Thought content (hallucinations, delusions, unusual beliefs,

      suspiciousness, grandiosity, somatization, helplessness):

      _____

    Opinion of self-worth/self-esteem: _____

    Attitudes toward value of own life: _____

    Feelings of hopelessness: _____

    Guilt & source: _____

    Degree & nature of ambivalence: _____

    Decision making abilities/limitations: _____

    Affect (normal, flat, blunted, constricted): _____

    Type & change of mood (depressed, excited, anxious, aggressive, hostile):

    _____

(continues)

FIGURE 3-2. (Continued)

Unusual sensations & perceptions: _____

Level of insight and judgment (including degree of denial):

_____

ASSESSMENT OF EDUCATIONAL FACTORS

Cognition impacting learning: _____

Affect impacting learning: _____

Ability to follow instructions: _____

Dominant language: _____

Occupational history: _____

Current employment history: _____

Education: _____

Educational goals: _____

Knowledge & perception about present illness (cause, prevention,
treatment, self-care responsibilities): _____

_____

Knowledge about current medications: _____

Knowledge & beliefs about illness, & health: _____

Knowledge about & attitudes/beliefs toward treatment & health care

personnel: _____

Expectations & goals for current hospitalization: _____

Personal long term health goals: _____

Past & current compliance with prescribed treatment & health instructions:

_____

ASSESSMENT OF ENVIRONMENTAL FACTORS

Previous & current use of health care resources: _____

Home environment (e.g., safety, weapons, transportation): _____

_____

Community environment: _____

Cultural factors

Influence of cultural factors: _____

Community values & beliefs about mental health: _____

(continues)

FIGURE 3-2. (Continued)

Customs related to verbal & non-verbal communication: _____

Customs related to decision making: _____

Religious customs: _____

Customs related to foods: _____

Customs related to family roles: _____

Social structure components (family structures, religion, economics,

available health systems): _____

Physical environment: _____

DISCHARGE PLANNING FACTORS

Level of achieving client's health care expectations: _____

Client teaching (signs/symptoms of mental condition; effect, dosage, side

effects of medications): _____

Current living arrangements: _____

Community resources: _____

Financial resources: _____

Medication prescriptions: _____

Treatment prescriptions: _____

Self-care assistance needed following discharge: _____

Follow-up appointments: _____

Referral to community resources: _____

FIGURE 3-2. (Continued)

> Observe client for levels of alertness (drowsiness, hyperalertness, somnolence, intermittent alertness, drowsiness and stupor)
> 2. Orientation
>   a. Orientation to time
>   Ask the client to name the month, day of the week, time and to state how long the client has been in the hospital.
>   b. Orientation to place
>   Ask the client: Where are you now located? What is the name of this place?
>   c. Orientation to person

Does client know own name? Does client know who
the conductor of the interview is?

3. Memory
   a. Memory of remote events—ask the client the fol-
      lowing:
      (1) Dates of marriages and divorces, if any
      (2) Birth dates of children, if any
      (3) Own birth date
      (4) Name of grade school, high school and/or col-
          lege attended
      (5) Type of position, the month and year of first
          job after high school or college graduation
   b. Memory of recent past events—ask the client the
      following:
      (1) Where did client live during past three
          months? With whom did the client live? Where
          did the client work?
      (2) What types of recreational activities did the
          client engage in?
   c. Memory of recent events—ask the client the fol-
      lowing:
      (1) What did the client eat for breakfast, lunch,
          and dinner today?
      (2) What activities did the client engage in yester-
          day and today?
   d. Immediate memory and recall
      (1) Give client the names of three unrelated
          objects, ask client to repeat; wait 3–5 minutes
          and ask client to repeat again.
      (2) Administer digit span test. Ask client to repeat
          numbers in sequence, increasing to as large a
          span as client can repeat. Repeat process, ask
          client to repeat numbers in reverse order.
      (3) Ask client the same questions several times
          during the interview to determine whether
          the same or a different answer is given.
      (4) Examine for the presence of impaired mem-
          ory, such as amnesia, anterograde amnesia,
          psychogenic amnesia.

4. Attention and calculation
   Instruct client to subtract 7 from 100 and to keep subtracting 7's, allowing up to 30 seconds between calcu-

lations. If the client is unable to complete this activity, have the client spell "world" forward and backwards.

  5. Level and fund of knowledge

    a. To determine fund of knowledge, ask such questions as: What are the names of three countries in Europe? The colors in the American flag? The distance between any two major U.S. cities?

    b. Request listing of three items in different categories, such as U.S. state capitals and fruits.

    c. Overall responses to all interview questions are used to assess level of knowledge appropriate to client's age, socioeconomic level, and cultural, occupational and educational background.

  6. Ability to think abstractly or to make generalizations

    a. Ask client to interpret a proverb or to find the inherent similarity between two objects, e.g., a bicycle and a train, an apple and an orange.

    b. Use object sorting test—have the client group toy objects according to use.

F. Perception

Observe for signs of altered or abnormal awareness of self or environment, such as the following:

  1. *Hallucinations*—false sensory experiences, reactions to non-present stimuli that may be triggered by another external or internal stimulus. These can be visual, olfactory, auditory, tactile, gustatory, or kinesthetic.

  2. *Hypnagogic hallucinations*—misperceptions occurring as a client is falling asleep for which there is no basis in reality.

  3. *Hypnopompic hallucinations*—misperceptions occurring as client is waking up for which there is no basis in reality.

  4. *Illusion*—misinterpretation of an actual, existing external stimulus by any of the senses.

Observe for the following changes in the client's general manner of feeling, thinking or behavior during the interview: cooperative, outgoing, withdrawn, evasive, sarcastic, aggressive, perplexed, hostile, arrogant, dramatic, ingratiating, submissive, fearful, seductive, impatient, uncooperative, remote, resistant, unfeeling, apprehensive, or apathetic.

G. Mood and affect

Observe for unusual mood or expression of emotion, such as the following:

1. *Euphoria*—excessive feeling of emotional and physical well-being inappropriate to actual environmental stimuli
2. *Flat affect*—less than normal expression of feelings
3. *Blunting*—loss of affective depression
4. *Elation*—high degree of confidence, boastfulness, uncritical optimism and joy, accompanied by increased motor activity
5. *Exultation*—affective reaction extending beyond elation and accompanied by feelings of grandeur
6. *Ecstasy*—overpowering feeling of joy and rapture
7. *Anxiety*—apprehensive, uneasy and worried feeling usually of unconscious, intrapsychic origin
8. *Fear*—apprehensive, uneasy and worried feeling related to a known source of danger, usually externally based
9. *Ambivalence*—expression of the existence of two opposing feelings or emotions at the same time
10. *Depersonalization*—feeling that oneself or one's environment is unreal
11. *Irritability*—feeling characterized by impatience, annoyance and easy provocation to anger
12. *Rage*—furious, uncontrolled anger
13. *Lability*—quick change of expression of mood or feelings
14. *Depression*—feeling characterized by sadness, dejection, helplessness, hopelessness, worthlessness and gloom.

H. Thought processes and content

Observe for the following:

1. *Blocking*—sudden cessation of flow of thinking and speech related to strong emotions
2. *Flight of ideas*—rapid conversation with logically unconnected shifting of topics
3. *Word salad*—combination of phrases, words and sentences that are disconnected or incoherent
4. *Perseveration*—pathological repetition of a sentence, phrase, or word
5. *Neologisms*—use of new expressions, phrases or words (See speech)

      6. *Circumstantiality*—interjection of great detail and incidental material

      7. *Tangentiality*—deviation from central theme of conversation

      8. *Echolalia*—repetitive imitation of another person's conversation

      9. *Condensation*—process of reducing several ideas into one symbol

     10. *Delusion*—false belief kept despite nonsupportive evidence

     11. *Phobia*—strong, persistent, abnormal fear of an object or situation

     12. *Obsession*—persistent, unwanted, recurring thought

     13. *Hypochondriasis*—morbid concern for one's health and feeling ill without any actual medical basis

I. Judgment
Observe client's ability to solve problems and choose among real alternatives (e.g., What would you do if you were in a theater and smelled smoke?).

■ The Multiaxial Evaluation System of the Diagnostic and Statistical Manual of Mental Disorders (Fourth Edition, Revised) (DSM-IV)

A. The purpose of the DSM-IV "is to provide clear descriptions of diagnostic categories in order to enable clinicians and investigators to diagnose, communicate about, study and treat the various mental disorders."[2, p. xxvii]

B. The DSM-IV recommends the evaluation of a client's psychological and physical functioning, stressors contributing to the development of a psychological disorder, strengths, and limitations.

C. In using the DSM-IV, the clinician looks at specific behaviors and takes into consideration prior history of illness and family history. In order to arrive at a differential diagnosis, the clinician views the client both longitudinally and cross-sectionally.

D. The five axes of the DSM-IV on which the client is evaluated are as follows:[2, p.25]
Axis I—Clinical Disorders

Other Conditions That May Be A Focus of Clinical Attention

Axis II—Personality Disorders

Mental Retardation

Axis III—General Medical Conditions

Axis IV—Psychosocial and Environmental Problems

Axis V—Global Assessment of Functioning

Administration of Drug Therapy

▌Medication Administration

A major responsibility of the nurse is to administer medication in collaboration with the physician, pharmacist, and client. The degree of involvement in the administration of psychiatric medications is influenced by the varying conditions of the clients, the health care systems, and the qualifications of the nurse. Careful assessment, diagnosis, and evaluation contribute to the effectiveness of medication administration, client and family education, and supportive processes.

Areas for Nursing Assessment and Monitoring

The nurse should observe and evaluate the following areas:

Physiological

- Baseline data for future assessment of changes: blood pressure in standing and sitting positions, temperature, pulse, respiration, weight, CBC, urinalysis, blood chemistry screens, ECG, and other tests as indicated and ordered by physician/psychiatric nurse
- Signs/symptoms of other medical problems
- Changes in intake
- Changes in elimination pattern, particularly constipation and polyuria

- Changes in activity
- Changes in sleep
- Changes in sexual functioning (e.g., impotence and changes in libido related to drug use may be quite frightening)

Medication
- Past responses to medication
- Use of other prescribed and over-the-counter drugs (OTCs), alcohol, and street drugs: many potentially dangerous drug interactions may occur
- Signs/symptoms of side effects, toxicity
- Effect of medication on work, e.g., not being as alert
- Dysphoric responses to the medication, e.g., feelings of being in space, slowed down, confused, fearful, and nervous
- Changes in feeling, thought, and perception

Education
- Client preferences for learning new material
- Areas for client education, including readiness for self-medication
- Client's ability to ask specific questions about medications

Psychosocial
- Support network; beliefs of others about taking medication
- Changes in important interpersonal relationships, including ability to communicate with nurse and others
- Changes in social functioning
- Occurrence of major stressful life events that result in changes in daily routine
- Impact of leveling mood swings
- Ability of client to afford medication and laboratory tests

▌ Antipsychotic Drugs (Table 4-1)*

Indications

Schizophrenia
Psychotic mood disorder (with either depression or mania)
Bipolar disorder, mania
Psychosis related to medications or medical condition
Nausea, vomiting

*References 8–10,16,17,22–24,32,36–39,43–45,48,56,57,60,64,66,69,76,77

TABLE 4-1 Antipsychotic Agents

Major Groups	Generic Name	Trade Name	Daily PO Dose (Range)	PRN IM Dose (Range)	Depot IM Dose (Range)
Phenothiazines					
Aliphatics	chlorpromazine	Thorazine	300–2,000 mg	12.5–50 mg	
	trifluopromazine	Vesprin	100–300 mg		
	promazine	Sparine	50–800 mg	50–300 mg	
Piperazines	fluphenazine HCl	Prolixin	2.5–30 mg	2.5–5 mg	
	decanoate	decanoate			12.5–100 mg q 1–4 wks
	enanthate	enanthate			12.5–100 mg q 1–2 wks
	perphenazine	Trilafon	16–64 mg		
	trifluoperazine	Stelazine	10–100 mg		
Piperadines	mesoridazine	Serentil	75–400 mg		
	thioridazine	Mellaril	50–800 mg		
Non-Phenothiazines					
Butyrophenones	droperidol	Inapsine		0.625–10 mg (IV/IM)	
	haloperidol	Haldol	2–100 mg	2–5 mg	
	decanoate	decanoate			100–300 mg q month
Thioxanthene	thiothixene	Navane	6–60 mg		
Dibenzoxazepine	loxapine	Loxitane	25–250 mg		
Indolone	molindone	Moban	25–400 mg		
Dibenzazepine	clozapine	Clozaril	100–900 mg		
Benzisoxazol	risperidone	Risperdol	2–6 mg		

Pharmacodynamics

- Antipsychotics block dopamine receptors in the pathways concerned with psychotic, extrapyramidal, and endocrine activities, and block presynaptic alpha (α) and cholinergic receptors. The mechanism for the benefit of these drugs in reducing psychosis is not clearly established.
- High potency and low potency refer to an antipsychotic drug equivalency to 100 mg of chlorpromazine, e.g., high potency: fluphenazine, haloperidol, trifluoperazine, thiothixene; low potency: thioridazine, chlorpromazine (CPZ).

Pharmacokinetics

- These drugs are absorbed erratically from GI tract and have extensive first pass liver metabolism.
- Serum levels peak in 30 minutes following IM injection and 90 minutes after oral dosage.
- Half-life: 1–2 days; steady state reached in 5–10 days.
- Drugs are stored in body fat; this leads to prolonged duration of side effects after drug is discontinued.
- Serum levels to guide administration of drugs are not useful due to their complex metabolism, storage in body fat, and individual unknown factors.

Contraindications

Comatose states, severe CNS depression, brain damage, bone marrow depression, or history of neuroleptic malignant syndrome (NMS).

Precautions

Closed angle glaucoma, recent myocardial infarction or other severe cardiac problems, seizures (all antipsychotic drugs will lower seizure threshold).

Side Effects (Table 4-2)

A. Life-Threatening Effects
   1. Hyperpyrexia

TABLE 4-2 Comparison of Relative Side Effects of Antipsychotic Drugs

Side Effects	Drugs With Highest Effect	Drugs With Least Effect
Sedative and hypotensive	chlorpromazine thioridazine	haloperidol thiothixene
Extrapyramidal (EPS)	haloperidol droperidol thiothixene fluphenazine	thioridazine mesoridazine chlorpromazine clozapine risperidone
Anticholinergic	thioridazine mesoridazine chlorpromazine	haloperidol droperidol thiothixene

Client is vulnerable to hyperpyrexia induced by heat, humidity, and exercise caused by suppression of hypothalamus by antipsychotic drugs. Occurs rarely. Treatment: Follow guidelines for management of heat stroke, using techniques to lower body temperature and to maintain respiratory and cardiovascular systems.

2. Agranulocytosis
   Occurs rarely.
   Most frequently occurs with chlorpromazine, thioridazine.
   Symptoms: rapid onset of sore throat and fever.
   Occurs in first 3 to 8 weeks of treatment.
   Prevention: Advise the client to report sore throat/fever promptly. CBC ordered to rule out disease.
   Treatment: Stop the drug immediately; use reverse isolation technique; administer antibiotics.
   Mortality rate is 30%.

3. Neuroleptic malignant syndrome (NMS) (differentiate from catatonia)
   Occurs within 2 weeks to months after starting drug.
   Frequency is 0.5% to 1%.
   Differentiate from lethal catatonia: extreme psychotic excitement (initial), fever, muscular rigidity, which is treated with antipsychotic medication and supportive measures.

Symptoms: Initial muscular rigidity (described as "lead-pipe" as opposed to cog-wheel type), hyperpyrexia (>40°C), autonomic nervous system dysfunction (e.g., hypertension, hypotension, diaphoresis, mental status changes); evolve over 24 to 72 hours.

Risk factors: Young, male, dehydration, prolonged agitation, prior treatment with lithium, prior occurrence of NMS (especially within the prior 14 days); current lithium treatment combined with high-dose, high-potency antipsychotic drugs.

Although some clients reverse completely, mortality is reported at 12% to 25% and is related to respiratory failure and cardiovascular collapse. If untreated, may last 10–14 days.

Treatment: Stop all antipsychotic drugs; maintain electrolyte balance, treat complications, control behavior; administer bromocriptine po 15-80 mg/day, dantrolene 60 mg IM q6h; 1–5 mg/kg IV or 1 mg/kg po qid.

4. Laryngeal spasm: treat with IM diphenhydramine or IV benztropine

B. General Side Effects

1. Drowsiness and sedation

Tolerance to drowsiness develops in about 2 weeks. Alertness and muscular coordination are impaired: activities such as driving a car or repairing delicate equipment should be avoided.

Give at bedtime to take advantage of sedation.

2. Orthostatic hypotension

Symptoms: ≥20/10 mm Hg fall in BP or pulse increase of >20 bpm, dizziness, weakness; although tolerance develops rapidly in some clients, orthostatic changes may persist with continued therapy. The danger exists that the client could fall and sustain injuries.

Monitor BP standing and sitting before and after the first dose and the first few days of treatment—and periodically, if problems persist.

Instruct the client to change positions slowly to prevent hypotension.

Lower head and raise feet slightly if hypotension occurs.

Be aware that other drugs may affect blood pressure.

3. Anticholinergic effects

Dry mouth: Rinse mouth frequently with water, use sugarless candy or gum.

Blurred vision: Physostigmine drops may be ordered.

Bowel problems range from constipation to paralytic ileus: increase fluids and bulk in diet and exercise. Laxative or stool softener may be indicated.

Urinary problems may range from urinary retention to bladder paralysis: advise the client to empty bladder every 3 to 4 hours. Bethanechol may be prescribed, although it has not been found to be very effective.

Central anticholinergic syndrome: Caused by ingestion of excess anticholinergic drug(s). Client exhibits dilated pupils, flushed and dry skin, fever, restlessness, delirium, hallucinations, and/or coma. Treat by stopping drug(s) and supporting client; physostigmine 2 mg slow IV infusion may be used.

4. Extrapyramidal symptoms (EPS): Highest incidence with the high-potency drugs.

a. Dystonia: Spasms of muscles of jaw (most common), face, neck, back, eyes, arms, and legs.

Most common in younger male clients.

Occurs within 5 minutes to first few days of treatment in about 10% of clients.

Risk decreases after about 1 month of therapy.

Symptoms: Opening of jaw, protrusion of tongue, oculogyric crisis (fixed upward gaze from spasm of the oculomotor muscles), torticollis (pulling of head to the side from spasms of cervical muscles), opisthotonus (hyperextension of back from spasms of back muscles).

Treatment: Administration of anticholinergic agent, e.g. benztropine, or an antihistaminergic agent, e.g. diphenhydramine, orally or parenterally (for more rapid relief).

Prophylaxis: Administration of anticholinergic agent for 7–10 days in high risk patients. Continue for 3 months if symptoms continue/recur.

b. Akathisia

Occurs within 6 hours to 60 days.

Symptoms: Feelings of inner tension, continuous motor restlessness that may not be noted because restlessness may be erroneously attributed to psychosis or resistance to antipsychotic drug.

Treatment: Reduction of dose; perhaps use of lipophilic beta-blocker, e.g., propranolol 30–120 mg daily, clonidine 0.1–0.5 mg daily, lorazepam 2–8 mg daily; change to low-potency antipsychotic or clozapine.

c. Parkinsonism

Most common in clients over 40 years of age, and more common in women than in men.

Occurs in about 15% of clients in 1 to 4 weeks and in 30% with chronic use.

Symptoms: Shuffling gait, masklike facies, drooling, tremor, brady/akinesia (low or no body movement), cogwheel rigidity (overlying racheting during passive flexion at a joint), rabbit syndrome (chewing tremor).

Treatment: Withdraw drug; change to low-potency antipsychotic or clozapine; add anticholinergic drug or amantadine.

d. Tardive Dyskinesia (TD)

Generally occurs after at least 3 months to years of use of antipsychotics.

Incidence of 3% to 5%; 25% incidence in clients on drug for more than 3 months.

Irreversible in about 50% of clients.

Risk is associated with high-level antipsychotic drug dosage, female sex, age of 50 years or older, and history of acute EPS.

Symptoms: Repetitive, involuntary, abnormal movements, most commonly of jaw, tongue, lips. May also involve neck, trunk, pelvis or diaphragm.

Management:

No known effective treatment.

Discuss advantages and disadvantages of antipsychotic drugs with client before use; document informed consent.

Use antipsychotic drugs only as necessary and at minimum dose.

Monitor for symptoms using a TD rating instrument, e.g., Abnormal Involuntary Movement Scale (AIMS) or Dyskinesia Identification System: Condensed User Scale (DISCUS).[17,23]

Evaluate use every 6 months for possible dose reduction.

When symptoms appear, reduce and/or discontinue antipsychotic drug. Some clients experience disappearance of symptoms within months after discontinuation.

Change to clozapine.

Add carbamazepine, lithium, or benzodiazepine to reduce intensity.

Concurrent use of α-tocopherol (vitamin E) may reduce incidence.

5. Endocrine or metabolic effects

Symptoms: Glycosuria; weight gain (indicates need for exercise and dietary adjustments or change to loxapine or molindone); menstrual irregularities, galactorrhea (indicates need for dose adjustment); decreased libido, impotence, impaired ejaculation in males (which client may be too embarrassed to report); decreased thermoregulatory ability (client complains of being too hot or cold—care should be taken in use of ice bag or hot water bottle and in regulation of temperature of seclusion room).

Treatment: Generally consists of changing to another drug or lowering dose; maintain respiratory and cardiovascular systems.

6. Dermatologic effects

Symptoms: Rashes that generally clear up after a few weeks; phototoxicity or severe sunburn occurring with use of phenothiazines, particularly chlorpromazine.

Treatment: Sunscreens and adequate clothing recommended for clients on phenothiazines.

7. Opthalmologic effects

Phenothiazine lens disease is partially reversible and does not affect visual acuity (e.g., chlorpromazine).

Irreversible retinal pigmentation that can progress to blindness occurs with doses of thioridazine over 800 mg/day or mesoridazine over 400 mg/day.
Prevention: Eye examination every 3 to 12 months; stay under maximum doses of above drugs.

8. Jaundice
   Occurs in first 5 weeks of treatment; seen particularly with use of chlorpromazine.
   Preceded by flulike symptoms, nausea, vomiting.

9. Seizures
   All antipsychotic drugs can lower seizure threshold.

Overdose

- Symptoms: Increased sedation, decreased deep tendon reflexes, hypotension, delirium, extrapyramidal signs, seizures, death secondary to ventricular fibrillation.
- Treatment: Gastric lavage, activated charcoal, antiparkinsonian drugs, IV fluids, norepinephrine or dopamine for decreased blood pressure (do not use epinephrine), anticonvulsants (IV diazepam, phenytoin).

Drug Interaction Examples

- Alcohol, barbiturates, opioids, and other CNS depressants: Potentiate sedation, hypotension.
- Antiparkinsonian drugs and tricyclic antidepressants: Increase anticholinergic effects.
- Antacids: Interfere with absorption. Give antipsychotic drug 2 hours before antacid.
- Epinephrine: Decreases blood pressure.
- Chronic cigarette smoking: Induces liver metabolism and lowers blood levels.

General Responses to Treatment

- Sedative effect may be noted 30 to 60 minutes following IM administration; it lasts 2 to 3 hours.
- Client's ability to cooperate increases and disruptive behavior decreases within a day to a week of administration of drug.

- Thought disorder generally does not disappear until 6 weeks or more following initial dose.
- Failure to respond may be caused by the following:
  - underdosage
  - insufficient trial of drug (minimum 2 weeks)
  - undiagnosed medical disorder
  - noncompliance
- Positive symptoms (hallucinations, delusions, thought disorganization) respond better than negative ones (blunted affect, decreased social interactions).

Administration Considerations

- All antipsychotic drugs are equally effective in relieving psychosis.
- Target or positive symptoms are hallucinations, delusions, assaultiveness, agitation, and sleep alteration.
- The effectiveness of low-potency versus high-potency drugs in agitated or withdrawn clients is a myth and not supported by research.
- Allow 4 to 6 weeks for adequate drug trial.
- The choice of drug for treatment is related to side effect profile, psychiatrist preference, and what has worked for client in the past.
- Dosage may be divided throughout the day or given at bedtime. Compliance is better when given at bedtime because the sedative effect assists in establishing a normal sleep pattern.
- Use of more than one antipsychotic drug has not proved to be effective or harmful; it is not recommended.
- Concentrate forms are light-sensitive; keep in dark bottles or packaging.
- Add concentrate to liquid or food just before administration to ensure potency; avoid using liquids containing tannic acid (tea), caffeine (coffee, cola), and pectinates (apple juice).

Treatment of Acute Psychosis

- Treat secondary causes of psychosis.
- Obtain baseline vital signs.
- Administer antipsychotic drug in a small test dose.
- Observe for 1 hour and then give daily.

- Increase dosage every 3 to 4 days, remembering that most clients respond to doses equivalent to 1500 mg CPZ.
- Rapid neuroleptization is achieved by the hourly administration of haloperidol 5 mg IM until sedation or control of violent behavior is achieved. Total dosage should not exceed 50 mg in 12 hours. This is believed now to be no more effective than using 10 mg po daily.
  - Monitor blood pressure for hypotension before each dose; withhold dose if BP is ≤90 systolic.
  - Monitor for dystonia occurring 1 to 48 hours after beginning of treatment; treat with an anticholinergic or antihistaminergic drug.
  - Monitor sleep state to achieve a 6- to 7-hour period.
  - Monitor the client for a decrease in danger to self and others.
- For sedation, lorazepam 2 mg IM or amobarbital 50–250 mg may be added.

Maintenance Antipsychotic Drug Treatment

- Recommended time periods:
  - First or second psychotic episode: 6 months
  - Three or more psychotic episodes: indefinitely, with trial withdrawal every 4 to 5 years
- To prevent dyskinesia or relapse the drug is tapered slowly.
- Compliance is a major problem in long-term treatment.
- Long-acting (depot) antipsychotic drugs:
  - Indicated in maintenance treatment of schizophrenia to deal with problems of compliance
  - Administered every 1 to 4 weeks
  - Given deep IM or using Z-track injection technique to prevent tissue irritation
  - Do not have a higher incidence of NMS, EPS, or TD.

Antipsychotic Drug: Clozapine[*]

INDICATIONS

- Treatment-resistant Schizophrenia: may improve both positive and negative symptoms
- Clients with severe EPS or TD

[*]References 4,16,24,44,60

- Hallucinations, delusions, and paranoia in clients with Parkinson's disease

PHARMACODYNAMICS

- Blocks serotonin, histaminergic, adrenergic, and cholinergic receptors to a greater extent than dopamine receptors
- Is classified as a dibenzazepine

PHARMACOKINETICS

- Absorbed almost completely from GI tract; completely liver metabolized
- Half-life: 8 to 12 hours

CONTRAINDICATIONS

Blood dyscrasias, bone marrow suppression, previous agranulocytosis from clozapine, pregnancy

SIDE EFFECTS AND MANAGEMENT

Of note, no EPS or TD has occurred to date. May actually cause remission or decrease severity of TD caused by other antipsychotics.

- Agranulocytosis: 1–2% incidence
  ○ Symptoms: Sore throat, fever
  ○ Monitor WBC weekly
  ○ Treatment: Discontinue drug if WBC < 3000 cells/mm^3 or granulocytes < 1500 cells/mm^3
- Sedation: Is dose limiting. Warn client about driving vehicles or operating other equipment that requires alertness.
- Seizures: Dose related; 1% to 5% incidence. Use seizure precautions. (See Protective Interventions: Seizure Management in Chapter 5.)
- NMS: Few case reports—in combination with lithium or carbamazepine.
- Hypotension: Orthostatic vital sign monitoring 3 times per day.
- Hypertension: Common in the first 2 weeks.
- Tachycardia: Dose dependent.
- EKG changes: Increase in PR interval. Use cautiously in clients with preexisting bundle branch block (BBB) or AV block.

- Pruritus: Cool water bath.
- Nausea: Provide crackers, have client focus on deep breathing.
- Hypersalivation: Occurs in 1/3 of clients. Reduce dosage; use anticholinergic drug.
- Hypothermia/hyperthermia: As with other antipsychotics, disruption in thermoregulatory mechanism may occur. Monitor room temperature, provide warm blankets and clothing as needed.
- Fever: Occurs in first 3 weeks in 10% to 20% of clients. Give antipyretic.
- Dizziness: Occurs in 20% of clients; higher incidence in elderly.
- Weight gain.
- Priapism.

COMMON DRUG INTERACTIONS

- Carbamazepine, sulfonamides, captopril: Are associated with agranulocytosis, therefore avoid concurrent use.
- Benzodiazepines: Possible increased risk of respiratory arrest. If an outpatient client, observe for 2 to 4 hours after initial administration. May see increased sedation, sialorrhea, ataxia.
- Anticonvulsants: Induce liver enzymes, therefore will enhance clozapine metabolism and reduce clozapine levels.

ADMINISTRATION CONSIDERATIONS

- Must be registered in the Clozapine Patient Management System (CPMS) for hematologic monitoring.
- Weekly CBC. Drug is dispensed following analysis of test results and clinical change.
- Do not exceed 900 mg/day.
- After 6 weeks 30% of clients respond.
- Levels may be clinically useful. Therapeutic = 4–500 ng/ml. Check after 5 to 7 days at steady dose.

Antipsychotic Drug: Risperidone[*]

INDICATIONS

Schizophrenia, Psychotic Disorders

[*]References 12,14,16,33,43,44,46,47,53,54,61,71

PHARMACODYNAMICS

Blocks serotonin (5HT), dopamine (weakly), alpha$_1$, histamine (strongly) receptors

PHARMACOKINETICS

- Metabolized in liver to one active metabolite
- Half-life, 3 to 4 hours; with both parent and metabolite 24 hours

CONTRAINDICATIONS

Hyperprolactinemia

SIDE EFFECTS

- Insomnia, sedation, agitation, dizziness, orthostatic hypotension (usually not clinically significant), weight gain
- Dose-related EPS: rare akathisia
- Possibly less TD with doses < 6 mg/day; may decrease symptoms of existing TD
- NMS: Several case reports

DRUG INTERACTION EXAMPLES

- Carbamazepine, phenobarbital: Induce liver metabolism and decrease risperidone levels.

ADMINISTRATION

- Begin dosing at 1 mg bid; may increase up to 3 mg bid after 6 to 8 weeks.
- In elderly begin at 0.5 mg bid.

▎ Anticholinergic/Antiparkinsonian Drugs (Table 4-3)[*]

There are three major categories of drugs used to alleviate the side effects of antipsychotic drugs: anticholinergic, antiparkinsonian (amantadine), and antihistaminic drugs. These drugs are used if it is impossible to decrease antipsychotic dosage or if client is at high risk for developing EPS.

[*]References 32,37,39,43,44,57,66,76

TABLE 4-3   Anticholinergic/Antiparkinsonian/Antihistaminic Agents

Major Classes	Representative Drug	Trade Name	Daily PO Dose (Range)	One-Time PRN Dose IM or IV (Range)
Anticholinergic	benztropine	Cogentin	0.5–6 mg	2 mg
	biperiden	Akineton	2–10 mg	
	procyclidine	Kemadrin	5–30 mg	
	trihexyphenidyl	Artane	2–15 mg	1–2 mg
Antiparkinsonian	amantadine	Symmetrel	100–300 mg	
Antihistaminic	diphenhydramine	Benadryl	25–100 mg	10–50 mg

Anticholinergic Drugs

INDICATIONS

Antipsychotic drug–induced EPS (acute dystonic reactions, akathisia, parkinsonism)

PHARMACODYNAMICS

Reduce cholinergic activity by inhibiting the effect of acetylcholine.

PHARMACOKINETICS

- Excreted in the urine.
- Effects of benztropine or biperiden are seen within 30 minutes after IM or IV injection and in 30 to 60 minutes after oral dose; they last up to 24 hours. (There is no significant difference in rate of effect between IM or IV administration.) Effect of trihexyphenidyl is seen at 1 hour after oral dose and lasts 6 to 12 hours.

CONTRAINDICATIONS

Closed angle glaucoma, bladder outlet obstruction (not absolute contraindication), delirium

PRECAUTIONS

Pregnancy, lactation

SIDE EFFECTS

Dry mouth, blurred vision, constipation, drowsiness, nausea, nervousness, urinary retention

OVERDOSE ("ATROPINE PSYCHOSIS")

- Symptoms: Dilated pupils, flushed face, hypotension, tachycardia, decreased bowel sounds, urinary retention, confusion, anxiety, hallucinations, picking motions by upper extremities, coma.
- Treatment: Lavage, supportive measures (administration of physostigmine is controversial).

ADMINISTRATION

- Dose is kept at a minimum level because of side effects. If symptoms of dry mouth and blurred vision are experienced, dose is not increased.

- Use for first 3 months of antipsychotic agent therapy; may use for 6 to 12 months if symptoms of EPS recur.
- Drug is discontinued slowly so as not to produce EPS.

Antiparkinsonian Agent: Amantadine

INDICATIONS

Parkinson's disease, counteract EPS caused by antipsychotic drugs, antiviral against influenza Type A.

PHARMACODYNAMICS

Causes presynaptic release of dopamine.

PHARMACOKINETICS

- Cleared 90% via kidney. Dose must be adjusted based on estimated creatinine clearance.
- Half-life 24 hours; longer in the elderly.

PRECAUTIONS

Avoid use in seizure disorder, uncontrolled psychosis, CHF, orthostatic hypotension, renal dysfunction.

SIDE EFFECTS

- Dizziness, decreased concentration, nausea—inform client that these will diminish with time.
- Hallucinations—drug usually is discontinued.
- Livedo reticularis—purple mottling of lower extremities that is not harmful to client.
- Mental status changes—if dose is not adjusted for renal function.
- Insomnia—give early in day (at dinner time, not bedtime).

DRUG INTERACTIONS

Anticholinergic drugs—additive effects.

RESPONSE TO TREATMENT

Improvement in EPS occurs within 4 to 48 hours.

ADMINISTRATION CONSIDERATIONS

- Initial dose should be based on renal function.
- Discontinue drug slowly to avoid seizures.

Antihistaminic Agent: Diphenhydramine

INDICATIONS

Treatment of EPS, motion sickness, allergic conditions.

SIDE EFFECTS/CONTRAINDICATIONS

Similar to anticholinergic agents.

▌Antidepressant Drugs (Table 4-4)*

A number of different types of antidepressant drugs are used to treat affective disorders: tricyclics (TCAs), selective serotonin reuptake inhibitors (SSRIs), monoamine oxidase inhibitors (MAOIs), and several miscellaneous agents.

Tricyclics (TCAs)

INDICATIONS

Major depression
Bipolar disorder, depressed or mixed
Psychotic depression
Panic disorder
Agoraphobia
Obsessive compulsive disorder (OCD)
Post-traumatic stress disorder (PTSD)
Chronic pain (neuropathy, post-herpetic neuralgia)
Migraine headache prophylaxis
Childhood enuresis
Eating disorders

PHARMACODYNAMICS

Believed to cause an increase in norepinephrine and/or serotonin in CNS; exact mechanism not known yet.

PHARMACOKINETICS
- Liver metabolism, then excreted by kidney.
- Serum levels peak in 2 to 8 hours.
- Half-life may extend for 3 days (range 10 to 89 hours).
- Steady state plasma level may take 5 to 14 days to achieve.

*References 6,8,11,18,24,36–38,41,43,48,49,52,55,56,58,62,63,70,73,76,77

TABLE 4-4 Antidepressant Drugs

Major Groups	Generic Name	Trade Name	Daily PO Dose (Range)	Therapeutic Levels (Range)	Half-Life (Hours)
Tricyclic	amitriptyline	Elavil	25–300 mg	100–250 ng/ml	
	clomipramine*	Anafranil	25–250 mg		
	desipramine	Norpramin	25–300 mg	150–300 ng/ml	
	doxepin	Sinequan	25–300 mg	100–250 ng/ml	
	imipramine	Tofranil	25–300 mg	150–300 ng/ml	
	nortriptyline	Pamelor	25–200 mg	50–150 ng/ml	
	protriptyline	Vivactil	15–60 mg		
MAOIs	phenelzine	Nardil	15–90 mg		
	tranylcypromine	Parnate	10–40 mg		2–5
Phenylpiperazines	nefazodone	Serzone	200–600 mg		5–9
	trazodone	Desyrel	25–600 mg		36; 7–15 days for act.met.
SSRIs	fluoxetine	Prozac	20–80 mg		15
	fluvoxamine*	Luvox	50–300 mg		21
	paroxetine	Paxil	20–40 mg		25
	sertraline	Zoloft	50–150 mg		4
	venlafaxine	Effexor	75–375 mg		8
Dibenzoxazepine	amoxapine	Asendin	50–300 mg		50
Tetracyclic	maprotiline	Ludiomil	50–225 mg		10–21
Unicyclic	bupropion	Wellbutrin	300–450 mg		
Aminoketone					

*Not FDA approved for depression; for use in OCD only.

CONTRAINDICATIONS

Closed-angle glaucoma, agitated states, urinary retention (bladder outlet obstruction), cardiac conduction disorders (e.g., bifascicular block, bundle branch block, second- or third-degree AV block), acute MI, orthostatic hypotension, delirium.

PRECAUTIONS

- Urinary retention: Monitor closely.
- Surgery: Discontinue prior to elective surgery.
- Myocardial infarction: Discontinue during acute period.
- Suicide: Potential for suicide is greater as the client begins to feel more energetic and as depression lifts as a result of drug therapy.
- Plasma concentrations > 1000 ng/ml will increase the QRS interval (may occur earlier).
- Abuse of amitriptyline by drug abusers.
- Seizure disorder: All antidepressants lower seizure threshold.
- Pregnancy: Avoid use, or use with caution during first trimester and while nursing because of potential harm to fetus or newborn.
- Ongoing therapy with MAOI.
- May potentiate preexisting psychosis.

SIDE EFFECTS

- May be partially treated by dose adjustment.
- Sedation: Greatest with amitriptyline, doxepin, imipramine.
- Anticholinergic effects: Greatest with amitriptyline, doxepin, imipramine. Treatment: Sugarless candy and gum, increased fiber and fluids. Bethanechol may be prescribed in some cases but is usually ineffective.
- Orthostatic hypotension, frequently resulting in falls, particularly in the elderly; clients do not become tolerant to this effect. Discontinue drug. Nortriptyline has least effect.
- Cardiovascular effects: Tachycardia, arrhythmia, conduction delays (quinidine-like effect).
- Precipitation of manic episode: Drug should be discontinued.
- Skin rashes.
- Weight gain: Caloric restrictions and increased exercise may be recommended.

OVERDOSE

- Symptoms (occur within 1 to 6 hours): cardiac arrhythmia and/or heart block, convulsions, hypotension, respi-

ratory depression, mydriasis, delirium. TCAs concentrate in heart, and owing to anticholinergic delay in drug absorption, client is at risk for arrhythmias for 3 to 4 days after the overdose. Close monitoring in hospital is required.
- Death may ensue with plasma levels > 1000 ng/ml.

COMMON DRUG INTERACTIONS

Many interactions are reported; therefore, refer to a current list of drug interactions or to a pharmacist when other drugs are being given.

- Antipsychotic drugs: Increased anticholinergic and sedative effects.
- Alcohol, barbiturates, cold medications, opioids: Additive CNS depression.
- Heavy smoking, birth control pills, lithium, chronic alcohol, carbamazepine, chloral hydrate: Decreased TCA plasma levels.
- Antihypertensives: Blocking of antihypertensive effect when used in conjunction with clonidine, methyldopa.
- Anticholinergic drugs: Anticholinergic-induced delirium.
- Anticoagulants: Increased anticoagulant effect.
- Procainamide, quinidine: Additive cardiac conduction delays.
- SSRIs: Increased TCA levels by a decrease in liver metabolism.
- MAOI: With clomipramine, Serotonin Syndrome can occur (see SSRI section).

GENERAL RESPONSES TO TREATMENT
- Drowsiness may occur and subside after initial period. Warn client about driving a car or operating a vehicle that requires alertness during the initial period of adjustment to medication.
- Maximum clinical response is noted in 2 to 4 weeks (up to 6 weeks in some clients):
  ○ Sleep pattern and appetite improve first.
  ○ Psychomotor activity increases before the client speaks about feeling better.
  ○ Mood and other symptom improvement occurs approximately 3 weeks later.

- Drug dose frequently is lowered or discontinued prematurely, causing a relapse, or not increased to therapeutic dose.
- Abrupt discontinuation of drug may lead to withdrawal symptoms (GI or sleep disturbances, movement disorder, hypomania or mania).
- Minimal potential for abuse; serious potential for overdose and sudden occurrence of cardiovascular reactions that can cause acute heart failure.
- Need for lag time of minimum of 14 days when changing from TCA to MAOI, to avoid potential hypertensive crisis. For treatment-resistant depression, however, both may be used together; they must be started together.
- Need for attentiveness to overall anticholinergic effects from all medication prescribed for client to minimize "atropine poisoning" effect; elderly are particularly vulnerable to interaction from central and peripheral effects of anticholinergic medication.

ADMINISTRATION CONSIDERATIONS

- Initial dose is low to minimize side effects and gradually increased as tolerated by client.
- For young client: Increase dose every 2 to 3 days.
- For clients over 65 years: Increase every 5 to 7 days.
- A maintenance dose may be given at bedtime, thereby reducing daytime drowsiness, dry mouth, etc., while assisting sleep at night.
- Generally, prescriptions are written for short intervals initially (e.g., 1 week) to decrease overdose potential, then monthly, then at 2- to 3-month intervals.
- Antipsychotic medications may be added when treating psychotic depression.
- Lithium may be continued when treating bipolar disorder.
- Six weeks or longer should be allowed for drug trial.
- Medication should be continued for 3 to 4 months after the client is free from depression because of the risk of relapse in first 4 months. For those clients with relapse history, long-term treatment may be recommended.
- Following the acute phase, the dosage is tapered slowly to prevent cholinergic reversal, i.e., nausea, vomiting, headache, sweating, pain in neck area.

Selective Serotonin Reuptake Inhibitors (SSRIs):
Fluoxetine, Fluvoxamine, Sertraline, Paroxetine,
Venlafaxine*

INDICATIONS

> Major affective disorders
> Obsessive-compulsive disorder (fluvoxamine only indi-
>   cated for this condition)
> Bulemia
> Panic disorder
> PTSD

PHARMACODYNAMICS

- Inhibit serotonin (5HT) reuptake in presynaptic neuron,
  selectively block neuronal uptake of 5HT, thus enhancing
  serotonergic neurotransmission at synaptic binding
  sites. Venlafaxine also inhibits norepinephrine (NE)
  reuptake.
- Decrease REM sleep (possibly the reason for its benefit
  in PTSD).

PHARMACOKINETICS

- Fluoxetine metabolized to active metabolite, norfluoxetine.
- Paroxetine metabolized in liver; no active metabolites.
- Sertraline absorption increased with food; food
  decreases nausea.
- Venlafaxine: In renal failure, decrease dosing interval
  from bid to qd. Food decreases nausea, has no effect on
  absorption.
- All inhibit liver isoenzyme CYP2D6; paroxetine > fluoxetine > sertraline > fluvoxamine > venlafaxine, leading to
  many drug interactions. Watch for drugs with narrow
  therapeutic index used concurrently: flecainide, quinidine, carbamazepine, propafenone, TCAs.

CONTRAINDICATIONS

Concurrent use or use within 5 weeks of MAOI.

PRECAUTIONS

- May cause hypomania or mania.
- May cause hyponatremia.

*References 6,7,8,15,22,24,27,28,30,35,36,40,43,38,39,55,56,58,60,62,63,65,
  68,70,72–74

SIDE EFFECTS

- Sexual dysfunction, anorgasmia.
- Headache, insomnia, somnolence, dry mouth.
- GI: Nausea (usually decreases after few weeks), anorexia, diarrhea.
- EPS: Highest risk in Parkinson's Disease or Bipolar Disease; parkinsonism, akathisia.
- Cardiac: No conduction effects or orthostasis seen (fluoxetine has been used to treat orthostatic hypotension)[21]
- Hypertension, agitation, tremor, dizziness (venlafaxine). Monitor blood pressure closely.
- Hypomania.
- Decrease in seizure threshold.

OVERDOSE

- Fluoxetine: Tachycardia, sedation, tremor, nausea, vomiting, agitation; 2+ suicide deaths.
- Fluvoxamine: Drowsiness, convulsions, tachy/bradycardia, hypotension; 2 suicide deaths.
- Paroxetine: Nausea, vomiting, CNS symptoms; 3 suicide deaths.
- Sertraline: Nausea, vomiting; no suicide deaths.
- Venlafaxine: Tachycardia, somnolence, convulsions, EKG changes; no suicide deaths.

COMMON DRUG INTERACTIONS

- MAOI—Serotonin Syndrome:
  - Caused by overactivity of central 5HT receptors leading to abdominal pain, diarrhea, fever, hyperreflexia, tremor, tachycardia, hypertension, delirium, myoclonus, irritability, hostility, cardiogenic shock, death.
  - Treatment: DC SSRI, supportive measures: anticonvulsants for seizures, clonazepam for myoclonus, nifedipine for hypertension.
  - May be divided into three types of symptoms:
    1. CNS changes: Agitation, restlessness, incoordination, hypomania, coma, seizures, confusion.
    2. Muscle tone changes: Myoclonus, tremors, shivering, rigidity, hyperreflexia.
    3. Autonomic instability: Hyper- or hypotension, tachycardia, sweating.

- ○ May look like NMS. Differences: NMS evolves over 2 to 8 days; has more autonomic symptoms, rigidity, pallor. Serotonin Syndrome evolves over hours and has more hyperreflexia, restlessness, unstable gait, myoclonus.
- Paroxetine: No change in any anticonvulsant levels.
- Haloperidol: Increased toxicity with fluoxetine.
- Cimetidine: Increases levels of paroxetine, venlafaxine.
- Metoprolol, propranolol: Fluoxetine, fluvoxamine decrease metabolism leading to bradycardia.
- Diazepam, alprazolam, theophylline: Clearance is decreased, half-life increased to 2 to 4 days by fluvoxamine
- TCAs: Increased levels by fluoxetine, fluvoxamine.
- Valproate: Increased levels by fluoxetine; decreased paroxetine levels.
- Clozapine: Increased levels by fluoxetine, fluvoxamine.
- Bupropion: Increased levels by fluoxetine.
- Phenytoin: Increased levels by fluoxetine; decreased paroxetine levels.
- Benzodiazepines: Increased levels by fluoxetine.
- Carbamazepine: Increased levels by fluoxetine, fluvoxamine; no effect on other SSRI levels.
- Pentazocine: Central excitatory syndrome in one case report: do not use together.
- Warfarin: Increased bleeding time by fluoxetine, fluvoxamine, paroxetine.
- Quinidine: Increased levels by fluoxetine, paroxetine.
- Astimazole, terfenadine: Use contraindicated.

ADMINISTRATION CONSIDERATIONS

- For OCD: Effect is seen in 4 to 6 weeks. May take 8 to 16 weeks for maximum effect.
- Discontinue venlafaxine slowly over 2 weeks or else dizziness, insomnia, nervousness and weakness can occur.

DOSING

- For depression: See Table 4-4.
- For OCD: Clomipramine 100–250 mg qd (200 mg in elderly) FDA approved.
- Fluoxetine: 40–80 mg qd (60 mg in elderly) FDA approved.

- Fluvoxamine: 100–300 mg qd (200 mg in elderly) FDA approved.
- Sertraline: 100–200 mg qd.
- Paroxetine: 20–40 mg qd (least amount of data).

Monoamine Oxidase Inhibitors (MAOIs)*

INDICATIONS

Atypical depression
Treatment failures with TCAs
Panic disorders
Chronic atypical facial pain
Bulimia
Migraine, cluster headache prophylaxis

PHARMACODYNAMICS

Block the MAOI enzyme that inactivates catecholamines (norepinephrine, 5HT, dopamine), thus resulting in higher levels in the nerve synapse; the process is irreversible and the body takes 2 weeks to produce more MAOI enzyme.

PHARMACOKINETICS

Metabolized in liver; unclear if distributed into placenta, breast milk.

CONTRAINDICATIONS

Liver disease, hypertension, CHF, pheochromocytoma, cerebrovascular disease, pregnancy and lactation, history of CHF.

PRECAUTIONS

- Discontinue prior to elective surgery.
- Begin diet restriction 2 days before therapy starts; continue for 2 weeks after therapy ends. (See Tyramine-Induced Hypertensive Crisis under Side Effects.)
- Seldom initially prescribed for children under 16 years of age or adults over 60.
- May cause excessive stimulation in clients with preexisting agitation or psychosis.
- Additional cautions include clients who are suicidal; history of seizure disorders, diabetes mellitus, hyperthyroidism.

*References 6,8,22,24,30,31,37,41,43,48,55,58,60,62,63,70,73,76,77

SIDE EFFECTS

- May be partially treated by adjustment of dosage.
- Drowsiness (and in some cases, brief stimulation): Warn client about driving a car or operating other equipment that requires alertness during initial adjustment to medication.
- Insomnia: Arrange dosage schedule so that drug is not given after dinner.
- Orthostatic hypotension: Advise client to change positions slowly, wear support hose, and maintain adequate fluid intake; warn client of potential danger from falls.
- Sexual dysfunction, impotence, anorgasmia in women (20%): May decrease with time; refer to physician for dosage adjustment.
- Constipation: Increase bulk and fluids in diet; exercise.
- Weight gain, edema: Instruct in dietary and exercise management. (Tranylcypromine causes least weight gain.)
- Precipitation of manic attack: Monitor closely.
- Hepatotoxicity: Monitor by periodic liver function tests.
- Neurologic: Myoclonic jerks (may respond to cyproheptadine), neuropathy, paresthesia (hard to treat).
- Pyridoxine (vitamin B_6) deficiency: May be treated with supplemental pyridoxine.

TYRAMINE-INDUCED HYPERTENSIVE CRISIS

- Prevention: Advise avoidance of certain OTC medications (see Sympathomimetic Drugs under Drug Interactions) and dietary restriction of tyramine-rich foods (aged cheese, beer or wine, MSG, liver, fava beans, packaged soups, meat extracts, pickled and smoked meats, fish, and poultry). Advise client to eat only cottage or cream cheese and only moderate amounts of coffee, tea, soy sauce, chocolate, bananas, and avocados. Teach recognition of signs and symptoms of hypertensive crisis and emphasize importance of immediate reporting if these should occur.
- Symptoms:
  - Occur 30 minutes to 24 hours after eating foods containing tyramine.
  - Headache, neck stiffness, nausea, vomiting, flushing or photophobia: Advise client to seek medical treatment immediately.

- ○ As crisis progresses, symptoms of severe headache, increased BP, chest pain, and collapse occur.
- Treatment:
  - ○ Chlorpromazine or sublingual nifedepine may be given to client to take as an emergency treatment. Teach client that headache may be caused by the hypotension from chlorpromazine as well as by hypertension from tyramine-rich foods.
  - ○ Phentolamine 5 mg IV is given to lower BP.

OVERDOSE

- Symptoms: Coma, increased respirations, tachycardia, hyperthermia, hypertension, hypotension, agitation, hyperreflexia, rigidity. Arrythmias, coma, and death rarely occur. Note that there is a 1- to 6-hour lag before serious symptoms appear.
- Treatment is symptomatic; dialysis can also be used.

COMMON DRUG INTERACTIONS

- Sympathomimetic drugs (ephedrine, phenylpropanolamine, pseudoephedrine, phenylephrine and amphetamines), foods rich in tyramine or tryptophan or excessive ingestion of chocolate or caffeine may cause hypertensive crisis and CNS stimulation.
- SSRIs (refer to SSRI section).
- Drug-free intervals of 1 to 2 weeks are recommended before changing from one MAOI to another MAOI, from an MAOI to a TCA, or from a TCA to an MAOI to prevent hypertensive crisis or seizures. However, TCAs and MAOIs have been used in combination for treatment-resistant clients.
- Psychotropic agents: Potentiation of MAOI effect.
- Anticholinergic agents: Additive anticholinergic effects.
- Antihypertensive drugs: Additive hypotension.
- Insulin or oral hypoglycemics: Additive hypoglycemic effect.
- Levodopa: Potentiates MAOI effect.
- Meperidine, dextromethorphan: Increase in temperature, hypertension, coma, or death. Use other opioids for analgesia and other cough suppressants for cough.

RESPONSE TO TREATMENT
- Clinical response may not be seen for 4 weeks.
- Positive response is seen by 50% of TCA non-responders.

ADMINISTRATION CONSIDERATIONS
- Advise dietary restriction of tyramine-rich foods (see Tyramine-Induced Hypertensive Crisis).
- Initial dosage is low and is gradually increased as tolerated by the client.
- Administer before 3 or 4 PM to avoid insomnia.
- Advise client of lag time before desired therapeutic effect achieved; allow at least 4 weeks for drug trial.

▌Miscellaneous Antidepressants*

Includes the two phenylpiperazines nefazodone and trazodone, along with the unicyclic aminoketone, bupropion, the dibenzoxapine amoxapine, and the tetracyclic maprotiline.

Trazodone, Nefazodone

INDICATIONS

Major depression
Sleep disorder
Chronic pain (neuropathic)
Agitation in dementia

PHARMACODYNAMICS
- Inhibition of 5HT reuptake, 5HT blocker.
- Increase in REM sleep, no change in REM latency; increases sleep time.

SIDE EFFECTS
- Nefazodone: Somnolence, dizziness, dry mouth, blurred vision.
- Trazodone: Sedation, GI distress, orthostatic hypotension (dose related), headache, priapism (prolonged erection–prompt treatment is needed).

COMMON DRUG INTERACTIONS
- Triazolam, albuterol: Half-lives increased by nefazodone.

*References 6,11,22,24,43,48,49,51,55,58,60,62,63,73,76,77

- Astemizole, terfenadine: Avoid use; no adverse events noted yet.

GENERAL RESPONSES TO TREATMENT
- Therapeutic effect may be noted in 4 to 6 weeks.
- Differs from TCAs in that the side effects do not include most cardiac or anticholinergic effects.

ADMINISTRATION CONSIDERATIONS
Must be given 2 or 3 times daily.

Bupropion

PHARMACODYNAMICS
Blocks dopamine reuptake; no effect on serotonin, norepinephrine, cholinergic or MAO systems.

CONTRAINDICATIONS
Seizure disorder

SIDE EFFECTS
- Insomnia, headache
- No anticholinergic, sedative, orthostatic effects

COMMON DRUG INTERACTIONS
- Carbamazepine, phenytoin, phenobarbital: Decrease plasma concentration of bupropion.
- Alcohol, antipsychotics, other antidepressants: Additive effects on lowering seizure threshold.
- MAOI: Increased toxicity of bupropion.

ADMINISTRATION CONSIDERATIONS
Do not exceed 150 mg per dose or total of 450 mg daily (avoid seizure possibility).

Amoxapine, Maprotiline

- Prescribed for major affective disorder.
- These have limited use because of their side effect profile: both have high incidence of seizures in overdose; amoxapine causes EPS and TD; maprotiline has high incidence of rash.

▌ Antimanic Drugs*

A number of different drugs are used to stabilize mood: lithium salts, anticonvulsants (carbamazepine, valproate, and clonazepam) and rarely, verapamil and clonidine (minimal supportive literature).

Lithium Salts: Lithium Carbonate, Lithium Citrate (Liquid)

INDICATIONS

    Bipolar disorder, manic phase
    Prophylaxis for schizoaffective disorder
    Major depression; potentiation of antidepressant response
    Periodic impulsive aggressiveness
    Cluster headache prophylaxis

PHARMACODYNAMICS

The mechanism of action is believed to be related to a group of neurotransmitters acting through a second messenger system.

PHARMACOKINETICS

- Eliminated by kidneys.
- Excreted in breast milk and may be found in sweat and feces.
- Serum levels peak in 2 hours; half-life is about 24 hours.
- Steady state plasma level reached in 5 to 8 days.
- Therapeutic index (narrow): Adult 0.6 to 1.2 mEq/L; elderly 0.4 to 0.6 mEq/L.
- Ethnic difference: Asian clients may have increased CNS response; lower doses needed in black clients.

CONTRAINDICATIONS

Cardiovascular disease, renal disorders, epilepsy, dehydration, pregnancy (high fetal risk, but benefit may be acceptable despite risk).

PRECAUTIONS

- Fever and/or diarrhea: The amount of lithium required will be less and danger of toxicity will be greater.

*References 5,8,19,24,29,34,36,42,43,48,52,60,63,76

- Breast-feeding: Infant may develop toxicity.
- Surgery: Lithium may be restarted the following day.
- Hyponatremia/sodium-wasting diuretics: Will cause increased toxicity by increase in lithium reabsorption with sodium in the kidney.
- Not FDA approved for use in children under 12.

SIDE EFFECTS

- Subsiding after 1 to 2 weeks: nausea, vomiting, diarrhea, thirst, weight loss, hand tremors, muscle weakness, polyuria (may wet the bed at night), swelling in hands and feet, decrease in sexual functioning.
- Related to long-term use:
  ○ Fine hand tremor: Lithium-induced tremor is related to voluntary movement and is not relieved by antiparkinsonian drugs. Treatment consists of decreasing lithium dosage in cases where tremor is more troublesome. Beta-blockers have also been effective, i.e., propranolol 10 to 40 mg bid; atenolol 50 mg qd, nadolol 80 to 240 mg qd.
  ○ GI distress, pain, and diarrhea: Caused by presence of unabsorbed lithium irritating the large intestine. Treated by changing type of lithium product to extended release, by having smaller, more frequent doses, and by taking the drug with meals.
  ○ Weight gain: Approaches include dietary instruction about avoiding high-calorie drinks/foods, having a sufficient amount of sodium intake, and increasing exercise.
  ○ Nephrogenic diabetes insipidus: Due to cumulative lithium use. Symptoms are polyuria, thirst, weight gain, and nocturia; not considered a reason to discontinue lithium. A diuretic, such as amiloride, may by used as treatment. Usually reversible with discontinuation of lithium.
  ○ Nephrotic syndrome: Case reports, caused by glomerular nephritis; is reversible.
  ○ Neurologic symptoms: Parkinsonian symptoms, cognitive dysfunction.
  ○ Depressed thyroid function: There is an asymptomatic enlargement of the thyroid after long-term use of lithium. Symptoms of hypothyroidism are tiredness, coldness in extremities, headache, myxedema,

decreased T_3 and T_4, and increased TSH. Most commonly occurs within first 6 months of therapy. Higher incidence with women. Treat by addition of thyroid medications or discontinuing lithium.

○ Dermatologic effects: Hair loss, acne, exacerbation of psoriasis: may use topical dermatologic treatments.

○ Leukocytosis (13,000 to 15,000 cells/mm^3): is reversible, but often leads to unnecessary work-up for infection.

TOXICITY

• Causes: Kidney disease, severe dehydration, overdosage of lithium.
• Symptoms (may occur at lower levels in elderly):
  ○ Early: Muscle weakness, diarrhea, nausea, lack of coordination, fine tremor, slurred speech, polydipsia, polyuria
  ○ Moderate (1.5 to 2.5mEq/L serum levels): Vomiting, severe diarrhea, coarse tremor, lack of coordination, hypotension, seizures
  ○ Severe (above 2.5 mEq/L serum levels): Nystagmus, seizures, coma, oliguria, anuria, cardiac arrhythmias, muscle hyperirritability
• Treatment: Discontinue lithium, administer fluids, correct fluid and electrolyte imbalance, and protect kidney function; hemodialysis when lithium level is > 3.0 mEq/L.

NEUROTOXICITY

• Life-threatening.
• Causes: Antipsychotics, anticonvulsants.
• Symptoms: Confusion, slurred speech, absence of nausea, vomiting and diarrhea; lithium level is low to moderate.
• Treatment: Discontinue lithium or other drug.

DRUG INTERACTION EXAMPLES

• Antipsychotic drugs: Increase in EPS with high-potency agents. Questionable increased incidence of NMS.
• Diuretics or steroids: Electrolyte imbalance secondary to a decrease in lithium clearance; increase in lithium plasma levels.

- Antidepressant drugs: Increased risk of manic relapse.
- Nonsteroidal anti-inflammatory drugs (e.g., ibuprofen, naproxen): Increased lithium level. *Note:* Aspirin, acetaminophen, and sulindac do not affect serum levels of lithium; however, because sulindac has not been studied adequately, it should be used cautiously in lithium patients.
- Succinylcholine: Increased effect by lithium.

ADMINISTRATION CONSIDERATIONS

- Carbonate product available as regular release, sustained release, controlled release; latter two products may produce less nausea, diarrhea, tremor.
- Obtain CBC, electrolytes, pregnancy test, data on renal function, cardiac states, thyroid function.
- Adequate kidney function, sodium balance, and hydration are essential to lithium excretion.
- Sodium balance is affected by low-salt diets, fad diets, and diet pills that lead to reduction in food and fluid intake. Excessive use of foods and drugs that are high in sodium (e.g., diet sodas, corned beef, antacids) also affect sodium levels.
- Encourage consumption of 2 to 3 quarts of fluids per day: urination may be more frequent as kidneys excrete lithium.
- Coffee, tea, and colas in large amounts (over 10 cups per day) may also promote the excretion of lithium because of the diuretic effect of the caffeine in these drinks. The stimulant effects from caffeine may interfere with mood stabilization.
- Usually given 2 to 4 times a day because of its rapid excretion; may be given at mealtime to minimize tendency to cause gastric upset.
- Periodic serum lithium levels are drawn as frequently as necessary (usually at 4 days when steady state is reached) to assure maintenance of therapeutic dosage level.
  - Serum levels are drawn 12 hours after last dose of lithium.
  - Initially serum levels are monitored weekly.
  - Maintenance serum levels may be monitored every 2 to 3 months.
- Serum creatinine and TSH (thyroid-stimulating hormone) levels are checked 2 to 4 times a year.

GENERAL RESPONSE TO TREATMENT

- Lag time of 5 to 10 days before therapeutic effect.
- In acute mania, because of the lag period, an antipsychotic may be administered to achieve psychomotor control and relieve psychotic symptoms. Observe for EPS, NMS.
- Recommended trial period of 4 to 6 weeks.
- Geriatric patients require less lithium, probably because of decreased renal excretion.
- Because drowsiness may be experienced, extra precautions need to be taken if client is driving or handling mechanical equipment.

Anticonvulsants: Carbamazepine

INDICATIONS

Convulsive disorders; bipolar disorder, manic phase (rapid cyclers), possibly for bipolar prophylaxis; trigeminal neuralgia

PHARMACODYNAMICS

Unknown; not via dopamine blockade

PHARMACOKINETICS

- Liver metabolism; metabolites eliminated in urine and feces.
- Induces own liver metabolism.
- Serum levels peak in 2 to 8 hours.
- Therapeutic range: 4 to 12 mcg/ml.
- Check levels 12 hours after dose.
- Half-life at steady state 5 to 26 hours. Steady state reached in 4 days.

ADMINISTRATION

- Initial dose is low, 200 mg bid, and is increased after 3 to 5 days to tid to reduce side effects (i.e., drowsiness, dizziness, nausea and vomiting).
- Maximum dose of 1,600 mg daily.

SIDE EFFECTS

- Drowsiness, dizziness, nausea, vomiting, blurred vision, ataxia and photosensitivity. Increasing dosage slowly, as tolerance develops, may help relieve these side effects.

- Blood: Leukopenia (10%), do not have to discontinue unless WBC < 3000 cells/mm^3, granulocytes < 1500 cells/mm^3. Development of aplastic anemia or agranulocytosis; recommended monitoring of CBC every 3 to 6 months; educate client about symptoms of fever, bruising, sore throat.
- Rash: 10% to 15% incidence; must discontinue drug.
- Development of hepatotoxicity: Recommended liver function tests every 3 to 6 months.

TOXICITY

- Symptoms: Altered level of consciousness, from drowsiness to coma; motor restlessness, from tremors to more gross movements; nausea; vomiting.
- Treatment: Induction of vomiting, gastric lavage up to 12 hours after drug taken; hemoperfusion.

PRECAUTIONS

Pregnancy: teratogenicity; can decrease neural tube defects by increasing folic acid ingestion before conception.

CONTRAINDICATIONS

History of bone marrow depression; renal, hepatic, or cardiovascular disease.

DRUG INTERACTION EXAMPLES

- Lithium: Case reports of neurotoxicity
- Anticoagulants (oral): Increased liver metabolism leading to decreased INR (international normalized ratio), PT (prothrombin time)
- Cimetidine, erythromycin, propoxyphene, diltiazem, verapamil: All can inhibit liver metabolism of carbamazepine leading to toxicity.

GENERAL RESPONSE

- Lag time of 7 to 10 days.
- Greater effect if used with antipsychotic.
- Onset of benefit for mania with carbamazepine is same as antipsychotic and may be slightly faster than lithium.
- May cause less memory impairment than lithium.
- Clients having poor lithium response may have favorable carbamazepine response, e.g., those with rapid

cycling, having more dysphoria or depression during mania, and a lower family incidence.

• Advise client to avoid alcohol or over-the-counter drugs; always use contraceptive techniques; notify health care provider of unusual bleeding, bruising, jaundice, abdominal pain, pale stools, darkened urine, impotence, CNS disturbances, edema, fever, chills, sore throat, or mouth ulcer.

Anticonvulsants: Valproic Acid/Valproate Sodium/Divalproex Sodium

INDICATIONS

Convulsive disorders
Bipolar disorder, manic phase (rapid cyclers)
Acute migraine headache

PHARMACODYNAMICS

Probably via inhibition of GABA metabolism.

PHARMACOKINETICS

• Valproic acid is the active component of all three products.
• In the stomach, valproate sodium is converted to valproic acid which is then absorbed
• Divalproex sodium (enteric-coated), once in the small intestine, dissociates into valproate, which is then absorbed.
• Liver—metabolized to one active metabolite.
• Half-life of 5 to 20 hours.
• Steady state reached in 3 days.
• Therapeutic levels: 50 to 150 mcg/ml.
• Inhibits liver enzymes.

CONTRAINDICATIONS

Liver disease

PRECAUTIONS

History of liver disease.

SIDE EFFECTS

• Dose related: Anorexia, nausea, vomiting, diarrhea, increased liver function tests (LFTs), tremor, sedation—all usually decrease with time or dose reduction.

- GI effects can be minimized by use of the enteric-coated divalproex salt.
- Tremor can be treated with beta-blocker.
- Hair loss is transient and may be minimized by use of multivitamin with zinc and selenium.
- Liver toxicity: Irreversible hepatic failure; greater risk if < 2 years of age, used with other anticonvulsants, and in presence of other neurologic abnormalities.
- Teratogenicity: Neural tube defects with use in first trimester. May be decreased with concurrent use of a multivitamin with trace metals and folic acid.

OVERDOSE

- Treat with hemodialysis to decrease plasma levels.
- Coma may be reversed with naloxone.

DRUG INTERACTION EXAMPLES

- Phenytoin, TCAs, phenobarbital: Increased levels secondary to inhibition of liver enzymes by valproate.
- Carbamazepine: Decreases valproate levels.
- Fluoxetine: Increases valproate levels.

GENERAL RESPONSE TO TREATMENT

- Educate client to symptoms of liver or hematologic dysfunction.
- Therapeutic drug monitoring required only every 6 to 24 months when used for mania.
- Factors associated with positive response: Rapid cycling, dysphoric or mixed mania, later age at onset, mania secondary to illness, hyperarousal.

Benzodiazepine Anticonvulsant/Mood Stabilizer: Clonazepam

INDICATIONS

Seizure disorder
Acute mania
Nocturnal myoclonus

CONTRAINDICATIONS

- Pregnancy and lactation (effects are unknown), liver disease, closed angle glaucoma.

- Seizures: use cautiously—may increase seizures when seizure disorder exists.

SIDE EFFECTS

Drowsiness, ataxia.

OVERDOSE

- Symptoms: Drowsiness, confusion, decreased reflexes.
- Treatment: Gastric lavage, supportive measures.

DRUG INTERACTION EXAMPLES

Antipsychotics, anxiolytics, antidepressants: Additive CNS depression.

ADMINISTRATION CONSIDERATIONS

- May be used in acute mania to achieve behavior control when an antipsychotic drug cannot be used.
- Discontinuation of drug may cause withdrawal symptoms (i.e., abdominal muscle cramps, sweating, nausea, convulsions).

GENERAL RESPONSE TO TREATMENT

- Decreased alertness: Advise care in driving or handling equipment where alertness is needed.
- Abruptly discontinuing the drug may cause status epilepticus.

Calcium Channel Inhibitor: Verapamil

INDICATIONS

Essential hypertension
Angina pectoris
Acute mania (no trials yet in maintenance therapy)

Note: Consult most recent literature for additional information.

SIDE EFFECTS

Constipation, congestive heart failure, atrial ventricular block

Alpha-adrenergic Agonist: Clonidine

INDICATIONS

Essential hypertension
PTSD
Acute mania (under study)

Note: Consult most recent literature for additional information.

SIDE EFFECTS

Constipation, drowsiness, hypotension, depression, urinary retention

▍ Antianxiety Drugs*

Antianxiety drugs (anxiolytics; Table 4-5) are used in the treatment of anxiety disorders and insomnia, in alcohol detoxification, to reduce preoperative anxiety and (certain drugs) as sleep aides. The major categories of anxiolytics include the benzodiazepines (BZDs) and buspirone; the sedative hypnotics include the BZDs, zolpidem, chloral hydrate, and certain antihistamines.

Benzodiazepines

Alprazolam, chlordiazepoxide, clonazepam, clorazepate, diazepam, lorazepam, oxazepam
Flurazepam, temazepam, triazolam (sleep agents)

INDICATIONS

Anxiety disorders
Relief of symptoms of anxiety associated with life crises (e.g., heart attack or other major medical conditions, death of a loved one)
Seizure disorders
Alcohol withdrawal
Panic disorder, PTSD
Skeletal muscle relaxation

PHARMACODYNAMICS

- Depressant effect on the CNS through the limbic system via the neurotransmitter GABA.
- Depresses Stage 3, 4 and REM sleep (making it useful for PTSD nightmares)

PHARMACOKINETICS

- Metabolized in the liver, some to active metabolites; excreted in urine.

*References 1–3,8,13,20,25,26,29,36,41,43,48,50,56,59,60,65,75,76

TABLE 4-5 Anxiolytic, Sedative-Hypnotic Agents

Major Classes	Generic Name	Trade Name	Daily PO Dose (Range)	Half-life (Hours) (includes metabolites)
Benzodiazepine	alprazolam	Xanax	0.5–10 mg	12–15
	chlordiazepoxide	Librium	15–200 mg	30–100+
	clonazepam	Klonapin	0.25–2 mg	34
(Anxiety)	clorazepate	Tranxene	15–60 mg	30–100+
	diazepam	Valium	2–40 mg	30–100+
	lorazepam	Ativan	2–6 mg	10–20
	oxazepam	Serax	30–120 mg	6–20
(Hypnotic)	flurazepam	Dalmane	15–30 mg	100+
	temazepam	Restoril	15–30 mg	10–20
	triazolam	Halcion	0.125–0.5 mg	1.5–5
Imidazopyridine	zolpidem	Ambien	5–10 mg	2–3
	chloral hydrate	Noctec	250–1000 mg	8–11
Azaspirone	buspirone	Buspar	15–60 mg	2–11

- Serum levels peak in 1 to 3 hours; 1 hour for diazepam.
- Steady state plasma level may take about 2 weeks.
- Lipid-soluble; effects of the drug may be noted for a longer period of time in the obese and in the elderly, who have less muscle tissue.
- Increased sensitivity and slower metabolism seen in Asian clients.
- Benzodiazepines are divided into two major groups based on their metabolism:
  ○ Short-acting: Oxazepam, lorazepam, alprazolam
  ○ Long-acting: Diazepam, chlorazepate, chlordiazepoxide, clonazepam

CONTRAINDICATIONS

Severe depression; closed angle glaucoma; psychosis.

PRECAUTIONS

- Confusion and memory impairment common in elderly.
- Suicide potential may increase as anxiety is reduced.
- Pregnancy and lactation: Increased risk of cleft palate when used in first trimester; safety not proved.
- Misuse or abuse, particularly after use for sedation.
- In continuous therapeutic dosing of long-acting BZDs, toxicity may develop due to slow liver metabolism.

SIDE EFFECTS

- Treat by dose adjustment.
- Faintness, dizziness, drowsiness, paradoxical reaction (i.e., violence related to disinhibiting effect); anterograde amnesia.
- Tolerance, dependence, withdrawal (return of symptoms at a greater intensity than before)
  ○ Generally does not occur when drug is taken for short time.
  ○ Withdrawal symptoms: Anxiety, insomnia, dizziness, headache, anorexia, hypotension, hyperthermia, psychosis, blurred vision, shakiness. Can use beta-blockers to manage the autonomic symptoms.

OVERDOSE

- Symptoms: Coma, confusion, diminished reflexes, hypotension.

- Treatment: Gastric lavage and maintenance of respiratory and cardiovascular functions. If other drugs (e.g., alcohol) are involved, the threat to life is more serious.

COMMON DRUG INTERACTIONS

- Tobacco: Induces liver metabolism, leading to decreased BZD efficacy.
- Alcohol, barbiturates, and other sedative-hypnotics: Potentiate sedative effects.
- Antidepressants: Potentiate symptoms such as sedation, dry mouth, blurred vision, rapid pulse, flushed face, urinary retention.
- Antihypertensives and diuretics: Potentiate antihypertensive effects.
- Sinemet: Loss of effect on Parkinson's disease symptoms.
- Fluoxetine: Decreases diazepam clearance.
- Digoxin: Increased half-life.

ADMINISTRATION CONSIDERATIONS

- Lorazepam is the only BZD consistently and rapidly absorbed by IM administration.
- Specific symptoms are targeted and treated for 1 to 3 weeks. Drug is usually tapered off in 1 or 2 weeks and discontinued; long-acting BZDs used for long periods of time are usually tapered off over 1 to 4 months.
- Recommend reevaluation if drug is being used for longer than 4 months.

GENERAL RESPONSES TO TREATMENT

- Sedative and calming effects are experienced 30 to 60 minutes after oral dose.
- IM administration of lorazepam produces sedation within 15 to 20 minutes. This drug is very useful in psychiatric emergencies.
- Anxiolytic effects are seen in first week.
- Sedation occurs at low dosage levels; therefore, client should be warned about handling machinery or engaging in activities requiring quick action.
- There is no antipsychotic effect.
- 20% to 30% of clients with Generalized Anxiety Disorder (GAD) do not respond.

Azaspirone: Buspirone[13]

INDICATION

Anxiety disorder: Useful in approximately 60% of GAD clients.

Not indicated for panic disorders.

This drug has less dependence and fewer drug interactions, particularly no additive effects with alcohol. It is preferred for initial anxiety presentations.

PHARMACODYNAMICS

Blocks 5HT both pre- and post-synaptically. Has no GABA effects.

PHARMACOKINETICS

- Absorbed in GI tract, metabolized rapidly and excreted in urine.
- Serum levels peak in 40 to 90 minutes.

PRECAUTIONS

Pregnancy and lactation.

SIDE EFFECTS

Nausea, headache, dizziness, ataxia, nervousness (treated by adjustment of dosage).

OVERDOSE

- Symptoms: GI symptoms, dizziness, drowsiness.
- Treatment: Gastric lavage, supportive measures.

COMMON DRUG INTERACTIONS

- MAOI: increased blood pressure; not absolutely contraindicated.
- Cyclosporine: Increased levels.
- Haldol: Increased levels, avoid concurrent use.

GENERAL RESPONSES TO TREATMENT

- There are *no* sedative, anticonvulsant, or muscle relaxation effects.
- Clients who have received prior treatment with BZD may complain because there are no sedative effects.

- Has no addiction, tolerance, withdrawal, decreased respiratory rate, or interference with complex tasks.

ADMINISTRATION CONSIDERATIONS
- Lag time for antianxiety effects may be 1 to 3 weeks; therefore, it cannot be used when reduction of anxiety is desired within hours.
- Need to administer for at least 6 weeks to determine efficacy.
- Take with food to increase absorption.

Antihistamines: Diphenhydramine, Hydroxyzine

INDICATIONS

Mild symptoms associated with anxiety (i.e., insomnia, nervousness).

SIDE EFFECTS

Drowsiness, anticholinergic effects, lack of tolerance to continued use.

Zolpidem

INDICATIONS

Sedative-hypnotic

PHARMACODYNAMICS
- Uses GABA receptors.
- Unlike BZDs, does not suppress REM, Stage 3 or 4.

PHARMACOKINETICS
- Half-life 2.5 hours.
- Absorption increased on empty stomach.

SIDE EFFECTS
- Nausea, vomiting at higher doses, drowsiness, dizziness.
- No tolerance or fatalities yet.

ADMINISTRATION
- Sleep onset 30 to 40 minutes.
- Short half-life may lead to limited duration of effect (3 to 4 hours); early morning awakening may occur.

- 5 mg HS for elderly.
- 10 mg HS for adults.
- Take on empty stomach.
- Use for short term only—7 to 10 days, although has been used effectively, without tolerance, for 1 year.

Chloral Hydrate

INDICATIONS

Sedative-hypnotic, alcohol withdrawal

PHARMACODYNAMICS

Unlike BZDs, does not suppress REM, Stage 3 or 4.

PHARMACOKINETICS

Liver metabolized to trichloroethanol, an active metabolite.

CONTRAINDICATIONS

Liver or renal dysfunction.

PRECAUTIONS

- Avoid use in clients with peptic ulcer disease (PUD).
- Pregnancy and lactation: Avoid use.

SIDE EFFECTS

- GI: Nausea, vomiting, and diarrhea are most common. Advise client to take with liquids.
- CNS: depression, daytime drowsiness, delirium, or dizziness may occur.

OVERDOSE

Can be lethal at doses as low as 4 gm.

COMMON DRUG INTERACTIONS

- Other CNS depressants: Additive effects.
- Furosemide: Blood pressure changes, diaphoresis, uneasiness. Avoid use together.
- Oral anticoagulants (warfarin): Increased PT/INR. BZD is preferred choice in clients on warfarin.

ADMINISTRATION CONSIDERATIONS

- Sleep onset 30 to 60 minutes.

- Tolerance occurs after 2 weeks of therapy.

See Table 4-6 for a list of generic medications and corresponding trade names.

TABLE 4-6 Generic Medications With Their Corresponding Trade Names

Generic Name	Trade Name
acetaminophen	Tylenol, Panadol, many others
alprazolam	Xanax
amantadine	Symmetrel
amiloride	Midamor
amitriptyline	Elavil
amobarbital	Amytal
amphetamine	Dexedrine
astemazole	Hismanol
benztropine	Cogentin
bethanechol	Urecholine
biperiden	Akineton
bromocriptine	Parlodel
bupropion	Wellbutrin
buspirone	Buspar
carbamazepine	Tegretol
chloral hydrate	Noctec
chlorothiazide	Diuril
cimetidine	Tagamet (now OTC also)
clomipramine	Anafranil
clonazepam	Klonapin
clonidine	Catapres
clorazepate	Tranxene
clozapine	Clozaril
chlorpromazine	Thorazine
chlorprothixene	Taractan
cyclosporine	Neoral, Sandimmune
cyproheptadine	Periactin
dantrolene	Dantrium
desipramine	Norpramin
dextromethorphan	Many OTC cough/cold products
diazepam	Valium
digoxin	Lanoxin
diltiazem	Cardizem, Dilacor, others
diphenhydramine	Benadryl, many OTC products
doxepin	Sinequan

(continued)

TABLE 4-6 *(Continued)*

Generic Name	Trade Name
droperidol	Inapsine
ephedrine	Tedral, Broncholate
erythromycin	E-mycin, many others
flecainide	Tambocor
fluoxetine	Prozac
fluphenazine	Prolixin
flurazepam	Dalmane
fluvoxamine	Luvox
furosemide	Lasix
haloperidol	Haldol
hydroxyzine	Atarax, Vistaril
ibuprofen	Motrin, Advil, Nuprin
imipramine	Tofranil
levodopa	Larodopa, Sinemet (in combo w/ carbidopa)
lithium carbonate	Lithobid, Lithonate, Eskalith, Lithotabs
lorazepam	Ativan
loxapine	Loxitane
meperidine	Demerol
mesoridazine	Serentil
methyldopa	Aldomet
metoprolol	Lopressor
molindone	Lidone, Moban
nadolol	Corgard
naloxone	Narcan
naproxen	Naprosyn, Anaprox, Aleve
nefazodone	Serzone
neostigmine	Prostigmin
nifedipine	Adalat/Procardia
nortriptyline	Pamelor
oxazepam	Serax
paroxetine	Paxil
pentazocine	Talwin
perphenazine	Trilafon
phenelzine	Nardil
phenylephrine	Neo-Synephrine
phenylpropanolamine	Dexatrim, many OTC cold products
phentolamine	Regitine
phenytoin	Dilantin
physostigmine	Antilirium (injection); Isopto-Eserine ophthalmic drops

(continued)

TABLE 4-6   *(Continued)*

Generic Name	Trade Name
procainamide	Procan SR, Pronestyl
procyclidine	Kemadrin
promazine	Sparine
propafenone	Rythmol
propoxyphene	Darvon, Darvocet, others
protriptyline	Vivactil
pseudoephedrine	Sudafed; in many OTC cold products
propanolol	Inderal
quinidine	Quinaglute, others
risperidone	Risperdol
sertraline	Zoloft
sulindac	Clinoril
temazepam	Restoril
terfenadine	Seldane
theophylline	Theodur, Slophylline, Theolair, Slobid, Uniphyl, etc.
thioridazine	Mellaril
thiothixene	Navane
tranylcypromine	Parnate
trazodone	Desyrel
triazolam	Halcion
trifluoperazine	Stelazine
triflupromazine	Vesprin
trihexyphenidyl	Artane
valproic acid	Depakene
valproate sodium	Depakene
divalproex sodium	Depakote
venlafaxine	Effexor
verapamil	Calan Verelan
zolpidem	Ambien

CHAPTER **5**

Major Nursing Interventions

▌ Abuse Protection*

Definition/Purpose

Abuse protection is the identification of clients who are at risk for or who have experienced physical, sexual, financial, or emotional harm in order to take appropriate action.

Specific Nursing Interventions

1. Identify clients who are at risk for abuse:
   a. Elders with limited resources who perceive themselves to be dependent on caretakers who have experienced abuse or neglect as children; elders with a history of being abusive to their children, who are now their caretakers; elders with extensive care needs who are dependent upon a single caregiver or family for help; mentally ill rural elderly;
   b. Developmentally disabled children and adults;
   c. Children whose parents have had another child removed from the home because of poor parenting, child neglect, or abuse; children whose parents have a history of Substance Abuse, mental retardation, or major psychiatric disorder; children who are the product of an unwanted or unplanned pregnancy; children who are perceived by a parent as the wrong sex or difficult and temperamental; children with a physi-

*References 7,18,22,24,43,63,65,73,76,79,82,102,103,110,116, 118,121,123, 130,131,136,146,151,153,163,172,178,181,183,188,205,210, 212,214,223

cal or mental impairment; children whose families experience social and kinship isolation, significant financial difficulty, high levels of family stress, and limited adaptation skills or resources; children who overrespond to negative emotional stimuli in the environment, have poor impulse control, display a sudden onset of temper tantrums, have difficulty in school adjustment, have problems with academic performance, social skills and competence; children in family foster care with younger foster mothers or who share bedrooms with other foster family members;

d. Children, elderly or dependent adults with persistent presentations for medical assessment and care that often results in multiple medical procedures, whose acute symptoms and signs of illness cease when separated from caregiver (possible Munchausen Syndrome by Proxy; see also Chapter 13);

e. Children or elderly whose caregivers are alcohol or substance abusers;

f. Clients with a history of domestic violence or history of "accidental" injuries; women whose partners feel entitled to dominate and control them and use verbal threats to reestablish or maintain dominance;

g. Women with "numerous physical problems that may be associated with battering, such as abdominal and gastrointestinal complaints, palpitations, dizziness, atypical chest pain, fatigue, decreased concentration and sexual dysfunction";[123,p.328] women with complaints that may also include choking sensations, hyperventilation, pelvic and back pain, insomnia, and nightmares.

2. Observe for signs of physical abuse in infant, child, elder, e.g., numerous injuries in various stages of healing; unexplained bruises, friction burns, fractures, facial lacerations and abrasions, indication of human bite marks.

3. Observe for indications of neglect:
   a. Children with poor or inconsistent growth patterns, failure to thrive, consistent hunger, poor hygiene;
   b. Elders with poor hygiene, inappropriate, torn, soiled clothing; untreated health problems, including mal-

nutrition, pressure sores, perineal excoriation; elders with evidence of medication deprivation or sedation; elders with lack of social contacts.

4. Observe for signs of sexual abuse:
   a. Children: "vaginal discharge, genital soreness, rashes, fear of the dark, sleep disturbances, nightmares, sexually provocative language, sexually inappropriate behavior"[65,p.236]; a child who has difficulty walking or sitting; child's underwear is stained or bloody; child with recurrent urinary tract infections, acquired sexually transmitted diseases.
   b. Elderly: genital, vaginal, anal, or penile injuries; presence of semen or dried blood; acquired sexually transmitted diseases; dramatic behavioral changes, health changes with undetermined etiology.

5. Note signs of emotional abuse in elderly—overly cautious behavior in presence of caregiver, apologetic about own behavior to health care provider, depression, humiliation, suicidal ideation/intent.

6. Inquire about history of emotional or sexual abuse in the pregnant client as appropriate.

7. Observe for presence of fearfulness toward spouse in women seeking treatment for marital difficulties.

8. Provide privacy for client prior to questioning and discussion of abusive relationship/situation; emphasize confidentiality of information, that it will not be shared with client's partner, caregiver.

9. Assess for presence of suicidal or homicidal ideation.

10. Inform client that intent to harm self or others will result in appropriate actions to protect client or others, e.g., admission or commitment to psychiatric facility, warning intended victim, notifying police.

11. Elicit information from female client about patterns of conflict resolution, e.g., who makes major decisions (money management, living arrangements), male use of aggressive strategies, verbal threats; disparity in relationship with male feeling entitled to dominate and control partner.

12. Validate seriousness of abuse by using statements such as "Did someone do this to you?" or "It sounds like he is being abusive to you"[121,p.11]; avoid reinforcement of denial in client who denies abuse but continues

to express concern; offer resources when client *can* acknowledge recognition of abuse; when a client is in an ongoing therapeutic relationship, periodically reintroduce topic (of abuse) to help the client to acknowledge recognition of abuse and to begin to explore options for ending violence.

13. Ensure accurate documentation in client's medical record, including verbatim statements from client (to the extent possible) to provide written communication for future health care providers as well as for future use by client who pursues legal recourse against abuser; include objective data, such as description of bruises or injuries, body chart that notes location of injuries and photographs (with client's permission); record assessment findings of client's descriptions of injuries that are inconsistent with severity and pattern of injury when client is unwilling to acknowledge actual abuse; follow agency protocol for collection and storage of evidence of abuse.

14. Emphasize importance of the client's conducting a danger assessment for recognition of escalation of abuse that puts her (and children) at risk for homicide, e.g., abuser's access to weapons, increased surveillance of client's daily activities, assaults on pets, threats to children, destruction of possessions of sentimental or monetary value.

15. Expedite development of a safety plan for client who chooses to remain with an abusive partner, e.g., "planning an escape route, arranging in advance for a safe place to stay, keep some money, house and car keys and important papers for herself and her children in a location where they can easily be retrieved."[76,p.52]

16. Ensure that client is provided with information for exploration of resources for independent living after leaving abusive relationship, e.g., housing, finances, job, child care, as well as information for accessing the criminal justice and law enforcement systems and legal counseling.

17. Based on individual assessment, collaborate with multidisciplinary team for evaluation and referral for further treatment of physical injuries or illness related to abuse, the need for referral to counseling, or treatment of Substance Abuse; consult legal counsel as appropriate.

18. Convey unconditional support to facilitate client's decision-making about actual or potential abusive situation.
19. In situations that involve potential or actual child or elder abuse, conduct a comprehensive family assessment that incorporates input from family members as well as other health care providers; review should be used to facilitate accurate problem identification and prioritization, to identify and use family's behavioral assets and strengths, and to set up achievable, measurable goals.
20. Emphasize concern for client safety when conducting family evaluation to verify suspected child/elder abuse; interview client and family members separately.
21. Inquire about cultural child-rearing beliefs and practices, discipline, and the use or tolerance of corporal punishment.
22. Inquire about the history of intra-family aggression.
23. Encourage family members or caregiver to describe their feelings, including discussion of frustrations and factors that could be associated with abusive and neglectful behaviors.
24. Encourage client's description about family's knowledge and ability to care for client.
25. Evaluate family's ability to meet client's care and safety needs.
26. Collaborate with multidisciplinary team for protection of child or elder who is a victim of Munchausen by Proxy (see also Chap. 13). Establish a plan of care that is based on the victim's age, level of dependence, and compliance toward the perpetrator. This plan will focus on protection of the client from injury (from family member) during hospitalization and may include close supervision of client when visitors are present with client in direct view of staff at all times; ongoing environmental assessment of client's room, including monitor alarm settings, IV infusion rates, items brought in from outside of the hospital, examination of wastebaskets for unusual items that may be associated with the client's symptoms; providing emotional support to family by keeping them informed of client's medical status; encouraging family to express their emotions; reinforcing positive family caregiver responses; developing a

discharge plan that maximizes the client's safety (this may mean that the client is not discharged home to the family).

27. Develop an individualized family treatment program that is culturally relevant.

28. Based on individual family assessment and availability of resources, use home-based services, e.g., a visiting nurse, to provide family education on topics such as maternal/infant health and care, to enhance informal support from close friends and other family, to establish linkages with formal health and human services, e.g., prenatal, well child care, Planned Parenthood, mental health counseling, legal aid.

29. Provide elderly client and family with information on community resources, e.g., access to senior services, visiting nurses, housing assistance, transportation, Meals on Wheels.

30. Teach client to avoid living with person with history of violent behavior or Substance Abuse.

31. Emphasize to elderly client the importance of having Social Security or pension checks deposited directly and of not signing documents or making financial arrangements prior to seeking legal advice.

32. Encourage families to maintain close ties with aging relatives and friends, to enable their monitoring of changes in health and ability to live independently.

33. Teach family to recognize warning signs of physical, sexual, or emotional abuse in child or elder.

34. Emphasize importance of careful scrutiny in hiring preschool program personnel or caregivers for elderly.

35. Acknowledge recognition of emotional suffering and trauma of parents whose children have been abused by another; offer individual or family therapy as deemed appropriate; provide referral to support group for parents whose children have been abused by others.

36. Based on individual assessment, refer parents who have been abusive to a self-help group such as Parents Anonymous.

37. Inform client's family of confidentiality limits as they apply to mandatory reporting of child/elder abuse to appropriate state agencies.

38. Follow agency guidelines for documentation and reporting of suspected or actual abuse; adhere to mandatory reporting of child and elder abuse as required by state statutes.

■ Assertiveness Training*

Definition/Purpose

Assertiveness training teaches clients, families, and groups communication techniques that enable them to directly express their opinions, thoughts, and feelings in a manner that fosters and maintains the dignity and self-respect of both the sender and the receiver of the communication.

Specific Nursing Interventions

1. Identify clients who are likely to benefit from assertiveness training, e.g., clients with passive or aggressive patterns of interaction.
2. Assist the client to identify behaviors that he or she would like to change.
3. Emphasize the importance of the client's recognition that he or she cannot change others but that the client *can* change *own* behaviors.
4. Suggest that the client focus on changing one behavior at a time.
5. Help the client formulate realistic goals that are achievable within a realistic time frame.
6. Teach the client to use statements that begin with "I" when expressing own viewpoint; to clearly convey information needs, expectations, or desired behaviors from others; how to deal with anger in self and in others; to differentiate passive, assertive, and aggressive behaviors; to become aware of nonverbal behaviors, e.g., facial expression, body posture, tone of voice that are congruent with the verbal message of the sender or the receiver.
7. Assist the client in learning to accept praise and to give compliments.
8. Use role-playing techniques and group feedback to increase the client's recognition of strengths and difficulties in using new communication techniques.

*References 8,33,129,131,134,139,140a,140b, 142,167,221

9. Provide opportunities for the client to practice self-praise and recognition.

▌ Contracting[*]

Definition/Purpose

Contracting is a method to obtain a mutually agreed-upon set of expectations, actions, or goals about the client's treatment or health care. Contracting is used to increase the client's adherence to a therapeutic regimen, to increase the client's motivation, to move the client to independence, to prevent violence, to minimize staff splitting, to set limits, and to maximize consistency among the treatment team.

Specific Nursing Interventions

1. Prior to contracting, establish rapport with the client (and family, as appropriate) to maximize potential for success in the intervention; assess client's cognitive ability to understand and to remember the contract; conduct a behavioral analysis that includes identification of events that precede the unwanted behavior, the smaller segments of the behavior, and the consequences that result from this behavior.
2. Assess the client's cognitive potential and motivation for participating in a treatment plan that includes contracting.
3. Respect the client's right to make informed decisions about psychiatric treatment.
4. Promote the client's participation in identifying desired behavioral changes and specific goals that are realistic, attainable, and measurable.
5. Use the client's own words, whenever possible, to describe target behaviors and goals.
6. Determine the need for including a reinforcer or reward in the contract.
7. Specify appropriate and unacceptable client behaviors, as well as consequences for breaching the contract.
8. Describe the responsibilities and expected activities of the client, the nurse, or other members of the interdisciplinary team.

[*]References 46b,106,107,127,131,143,185

9. Incorporate a time-dated component, e.g., specify when the client will begin to work on the behavioral changes, goals, and when the contract will be terminated.

10. Provide the client with a copy of the written contract after it has been signed by both the client and the nurse, and include a copy in the client's chart.

11. Collaborate with other members of the multidisciplinary team to ensure consistency in the implementation and adherence to the client's contract.

12. Review the contract with the client at agreed-upon time intervals, to evaluate the client's progress toward goal achievement and to determine the need for renegotiation and revision of the terms.

▌ Crisis Intervention*

Definition/Purpose

Crisis intervention uses crisis theory as the framework for applying structured problem-solving techniques (assessment, planning, intervention, and evaluation) to reduce the intensity of the crisis so that the client, family, or group experiences a perceptual-cognitive-emotional equilibrium that is equal to or better than their pre-crisis level. Crisis intervention is directed toward maximizing the potential for learning and growth while preventing or reducing ineffective and dysfunctional responses to biopsychosocial stressors.

Specific Nursing Interventions

ASSESSMENT

- Determine the client's level of anxiety, anger, and distress, including suicidal or homicidal intent, as well as the possible influence of alcohol and drug use on the current crisis.
- Help the client identify and describe the precipitating event.
- Help the client to maintain a focus on the here and now.
- Encourage the client to express thoughts, feelings, and behaviors aroused by crisis.
- Assist the client to describe the client's perceptions of client's ability to cope with current situation.

*References 2,6,11,19,46b,55,69,99,117,131,193,208

- Determine the client's current social support and available resources, e.g., family, community.
- Determine the client's ability to participate in planning for therapeutic interventions.
- Help the client identify, describe, and analyze past coping behaviors during problematic situations.

PLANNING

- Help the client explore various alternatives for coping with the current situation to maximize his or her support system.
- Help the client identify existing strengths and resources, e.g., spiritual beliefs, personal philosophy, and situational supports, e.g., family, friends, community, to minimize sense of isolation.
- Help the client develop realistic plans to cope with the current situation and to evaluate possible outcomes of proposed solutions.

INTERVENTION

- Initiate actions to minimize physical danger for client and/or significant others, e.g., arrange for protection from abusive spouse, notify appropriate persons of client's verbalization of intent to harm self or others.
- Facilitate the client's regaining emotional control by assisting him or her to redefine the situation by adding additional information or reorganizing existing information.
- Convey recognition of the client's contributions in generating possible solutions.
- Based on the individual situation, use the client's family or other support groups as a resource in the implementation of therapeutic strategies.
- Initiate referrals (specify dates, times, places) based on individual client need and desire to specific treatment programs, e.g., alcohol or drug treatment, marital or group therapy.

EVALUATION

- Facilitate the client's evaluation of the plan that was implemented, e.g., have client compare current level of psychological coping and comfort to level prior to the precipitating event.
- Help client develop realistic plans for the future.

• Consider the need for referral for a brief or long-term course of psychotherapy or for hospitalization.

▌ Decision-Making*

Definition/Purpose

Decision-making nursing interventions focus on the client's use of an organized, systematic process for choosing a specific course of action and for making informed decisions that are consistent with the client's personal beliefs, values, and goals. Decision-making interventions increase the client's sense of empowerment.

Specific Nursing Interventions

1. Determine if client wants or needs to make a decision or if client is seeking advice.
2. Conduct a cognitive assessment to determine the client's ability to comprehend and to make independent decisions, e.g., consistency in orientation, memory, reality testing, judgment; also, evaluate the impact of the client's level of anxiety and hopelessness on decision-making; if client's decision-making is impaired prior to treatment, collaborate with interdisciplinary team to ensure periodic re-evaluation of the client's decision-making ability after treatment has been initiated, to maximize the client's opportunities for making his or her own informed decisions.
3. Conduct a cultural assessment to determine the influence of the client's cultural background and values on decision-making.
4. Based on individual assessment and the client's preference, evaluate the benefit of including his or her family, significant others, other professionals, or resource persons in decision-making process.
5. Help the client to identify and clarify the problem that requires a course of action and to identify factors that interfere with decision-making process.
6. Encourage the client to prioritize and to focus on one decision at a time, to minimize feeling overwhelmed.
7. Have the client identify and describe desired goals and alternative goals.

*References 19,32,45,67,105,109,131,137,142,150,165,185, 213,222

8. Teach the client to consider a variety of approaches for arriving at a decision, by using techniques such as:

   brainstorming to generate a list of written potential solutions without taking time to evaluate how good or bad they are, in order to identify as many solutions as possible and to avoid rejecting any alternatives too hastily;

   changing point of view or frame of reference so that the client imagines advising another client or friend what to do;

   adapting or modifying a solution that has worked for client in previous similar situations.

9. Have the client prioritize alternatives according to his or her criteria of importance and input from others.

10. Avoid imposing own values and beliefs on the client's decision, selection, and ranking of alternatives.

11. Assist the client to compare and contrast the positive and negative consequences that could result from each alternative and to identify barriers or impediments for implementing decision or alternatives, e.g., client's knowledge, motivation, and availability of resources.

12. Help the client to develop contingency plans for dealing with consequences of chosen course of action.

13. Assist the client to communicate decisional needs, values, and plans to family and members of interdisciplinary team.

14. Support client's implementation of decision.

15. Provide opportunity for the client to evaluate effectiveness of decision by having him or her review original goals and compare current outcomes in terms of the successful achievement or failure to achieve original goals.

16. Support the client's analysis of decisional outcomes as preparation for selection of new solutions or modification of previous decision.

▎ Discharge Planning*

Definition/Purpose

Discharge planning comprises systematic nursing actions in collaboration with the multidisciplinary team, the client, and family (as appropriate) that focus on the process of

*References 35,60,91,111,124,131,133,135,149,176,180,190,198, 218

the psychiatric client's transition or termination from the current psychiatric mental health treatment setting to another environment within or outside the current health care community. Discharge planning reduces relapse or rehospitalization by ensuring continuity of health care.

Specific Nursing Interventions

1. Identify clients who are at risk for experiencing problems in their resocialization and reintegration into the community, e.g., clients with a history of Substance Abuse, the elderly living alone, the homeless, the unemployed, the chronically mentally ill, and clients with special education needs.
2. Collaborate with the multidisciplinary team in the development of an individualized discharge plan based on an assessment of client's discharge readiness to leave the current treatment setting. Assessment includes demographic information; the client's financial resources and past medical, psychiatric, and psychosocial history; the client's current level of functioning (ADLs); the client and family's information needs, e.g., understanding of diagnosis, medication monitoring, diet, call-back numbers.
3. Encourage the client and family to identify anticipated problems associated with discharge as soon as possible after entry into psychiatric treatment.
4. Have the client and family describe perceptions of current support system, e.g., family, friends, community resources.
5. Help the client describe plans for discharge and to develop measurable goals, including specific time frames, to be achieved prior to and following discharge.
6. Collaborate with the multidisciplinary team in the use of therapeutic passes to prepare the client for transition to community living.
7. Use the family as a resource in identifying problems associated with discharge and suggesting possible solutions for these problems; help family identify their needs and expectations.
8. Collaborate with the multidisciplinary team in the use of client/family meetings to formulate discharge plans and identify potential problems.

9. Contribute to discharge plans that are based on a realistic assessment of community resources for special populations, e.g., the chronically mentally ill, the homeless.

10. Maintain ongoing collaboration with the multidisciplinary team and other discharge planning resources, e.g., Advanced Practice Nurses or case manager, to clarify and coordinate discharge plans.

11. Coordinate referrals to appropriate and available mental health resources, e.g., individual or group therapy, halfway house, day treatment program, nursing home, visiting nurses, Meals on Wheels.

12. Based on the evaluation of outcome criteria, revise the client's plan of care prior to discharge.

13. Provide client and family with verbal and written information about available medical, social, and vocational community resources.

14. Assist the client and family in working through the termination process associated with the transition or discharge.

15. Provide client and family with specific information regarding mental health after-care appointments.

▌ Education: Client Education*

Definition/Purpose

Client education is goal-directed formal and informal teaching that is based on an assessment of the psychiatric client's learning ability, learning needs, and resources to meet these needs. Client education maximizes the client's understanding and management of health care and promotes adherence to treatment recommendations and plans.

Specific Nursing Interventions

1. Determine the client's learning needs and resources: identify the client's knowledge about psychiatric disorder (e.g., cause, treatment, symptoms, prevention, medication management); ask client to give examples of problems related to the management of psychiatric disorder; elicit client's desired information needs and learning goals; find out client's motivation for learning

---

*References 1,6,9,10,12,13,1,28,34,42,44,45,48,49,53,56,58,63,68,70,74,77,84,94, 122,131,147,159,160,215,218

(e.g., personal health beliefs and values, fears about mental illness, pressure from peers or family); find out the client's preferred style of learning (e.g., reading, individual or group education, television); identify possible impediments to learning (e.g., impaired vision or hearing, limited formal education, functional illiteracy, developmental or learning disabilities, presence of intrusive hallucinations, severe or extreme anxiety, memory loss); determine the influence of cultural factors or language barriers; obtain information about client's emotional support system and current living conditions.

2. Collaborate with the client in the development of realistic and measurable learning goals.

3. Develop an individualized teaching plan that is congruent with information obtained during assessment of learning needs and abilities, in addition to other information known about client's educational needs.

4. During initial, acute phase of treatment, collaborate with other members of the multidisciplinary team to assist the client to begin to recognize and learn that symptoms are manifestations of a disorder that can be treated; gradually provide the client with additional information about disorder and treatment.

5. Use simple words to explain treatment regimens; ask the client to use his or her own words to describe understanding of verbal and written instructions.

6. Use a variety of teaching tools, based on the availability of resources, that take into consideration the client's individual educational needs and learning abilities: consider using programmed and computer-assisted instruction to accommodate clients who are slow learners or those with poor tolerance for lengthy interpersonal contact; provide books and pamphlets that the client can easily read and understand; use printed materials that include questions to direct client's focus and maintain attention; use printed materials that primarily contain pictures for clients who have difficulty reading; use materials that are culturally relevant and written in client's own language; use techniques such as puppetry, artwork, and posters to enhance the teaching–learning process for children; use videotapes to enhance under-

standing and communication skills; use television for role-playing and social skills modeling; use audiotapes to provide client with ready access to review step-by-step processes in specific learning tasks; use bibliotherapy (e.g., books for laypeople and articles from current news magazines and journals) to explain psychiatric disorder and treatment in understandable terms and decrease some of the stigma that may be associated with mental disorders.

7. Use specific techniques to maximize client's self-care: use reframing to enhance client management of medication side effects, so that client views these effects as an indication that the medication is working; have client keep a journal to record medication side effects; use an individual or small group approach to teach the client the potential effects of psychiatric conditions and medical disorders as well as certain medications on client's sexuality; assign homework, e.g., specific reading assignment, television programs, practice of new skill, prior to individual or group meetings; use homogeneous groups for teaching self-monitoring and coping strategies and to provide psychological support, e.g., lithium group; use role-playing of potential problematic situations to prepare clients for re-entry into the community.

8. Collaborate with other members of the multidisciplinary team to provide classes that focus on activities of daily living such as the following: meeting self-care needs for grooming and personal hygiene, clothing selection, and care of clothing; planning and preparing meals, storing food, making grocery lists, and shopping for food and other basic necessities; money management, budgeting, using a bank, and managing a checking account; leisure planning and community resources for leisure activities; effective communication techniques and stress management.

9. Collaborate with Advanced Practice Nurses, e.g., Clinical Nurse Specialists and Nurse Practitioners, as well as members of the multidisciplinary mental health team to develop and implement health education programs that focus on issues such as healthy life-style practices, good nutrition, adequate sleep; regular

physical check-ups and self-exam (e.g., breast self-exam and Pap smears for women, testicular self-exam for men); management of existing health problems (e.g., hypertension, diabetes, obesity, emphysema and smoking-related disorders); risk for and prevention of AIDS and other sexually transmitted diseases and how to abstain from unwanted sex; assessment and management of safety hazards in the environment (e.g., group homes, private residences).

10. Evaluate the effectiveness of client education on an ongoing basis by asking him or her to provide a report of the achievement of identified learning goals (e.g., management of side effects of medication, ability to meet self-care needs, improved symptom management); directly observing the client's achievement of identified goals; using the client's family as a resource to provide additional information about his or her progress in achieving educational goals (when appropriate and with the client's consent); and by discussing mutual observations of the client's progress with the multidisciplinary team.

11. When the client's education goals are not met, evaluate the following: the client's acceptance of learning goals versus nurse's priorities for the client's learning needs; the clarity and appropriateness of goals in terms of the client's individual needs, learning readiness, motivation, and abilities; the effectiveness and appropriateness of teaching tools and techniques for the client (too complex, too elementary, culturally relevant, unrealistic time frame for accomplishment of educational goals).

12. Revise client teaching goals and plans, based on findings from evaluation.

▌ Education: Family Education*

Definition/Purpose

Family education encompasses goal-directed formal and informal teaching of the client's family or individual members within the family. Family education decreases anxiety about the client's health problems and treatment needs, clarifies misconceptions about the client's mental disorder,

*References 1,6,17,44,46a,49,68,69,77,81,88,100,108,122,128,131,132,154,157, 160, 218

promotes realistic expectations, promotes client/family adherence to treatment recommendations, reduces the client's risk of relapse, and improves family coping skills.

Specific Nursing Interventions

1. Conduct a learning assessment of the family's learning needs, abilities, and resources; include children in this assessment: find out the family's perception and personal beliefs about the client's psychiatric problems and mental disorder, e.g., causes, manifestations, course of disorder, and appropriate treatment; look for indications that the family is blaming themselves or client, stigmatization, denial, fears about hereditary aspects of mental disorder; observe for unrealistic expectations a family might have about the client's recovery and needs following discharge, e.g., living arrangements, financial support, emotional support, medication management; identify possible learning impediments of individual family members, e.g., impaired vision or hearing, limited formal education, functionally illiterate, developmental or learning disabilities; assess for influence of cultural factors on family learning needs and learning preferences.
2. Encourage the family to participate in decisions about the educational approach that would be most helpful to them, e.g., individual, group, meeting with or without client present.
3. Collaborate with the multidisciplinary team to implement a plan for psychoeducation that begins immediately following the identified client's entry into the psychiatric mental health care system: orient the family to the culture of the inpatient unit and its resources, e.g., physical environment, functions of different members of the client's mental health team and how they can be contacted; clarify roles of the client's mental health team; inform the family of inpatient unit rules and practices; provide family with basic information that also includes written information about the nature and anticipated course of the client's disorder and treatment, the expected outcome, and

the availability of institutional, local, regional, and national resources for the client and family.

4. Collaborate with the multidisciplinary team to offer psychoeducational groups to families, with a focus on interactive instructional activities, e.g., symptoms of disorder, communication skills that include facilitating contact with physician, medication management, and strategies for home management of stress and disruptive behavior.

5. Provide opportunities for family members to discuss the psychopharmacologic management of the client's disorder, e.g., target symptoms, dosage, side effects, resources for obtaining medication.

6. Prior to discharge, provide the family with information about the client's needs, responsibilities, and treatment plans, as well as information about day hospitals, day treatment programs, sheltered workshops, medication clinics, Alliance for the Mentally Ill.

7. Teach the family to differentiate between residual symptoms in the client and symptoms that are indicative of a recurrence of psychiatric disorder.

8. Teach the family to recognize and pay attention to their own needs in addition to the client's needs to prevent burnout in themselves.

9. Evaluate the effectiveness of family education on an ongoing basis by asking family members to report on fulfillment of their learning needs and goals, to identify additional learning needs, and to make direct observations of their ability to process and apply educational information to themselves and the identified client.

10. When family education goals are not met, evaluate the following: the family's identification, acceptance, and priority of learning goals versus nurse's identification and priority; clarity and appropriateness of goals in terms of family and client's needs, learning readiness, motivation, and abilities; effectiveness and appropriateness of educational approaches, e.g., too complex, too elementary, culturally relevant; unrealistic time frame for accomplishment of educational goals.

11. Evaluate need for referral to additional resources.

12. Revise family education goals and plans, based on findings from evaluation.

▌ Group Treatment*

Definition/Purpose

Group treatment is a therapeutic modality for achieving identified goals and measurable outcomes that are appropriate for the designated group.

1. The psychiatric nurse's leadership role in group treatment is influenced by his or her educational preparation and experience.
2. The psychiatric nurse can provide group treatment as a co-therapist with another nurse, another mental health professional, or a non-mental health professional; the psychiatric nurse can also function as the independent leader of a specified group.

Types of Therapies

GROUP THERAPY

Group therapy is "...a highly flexible psychotherapeutic modality...that can be adapted to a variety of settings, time constraints, goals, and techniques."[209,p.1148]

1. Setting: ranges from clients within long-term outpatient interactional groups to acute crisis drop-in groups.
2. Duration: as brief as one session (drop-in crisis group), time-limited sessions of 6 to 12 weeks, 1- to 3-year period for interactionally oriented outpatient groups.
3. Goals: achievable, measurable, and within capabilities of the specific group membership.
4. Selected therapy groups and goals:
   a. Acute inpatient psychiatric group: daily assessment, support, restoration of function
   b. Day hospital groups: deinstitutionalization
   c. Medication groups: support, education, maintenance of functions
   d. Behaviorally oriented group (Panic, Eating Disorders): specific behavior change
   e. Specialized groups for medical conditions: education, support, socialization

*References 3,5,6,12,16,28,29,36–39,47,62,69,93,113,119,120,128,132,140a,
145,155,157,158,162,166,175,177,185,196,207,209,211,217,219,220

f. Specialized groups for life events (bereavement, caregivers of persons with Alzheimer's disease): support, catharsis, socialization
g. Specialized support groups (Vietnam veterans' outreach, rape, crisis): support, catharsis

THERAPEUTIC GROUP

A therapeutic group provides a structured format for the encouragement of the client's natural healing potential.

1. Goal: to help client mobilize coping strengths to adjust to maturational or situational crises; enhancement of quality of life.
2. Selected therapeutic groups and brief description:
   a. Reality-orientation: often used with confused elderly to reduce or halt disorientation and to help maintain contact with their environment.
   b. Resocialization: used for withdrawn clients as part of their psychosocial rehabilitation; provides simple social setting with opportunity for modeling and guidance to improve social skills and self-esteem.
   c. Remotivation: uses a five-step technique to stimulate withdrawn or regressed clients to think about everyday life activities.
   d. Reminiscence: often used with elderly clients to help them recall past, personal life experiences that they can integrate in their current self-concept.

THERAPEUTIC ACTIVITY GROUPS

Therapeutic activity groups are a modality for expressing self through action and creative activities.

1. Goal: to improve self-esteem, express feelings and experience enjoyment and pleasure.
2. Selected therapeutic activity groups and brief description:
   a. Poetry and bibliotherapy: clients are invited to read and discuss books, poems, and newspapers.
   b. Recreational therapy: focuses on leisure activities that bring enjoyment and pleasure.
   c. Exercise therapy: stimulation of body movement and talking about effects of exercise on the mind and body.

SELF-HELP GROUPS

Self-help groups are small, face-to-face, informal, interactive units that are led by members themselves (there may be a professional person as an adviser).

1. Goal: focus on coping skills related to the purpose for the specific group.
2. Selected self-help groups: Alcoholics Anonymous, Al-anon, Ala-teen, Adult Children of Alcoholics, Compassionate Friends (parents who have experienced the death of a child of any age), Gamblers Anonymous, Narcotics Anonymous, Parents without Partners, Parents Anonymous (parents of child-abuse victims).

Therapeutic Factors[*]

Therapeutic factors that facilitate the client's development of more adaptive behavioral patterns are interdependent and do not occur or function separately. These factors exist in every type of therapy group; there is wide variation in their application and importance, according to the specific group. The emphasis of specific therapeutic factors in a given group is determined by the type of group therapy, stage of therapy, forces outside the group, and individual differences within the group. Therapeutic factors include the following:

1. Instillation of hope: The therapist works toward increasing clients' belief and confidence in the effectiveness of the group treatment. Clients develop hope for their own improvement as they see others in the group coping more effectively.
2. Universality: Clients discover that they are not alone and that others in the group may experience problems similar to their own.
3. Imparting information: Clients receive didactic instruction about mental health and mental disorder(s) and advice, suggestions, or direct guidance from the leader or other members in the group.
4. Altruism: Clients benefit from helping one another as they offer support, reassurance, and suggestions, often resulting in improved individual self-esteem.
5. Corrective recapitulation of the primary family group: Group experiences provide clients with the opportu-

[*]References 209,219

nity to correctively relive earlier family conflicts, to work through unfinished business from the past.

6. Development of socializing techniques: Clients have opportunity to experience direct learning, e.g., the development of basic social skills, as well as indirect social learning through the process of open feedback about maladaptive social behaviors.

7. Imitative behavior: Clients observe behavior of others in the group and have the opportunity to "try on and discard" specific behaviors for themselves.

8. Interpersonal learning: Clients display their behavior and gain an understanding of their impact on others through feedback, self-observations, and the opinion that others have of them. Clients also gain awareness of their own responsibility in developing their interpersonal world.

9. Group cohesiveness: Clients experience structure, warmth, and comfort in the group; are accepting of one another; are inclined to form meaningful relationships within the group; and develop the ability to express and tolerate inter-member hostility.

10. Catharsis: Clients are able to express strong feelings toward one another and work toward a genuine understanding of themselves and other group members.

11. Existential factors: Clients experience a sense of empowerment as they learn that there are limits to the guidance and support that they can receive from others and that they must take ultimate responsibility for the way in which they live their lives. They learn that no matter how close they get to others, there is also a basic aloneness in life that they must face.

Initiating Group Therapy

1. Decide on the type of group to be conducted: delineate the major emphasis and group goals.
2. In selecting group members for the type of group, consider the following:
   a. The diagnosis and the extent of the client's mental disorder
   b. Potential therapeutic value to client
   c. Client's motivation and willingness
   d. Factors such as age, sex, intelligence

e. The size of the group—depends to some extent on the type of group and the type of clients. A good range is from 6 to 10 members.
3. Select an adequate meeting area. It should be an adequate size for the group and free from interruptions, have good ventilation, and be attractively furnished.
4. Select the time and frequency of meeting:
    a. The actual frequency depends on type of group. A common frequency is once per week.
    b. Maintain consistency in meeting place, time, and frequency because changes can adversely affect the group process.

Therapist's Role in Client Preparation for Group

1. Role and interventions are influenced by the type of group, the type of clients, and the therapist's own theoretical orientation.
2. Preparation of the client for group can vary as follows:
    a. Client is referred for individual therapy prior to entering group therapy.
    b. Leader provides brief individual orientation that includes time, place, frequency; purpose of group; brief description of group members; ground rules, e.g., attendance, behavior that will not be tolerated.
    c. Client is informed if group session is to be videotaped or observed through viewing screen; client's permission is obtained prior to arrival at group.
    d. In an open group (one in which new members can be added at any time), the group leader introduces the client to the group and asks group members to introduce themselves; the group leader also summarizes what the group has been currently discussing.

Formative Stages/Phases of Group Development

1. Initial stage, orientation
    a. Tasks confronting the group include developing a method for achieving the purpose for which they joined the group and managing the social relationships so that all members gain comfortable roles for themselves.

b. Client behavioral characteristics include seeking to clarify the meaning of group therapy and what group membership entails; evaluating and testing other group members and seeking a viable personal role; seeking acceptance, approval, domination, or respect; demonstrating dependency on the leader and seeking guidance, approval, and direction; searching for member similarities; providing description of symptoms, medications, and former treatment; showing anxiety among members.

c. Specific interventions by group leader(s): serve as a role model for behavior expected in the group by demonstrating congruence, empathy, and unconditional positive regard for members; have members introduce themselves; discuss with group members what is expected of them in the group; offer structure and direction; answer questions in relation to time, place, frequency, and purpose of the group; foster and facilitate interaction by pre-empting monopolization; intervene to reduce social roles and interaction; avoid reinforcement of group need for dependency on leader.

2. Second phase

a. Client behavioral characteristics include: searching for power, control, and dominance; engaging in conflicts with members and between members and leader; expressing criticism and negative comments; giving advice, making judgments, and criticizing as a means of jockeying for position; expressing hostility and rebellion towards leader; engaging in fantasies of getting rid of leader.

b. Specific interventions by group leader(s) include: facilitate communication by reflecting or rephrasing group members' statements; permit expression of criticism and hostility toward leader; support the fragile group member, when needed, during inter-member conflict; foster and facilitate group interaction; continue to demonstrate congruence, empathy, and unconditional positive regard; focus on the here-and-now group experience; begin to explore group themes.

3. Third phase

a. Client behavioral characteristics include: development of group cohesiveness; increase in morale, self-disclosure, and mutual trust; suppression of expression of negative affect; increased concern about one another and missing members; increased awareness of interpersonal interactions as they evolve in the group; movement toward teamwork and focus on purpose and work of the group.

   b. Specific interventions by group leader(s) include: foster and facilitate communication; encourage exploration of behavior, interactions among members and topics discussed; provide feedback on group process; support development of group cohesiveness, self-disclosure, problem solving, and working towards group goals; offer the opportunity to work through feelings for loss or addition of group member (especially important for open groups); encourage members to respond to here-and-now experiences in the group.

4. Termination phase

   a. Client behavioral characteristics include: emergence of feelings about termination, e.g., mourning, reluctance to terminate; brief recurrence of earlier symptomatology; attempts to arrange for ongoing information about group; recognition of ability to constructively use resources in own personal environment.

   b. Specific interventions by group leader(s) include: regularly remind group of approaching termination; continue to focus on goal attainment; disclose own feelings about ending of group; facilitate members working through their feelings related to termination from the group or termination of the group.

▐ Protective Interventions: Activity Area Restriction*

Definition/Purpose

Activity area restriction is a therapeutic method of limiting the movement of a psychiatric client to a specific room or area, such as a client's room or unit, to protect the client from self-injury or injury to others; to assist the client to control impulsive behaviors; and to provide time for the client to re-evaluate the current situation and develop alternate responses for coping.

*References 83,97,101,131,143

Specific Nursing Interventions

1. Explain the procedure to the client; include the purpose and anticipated length of time of restriction.
2. Ensure that the client's treatment team is informed of rationale for the restriction.
3. Provide the client with support to remain within area, e.g., staff to help client focus on behaviors and actions that necessitated restriction.
4. Give client immediate feedback about inappropriate behavior; help client explore ways to modify behavior.

▌ Protective Interventions: Observation for Suicide Prevention[*]

Definition/Purpose

Observation for suicide is a method of prevention that employs continuous use of the nurse–client relationship to prevent suicide in a client who has been evaluated to be at risk for self-injury or suicide, to increase the client's control of self-destructive impulses, and to provide an opportunity for the client to talk about feelings associated with self-destructive behavior.

Specific Nursing Interventions

1. Provide a safe environment for the client: place the client in an area that permits constant observation, even in the bathroom, by nursing staff on a 24-hour basis; inspect the client's belongings in his or her presence and remove items that client could use to harm self, e.g., belts, scarves, pills, razors, glass, knives, matches; *remain within arm's length of client during waking hours; have the client sleep in a room or area that facilitates constant observation*; ensure that the client actually swallows oral medications; provide meals on a tray that contains no metal utensils or glass items, based on individual assessment of lethality potential with these items; if the client is allowed to have a regular tray, be sure to check for missing silverware or glass items when tray is collected.

[*]References 41,46b,57,61,80,85,131,165,179,187,216

2. Establish a dependable relationship with the client: introduce self, explain purpose for being with the client and ongoing availability; encourage description of thoughts and feelings about suicidal ideation or attempt; convey expectation of no self harm; develop a nursing plan of care with the client that includes (a) the client making a time-limited verbal or written "no self harm" contract and (b) a time-limited positive-action plan that facilitates increased client tolerance of emotional pain and development of "small constructive responses to suicidal ideation"[46b,p.162]; ensure presence of staff member at end of a specified time to evaluate need for continuation or revision of contract or action plan.

3. Monitor the following: current suicidal risk, presence of suicidal ideation, behavior, intent, change in suicidal plans; the client's perception of effects of suicidal ideation/attempt on others; presence of command hallucinations to harm self or others; prevailing feelings of hopelessness, helplessness, worthlessness, guilt; the client's perception of a support system, e.g., spouse, other family, friends, church; the client's ability to consider alternatives other than suicide as solutions for problems.

4. Help the client contact friend, spouse, parent, or other significant person; maintain one-to-one supervision during their visits; ensure that visitors do not inadvertently leave harmful objects with the client.

5. Collaborate with multidisciplinary team on a daily basis to discuss continuance of suicide precautions and observation.

▌ Protective Interventions: Seclusion*

Definition/Purpose

Seclusion is a therapeutic process of limit setting that involves the removal of a client from an open environment in contact with other clients, staff, or others to a private and secure room from which the client can be observed through a window. Seclusion prevents client harm to self or others, decreases stimulation from the immediate environment, helps the client regain control of unacceptable verbal and nonverbal behaviors, and prevents disruption of the ongoing treatment program and environment.

*References 4,50,54,64,75,80,97,112,114,131,143,152,171,191,200,202,208

Specific Nursing Interventions

1. Assess behaviors indicative of the need for the use of seclusion, e.g., increasing levels of agitation, hyperactivity, impulsivity, and intrusiveness; risk of client harming self or others, taking into consideration factors such as drug overdose or medical condition, that influence the client's medical and psychiatric status. *Seclusion is inappropriate for the client who is delirious or experiencing Acute Confusion, because the sensory deprivation may worsen the confusion.*

2. Provide protected room, e.g., empty cubicle with soundly constructed walls and floor, door that cannot be opened from the inside, protected window and ventilation equipment, recessed light fixtures, and no furnishings other than a durable mattress that is not flammable. A seclusion room cannot be used for clients on antipsychotics unless there is an adequate cooling system because of interference of medication with regulation of body temperature that could potentially result in death during hot weather. Try to have a clock and calendar within sight of client.

3. Ensure adherence to institutional and legal guidelines.

4. Clear immediate area of other clients and physical obstructions to seclusion room.

5. Select a designated leader to give client clear, brief explanations for seclusion, e.g., "Your behavior is out of control, and you must spend some time in a room by yourself to help you regain control."

6. Give the client the option of walking quietly to room, accompanied by staff. If client refuses, initiate seclusion procedure.

7. Use control and transport procedures as indicated in facility.

8. Assist the client, as necessary, in the removal of clothing, jewelry, and dangerous objects, e.g., belts, ties, scarves, knives, matches. Provide client with gown or shorts and tee-shirt.

9. Restate reason for seclusion and the necessary behaviors for release; inform client of the availability of the staff and how to ask for help with toileting or other additional needs.

10. The team should exit one at a time, releasing client's legs first and arms last. The last team member should quickly leave the seclusion room in a backward fashion, making sure that door to the seclusion room is securely locked.

11. Notify the client's physician immediately if this has not previously been done, keeping in mind that a physician's order is necessary for client to remain in seclusion.

12. Follow institutional guidelines for frequency of monitoring client—usually a minimum of every 15 minutes—and determine if constant observation is necessary.

13. Observe for client behaviors indicative of exhaustion or self harm as a result of agitation.

14. As soon as feasible, schedule time for staff to evaluate circumstances leading to the seclusion, discuss their reactions, and identify possible strategies for prevention of seclusion in the future.

15. Verbally signal nurse's presence at each check by calling client by name. Provide client with information such as time of day and when to expect next meal.

16. Collaborate with the multidisciplinary team to be sure that a direct visit in seclusion room is scheduled at least every 2 hours.

17. Provide for an adequate number of staff to accompany anyone who enters seclusion room, e.g., to talk with client, take vital signs, help with meals and toileting.

18. Take vital signs a minimum of every 2 hours.

19. Instruct client to sit in corner of seclusion room when serving food or providing fluids. Serve food in paper containers. Use blunt eating utensils. Promptly remove unused portions, containers, and utensils.

20. Offer fluids frequently to prevent dehydration.

21. Offer bathroom facilities every 2 to 3 hours.

22. Provide ongoing brief interactions to decrease client's feeling of abandonment.

23. Avoid exploration of conflicts, feelings, and ideas during initial period of seclusion.

24. Collaborate with physician and other team members regarding appropriate use of medication for agitation.

25. Check room on a regular basis for temperature, cleanliness, and safety of environment.

26. Provide for client's personal hygiene needs, e.g., daily bath, teeth brushing, and individual grooming needs.

27. Determine the client's need for continued treatment and ability to be weaned from seclusion by evaluating the client's responsiveness to verbal directions; behavior during feeding, bathing, toileting activities; level of agitation and aggression; ability to wait for things requested; behaviors indicative of hallucinatory experiences or delusional thinking.
28. Following removal from seclusion room, help the client describe issues that led to need for seclusion intervention, discuss benefits of the intervention, and identify ways to avoid use of this intervention in the future.

▌ Protective Interventions: Restraints*

Definition/Purpose

Use of restraints is the process of applying or maintaining specialized equipment that restricts and limits the physical activity and mobility of a client who is out of control, to prevent the client from harm to self or others, to prevent serious disruption of the treatment program or environment, as an ongoing behavioral treatment, or at the client's request. This intervention should never be used to punish the client or for the convenience of staff or other clients on the unit. Restraints consist of:

- Wristcuffs: wide, padded, leather cuffs secured with a leather strap and locking device that can be attached to wrists or ankles of client and then secured to client's waist or to the client's bed.
- Waist restraints: three belts, one of which is fastened around client's waist, with the other two being looped through each side of the waist belt and then secured to the bed frame.

Specific Nursing Interventions

1. Recognize behaviors indicative of a need for restraints, e.g., client inability or unwillingness to respond to staff attempts to control client's behavior with verbal interventions to prevent the client's injuring self or others; client in seclusion who is evaluated to be at high risk for harming self or others.

*References 4,15,54,75,80,97,126,143,152,184,191,200-202,208

2. Take into consideration the influence of factors such as drug overdose, medical condition, or self-mutilation because they may affect client's medical and psychiatric status.

3. Adhere to institutional guidelines for implementing intervention.

4. Clear immediate area of other clients and physical obstructions.

5. Use control and transport procedures as indicated in facility.

6. Search the client for potentially dangerous objects, e.g., matches, jewelry, belts, ties, and scarfs.

7. Notify the client's physician immediately, if this has not previously been done.

8. Follow institutional and legal guidelines for frequency of monitoring client's response to restraints—usually a minimum of every 15 minutes.

9. Convey recognition of the client's need for dignity and self-esteem.

10. Check skin areas for signs of irritation or impaired circulation; assure some movement of extremities every 15 minutes; check vital signs.

11. Release restraints one at a time as needed and at least every 2 hours (frequency is determined by institutional parameters—usually every 2 hours) or to allow the client to eat and go to the bathroom. Be sure that adequate staff are available during these times.

12. If the client's level of agitation does not permit an active exercise for limbs, then perform passive range of motion as the client's condition permits.

13. Provide one-to-one constant observation when the client is in four-point restraints.

14. Collaborate with physician and other team members regarding appropriate use of medication, to avoid overmedicating.

15. Schedule time with multidisciplinary team to evaluate circumstances leading to use of restraints, staff reactions to situation, and possible strategies for prevention in future.

16. Provide opportunity for other clients to verbalize their fears and concerns about the incident.

17. Collaborate with team to determine when restraints can be removed or if some type of restraint device is needed when client returns to open unit.
18. After removal of restraints, help the client to describe the issues that led to the need for this intervention, discuss benefits from use of restraints, and identify ways to avoid the use of this intervention in the future.

▌ Protective Interventions: Seizure Management[*]

Definition/Purpose

Seizure management is a nursing intervention for the psychiatric client who experiences, has had, or is at risk for having a seizure, to prevent and minimize injury during an actual seizure and to reduce or prevent the occurrence of seizure.

Specific Nursing Interventions

1. Identify clients who are at risk of having seizures, e.g., those taking antipsychotic medications that can lower the seizure threshold, those who are at risk for alcohol or drug withdrawal, those with previous seizure history, and those taking antiepileptic medication.
2. Assess the client's thoughts and feelings associated with risk factors for seizure, e.g., fears about injury during seizure, knowledge about seizure control, as well as thoughts and feelings associated with psychosocial issues of seizure management, e.g., social network, social isolation, discrimination.
3. Interventions for the client having actual seizure: assist client to lying position; protect and support head with pad or pillow if client is on floor; remove pillows if client is in bed; if possible, have the client lie on his or her side with head flexed forward, to allow tongue to fall forward and to promote drainage of secretions; do not attempt to force anything into the client's mouth; remove client's glasses; loosen clothing; remove furniture or objects that client might strike during seizure; do not attempt to restrain client (restraint during strong muscular contractions can cause fracture); provide privacy from onlookers; observe and report type of movements and body

[*]References 40,89,90,125,131,164

part affected, size of pupils, state of consciousness, duration, incontinence, and behavior following seizure.

4. Interventions after seizure: keep client on side to prevent aspiration; maintain patent airway; determine need for oxygen; check vital signs and neurologic status; do not offer liquids or solid food until client is fully awake; have staff member remain with client until he or she regains consciousness and is fully awake and oriented; reorient client to environment as necessary; help with oral hygiene as necessary for removal of secretions and blood; provide opportunity for client to discuss thoughts and feelings associated with seizure; ascertain if the client experienced aura prior to seizure.

5. Based on individual assessment, ensure that safety measures are taken to prevent injury from subsequent seizures, e.g., quiet environment for client who is at risk for seizures, a bed that is close to floor.

6. Monitor vital signs.

7. Collaborate with the client's physician regarding pharmacologic management for prevention of seizures.

8. Assess for possible contributing factors of seizure, e.g., history of alcohol and/or drug abuse or lack of understanding of importance of compliance with medication regimen.

9. Develop an individualized client education plan that incorporates information for prevention and control of future seizures, such as importance of abstinence from alcohol and drug abuse; importance of taking antiepileptic medication at optimal times; name of antiepileptic medication, purpose, and common side effects; keeping seizure record and using seizure calendar, e.g., name of health care provider and after-care plans for seizure management.

10. Ensure that the client with seizure disorder wears a Medic Alert bracelet.

▌Social Skills Training[*]

Definition/Purpose

Social skills training is a therapeutic group or individual approach that uses social learning principles to systemat-

[*]References 3,21,30,31,89,93,98,119,120,122,127,140a,140b,142,145,148,156, 162 , 192,203

ically teach psychiatric clients how to overcome illness-caused impairments, disabilities, and handicaps by developing interpersonal behaviors for successful social and community functioning. Social skills training reduces client relapse and rehospitalization and family stress and burden.

Specific Nursing Interventions

1. Identify clients who might benefit from social skills training: clients who have difficulty initiating and participating in routine day-to-day conversations; severely or persistently mentally ill clients who have difficulty initiating or maintaining relationships with others; clients who are socially ill at ease; clients whose expressions of disapproval or occasional aggression are embarrassing or frightening to others; clients with inappropriate sexual behaviors; clients who report having difficulties in specific interpersonal situations.
2. Collaborate with the multidisciplinary team in selecting clients who have similar deficits and in selecting the appropriate social skill group for the achievement of specified client outcomes.
3. Obtain specific information about the client's problematic social interactions: ask the client to give real-life examples to illustrate interpersonal problems; talk with the client's caregivers or family; compile observations from other team members; review client's previous medical records; ask client to keep daily diary to monitor difficult situations; use role-playing techniques to assess the client's social skills in specific situations; observe and evaluate client's social skills during unstructured interactions with others.
4. Have the client actively participate in the selection of specific and attainable goals that are relevant to his or her current life situation.
5. In a group setting, use techniques for group social skills training: begin and end group on time; welcome members and describe the purpose of the group; introduce new members; have returning clients introduce themselves and explain social skills training to new clients; allow for individual differences in learning new

skills; inquire about absent members, to convey the value of *all* members; have the clients describe the results of previous homework assignments; inquire about interpersonal difficulties during the past week or anticipated problems during coming week; help each individual client identify a specific problem and goal that will be focused on during the meeting; engage the group in a discussion of benefits associated with learning the identified desired skill; assist each individual client to select and plan the interpersonal situation for role play; enlist other clients in setting up role-playing scenes and participating as role players; help the client and other role player to focus on client's specific short- and long-term goals; give positive feedback through immediate praise and encourage group participation in giving positive feedback and praise; facilitate corrective feedback from members; use flip chart or blackboard to record ratings and general group feedback; ask the client to describe understanding of feedback, short- and long-term goals, and alternative approaches that could have been used (to validate the client's cognitive and perceptual comprehension). Select a client to model a "real" person in the client's life: ask the client to role-play response behavior to this person, concentrating on the targeted behaviors; coach the client on the desired behaviors. Give appropriate positive feedback on desired behaviors, encouraging group participation; at the conclusion of the training session, give the client specific homework that focuses on practicing the new responses in his or her actual environment.

6. In a one-to-one situation or family situation, use above techniques adapted for social skills training.

▌ Stress Management[*]

Definition/Purpose

Stress management is a nursing strategy that incorporates noninvasive, nonpharmacologic techniques and therapies to decrease the psychiatric client's counterproductive physiological and psychological responses to stressful sit-

---

[*]References 23,25,26,51,59,86,87,92,104,131,140,142,160,168,169,170,173, 174, 1 85,186,189,194,195,199

uations and life events. Stress management increases the psychiatric client's coping ability in managing internal and external stress.

Specific Nursing Interventions

1. Identify clients who would benefit from learning stress management techniques or therapies, e.g., clients who are experiencing difficulty in managing anger, anxiety, fear, Substance Abuse, or clients with Post-Trauma Response, Chronic Pain, Sleep Pattern Disturbance.
2. Conduct a careful review of the client's medical and psychiatric history and treatment to identify clients who are at risk for experiencing untoward effects from progressive relaxation or imagery techniques, e.g., depressed clients who might become more withdrawn, clients who hallucinate or are delusional who might experience loss-of-reality-contact reactions, clients whose pharmacologic regimen leaves them at risk for experiencing a temporary hypotensive or hypoglycemic state, clients with medical problems such as arthritis or lower back pain.
3. Collaborate with the client's mental health or primary care provider before initiating progressive relaxation techniques with these populations, and exercise caution in using progressive relaxation techniques with them.
4. Collaborate with the client to develop an individualized and appropriate plan for stress management. Have the client provide information that includes motivation for seeking help at this time; thoughts, feelings, and beliefs about stress; what has and has not helped in the past, including previous use of stress-management techniques; prescribed and over-the-counter medications; habits, e.g., dietary intake, caffeine, smoking, illicit drugs, alcohol intake; daily routines, including usual activities and sleep patterns; family history of similar difficulties; motivation for learning stress management; willingness to practice techniques in absence of direct supervision of nurse.
5. Use an individual or small group approach to discuss common maladaptive ways for dealing with stress or to teach specific relaxation techniques.

6. Teach the client that the relaxation response is a learned response requiring practice and work and that it can be elicited in almost any person.

7. Emphasize the importance of incorporating four essential elements needed to elicit relaxation response: a quiet environment with minimal distractions; the use of a mental device, word, or phrase that is repeated over and over in a consistent manner to help the client's mind shift from externally oriented thought; adopting a passive attitude that excludes worrying about how well the client is doing; and achieving a comfortable position (not lying down, which may lead to sleep).

8. Inform the client that relaxation techniques are tools for developing alternative responses to stress, that techniques are easy to use once they are learned, that it may take weeks or months before client experiences desired results, and that the overall goal is improvement and not the achievement of perfection.

9. Explain that the client needs to practice the techniques for 15 to 20 minutes one to two times a day.

10. Help client to recognize situations, interpretations, and self-talk that trigger a stress response and subsequent response patterns. Teach the client to begin to learn measures for control of these responses and patterns: control events by defining limits and refusing to become involved in situation that causes stress or by physically or emotionally removing self from stressful situation; control interpretation of stressful event by re-labeling the meaning of the experience; control of self-talk by replacing irrational ideas and beliefs with more realistic and accurate observations and statements.

11. Use visualization and imagery to decrease emotional intensity associated with an actual or potential stressful event or situation: confer with the client's mental health care provider prior to use of visualization and imagery; use caution in implementation of these techniques with psychotic clients; teach the client to create a positive mental picture of desired experiences and/or situations; have the client select a pleasurable image, e.g., lying on a warm beach, fishing at a secluded lake, walking through the woods on a sunny day, to create a relaxed state for visualization.

12. Engage the client in musical activities to decrease stress response: help the client to identify past associations with music that can influence the use of this modality for stress management; identify the role that music has played in the client's life; obtain information about music with which the client is familiar and the client's form of participation with music, e.g., singing, listening, playing an instrument; assess factors that can influence the client's response to music, e.g., cultural, spiritual, and religious beliefs, educational preparation, presence of delusional thinking and hallucinations; encourage the use of soothing, unobtrusive music as a pre-bedtime ritual for clients with sleep pattern disturbance that is associated with anxiety; use unobtrusive and preferably unrecognized background music in inpatient setting to create a calming effect during meal time; have the client use music as an adjunct for visualization and imagery in conjunction with chronic pain management and control; have the client monitor breathing while listening to music, emphasizing the importance of slow and deep breathing to enhance the relaxing effects from music; when appropriate, arrange for the client to have access to individual headset to use for listening to audiotapes for stress reduction; be judicious in use of headsets for clients who are actively experiencing auditory hallucinations.

13. Promote the use of humor as an emotion-focused coping strategy for relieving tension and anxiety: determine client's past use of humor to deal with stressful situations; identify topics the client finds amusing; when appropriate, facilitate the client's talking about events or topics that evoke humorous responses in the client, nurse, or others; facilitate the client's use of humorous audiovisuals, e.g., audiotapes of old radio comedies, movies, videotapes, or books.

14. Have the client keep a stress-awareness diary for a minimum of 2 weeks to track responses to stressful events and situations; have the client record information such as time of occurrence and physical and emotional responses; schedule time for client to review findings with nurse.

15. Coordinate referral for evaluation of biofeedback treatment for clients who are experiencing problems such

as job-related stress, tension or migraine headaches, sleep pattern disturbance, anxiety, and hypertension to help them gain conscious control over their unconscious body responses and to reduce or eliminate stress-related condition.

16. Evaluate the client's response to stress-management techniques and therapies by determining the extent to which client goals for stress reduction have been achieved, e.g., improved sleep pattern, reduced anxiety, increased sense of control, increased ability to cope with chronic pain.

17. Based on evaluation findings, collaborate with client, peers, and other members of the interdisciplinary team to revise and modify the original plan for stress management or to continue with current plan.

▮ Supportive Therapy: Offering Hope[*]

Definition/Purpose

Offering hope to the psychiatric client is a goal-directed nursing action that conveys the expectation that the client will be able to alter perceptions of futility or hopelessness associated with an actual or potential event or situation and that the client will be able to establish an interconnectedness with others.

Specific Nursing Interventions

1. Have the client describe perceptions of stressful life events.
2. Listen for themes that involve loss and change.
3. Evaluate the influence of psychiatric and medical problems, including illness management and interventions on the client's perceptions of hopelessness.
4. Determine the client's perception of current social support.
5. Have the client describe personal and formal spiritual beliefs, e.g., philosophy of life, religious activities, association with people with similar spiritual or religious beliefs.
6. Collaborate with appropriate clergy or spiritual counselors.
7. Collaborate with multidisciplinary team in appropriate medication management for symptom control.

[*]References 20,26,52,66,71,78,95,96,115,122,138,141,182,197

8. Convey hope that is grounded in the belief that client is able to prevent potential difficulties or overcome difficulties in current situation to normalize feelings.

9. Use statements that convey realistic hope for client, e.g,"One of the things that I have to offer as your nurse is that..."

"I can offer you hope that you will be able to return to your family."

"I can offer you hope that you will begin to feel better about yourself."

"I can offer you hope that you will be able to identify other solutions to your problems besides ending your life."

"I can offer you hope that you will recover from your loss and be able to find meaning in your life."

"I am spending time with you because I believe that you will be able to identify solutions that will help you to feel more optimistic about the future."

10. Use therapeutic humor to help the client reframe the actual or potential situation or event in more positive terms.

11. Encourage the client to emphasize strengths rather than weaknesses.

12. Convey recognition of client's past and present strengths and accomplishments.

13. Help the client identify irrational beliefs in self and others and to recognize self-defeating behaviors.

14. Encourage client to use affirmations that are congruent with current goals to overcome feelings of hopelessness, e.g., "I am hopeful for the future" or "I am feeling optimistic."

15. Encourage the client to set realistic daily goals.

16. Promote positive expectations of the future by having client identify problems that can be resolved; help the client develop realistic goals for resolving these problems and to recognize the potential for realistic future achievements.

17. Use the client's family as a resource in conveying hope for the present and the future, e.g., encourage client to share goals with family; encourage family to express positive feelings to client and to convey recognition of client's ability to change.

two

NURSING INTERVENTIONS AND PROCESS FOR MAJOR PSYCHIATRIC DISORDERS

Delirium, Dementia, and Amnestic and Other Cognitive Disorders

▋ Definition/Major Symptoms[*]

These disorders are characterized by memory deficits and/or deficits in cognition representing a major change from previous functioning level, frequent mood changes, anxiety, or psychotic symptoms. Etiology derives from a medical condition, effects of a substance (drug of abuse, toxin, medication), or a combination of both. Cognitive disorders are classified as irreversible or reversible.

▋ Definition/Major Symptoms of Selected Major Categories[†]

Delirium

Delirium is a transient, usually reversible dysfunction in cognition. It begins with an abrupt onset (hours to days) of an altered mental state that is characterized by distur-

[*]References 1,17
[†]References 1,4,8,17,31,36,39,45,47,52,59,60,63

bances in consciousness, cognition, attention, reduced or increased psychomotor activity, and disturbances in the sleep–wake cycle. There are variations in the specific symptoms over a 24-hour period; nocturnal exacerbation and fluctuations and "waxing and waning" are common.

- Attentional deficits include an impaired ability to mobilize attention, client is easily distractable, client has reduced or increased alertness.
- Cognitive changes include memory impairment (primarily recent), disorientation to time and place (disorientation to self is less common); language disturbances, e.g., dysnomia (inability to name familiar objects) or dysgraphia (impairment in ability to write); speech may be rambling, pressured, incoherent.
- Perceptual disturbances include impairment in perception of the passage of time, illusions, and hallucinations, with visual hallucinations more frequent than auditory or tactile ones.
- Psychomotor activity disturbances of hyperactivity (picking at bedding, attempting to get out of bed when it is unsafe to do so or hypoactivity (sluggish, apathetic, lethargic).
- Variation of emotional fluctuations such as anger, fear, cursing, screaming.
- Sleep disturbances include a reversal of sleep–wake cycle with inappropriate daytime drowsiness and napping, nighttime agitation, difficulty falling and remaining asleep, and vivid, frightening dreams while sleeping.

Subcategories of Delirium are differentiated according to their etiology; however, they share a common symptom presentation.

DELIRIUM DUE TO A GENERAL MEDICAL CONDITION

Delirium that is due to a general medical condition: metabolic disorder, e. g., hypoxia, hypoglycemia, hyponatremia; infection, e.g., viral encephalitis, bacteremia, pneumonia, and urinary tract infection (particularly in the elderly); cerebrovascular disease, e.g., transient ischemic attacks, cerebral embolism, subarachnoid hemorrhage; disorder of the brain, e.g., head injury, epilepsy, brain tumor.

SUBSTANCE-INDUCED DELIRIUM (SUBSTANCE INTOXICATION OR SUBSTANCE WITHDRAWAL)

Delirium that is due to drug abuse, e.g., alcohol, amphetamine, cocaine, hallucinogen; side effects from medications, e.g., antibiotic, anticholinergic, analgesic, sedative-hypnotic; exposure to a toxin, e.g., pesticide, solvent. Symptoms in this subcategory are in excess of those usually associated with the intoxication or withdrawal syndromes described in Chapter 8, and they require specific, independent clinical attention.

Examples of specific categories of drugs that carry a high risk for Substance-Induced Delirium include:

Anticonvulsants
Antiparkinsonian agents
Benzodiazepines
Centrally acting hypertensives
Corticosteroids
Digitalis
Opioids
Tricyclic antidepressants

Over-the-counter categories of drugs that carry a high risk for Delirium and are often overlooked include salicyates, antihistamines, and topical ophthalmic preparations.

DELIRIUM NOT OTHERWISE SPECIFIED

A designated category for Delirium that does not meet the criteria for previously referred to categories. This category is used when there is lack of evidence to confirm the specific cause of Delirium or for causes not listed in the DSM-IV criteria.

Dementia

Dementia consists of multiple cognitive deficits including impaired memory (a prominent early symptom, as well as a major source of the client's disability) *and* at least aphasia (language function deterioration), disturbance in executive functioning (complex thinking ability and execution of complex behavior), agnosia (inability to identify objects) *or* apraxia (impairment in motor activity execution); impaired social and occupational functioning representing a marked decline from previous functioning; can also be characterized by geographic disorientation, lack of awareness of cognitive deterioration, occasional violence and suicidal behavior, gait disturbances leading to falls, disinhibited behavior, slurred speech, mood disturbances, anxiety, sleep disturbances, delusions, and hallucinations (especially visual); stressors such as physical or psychosocial stressors can exacerbate symptoms.

Dementia is categorized on the basis of the etiology of the condition, i.e., whether it is a persistent effect of substance use, a medical condition, or a combination of these two, e.g., Dementia of the Alzheimer's Type, Dementia Due to HIV Disease, Substance-Induced Persisting Dementia, Vascular Dementia, and Dementia due to Head Trauma.

DEMENTIA OF THE ALZHEIMER'S TYPE

This disorder consists of multiple cognitive defects including memory impairment and one or more of the following cognitive disturbances: aphasia, apraxia, agnosia, and disturbance in executive functioning causing a significant reduction in social and occupational functioning. The disorder has a gradual onset with progressive cognitive decline; in addition, a client with Dementia can present with Delirium, delusions, depressed mood, and behavioral disturbances. Alzheimer's disease usually does not cause motor or sensory deficits until late in the course of the disease. The subtypes are based on age of onset and type of accompanying feature that is predominant.

Four types have been identified: "(a) benign, with little or no progression; (b) myoclonic, early onset, severe intellectual decline, and frequent mutism; (c) extrapyramidal, severe intellectual and functional decline with psychotic symptoms; and (d) typical, a gradual progression of intellectual and functional decline, but without other distinguishing features."[40, p. 29]

Amnestic Disorders

This category refers to a memory disturbance related to a general medical condition or to the effects of a substance. It describes prominent memory impairment with sparing of other cognitive functions, e.g., Amnestic Disorder due to a General Medical Condition and Substance-Induced Persisting Amnestic Disorder.

ALCOHOL-INDUCED PERSISTING AMNESTIC DISORDER

Korsakoff's syndrome often follows Wernicke's encephalopathy; the latter is characterized by confusion, abnormal movements of the eyes, ataxia, and other neurological signs. Wernicke's encephalopathy is caused by a thiamine deficiency; 84% of clients with Wernicke's develop Korsakoff's amnesia syndrome."The neuropathological substrate of both Wernicke's encephalopathy and Korsakoff's syndrome consists of punctate hemorrhages or, more commonly, necrotic lesions distributed around the ventricular system of the diencephalon and brain stem [which] suggest that these are facets of the same disease."[31, p. 682] Diencephalic lesions are probably responsible for memory disturbance. Korsakoff's psychosis exhibits shrunken mammillary bodies, severe neuronal loss, gliosis, and reactive astrocytosis.

▌ Incidence*

Delirium

Delirium is one of the most common mental disorders encountered in the general hospital population (incidence from 15% to 30%). It contributes significantly to morbidity and mortality of this population. It has been identified as a sign of impending death in 25% of cases; one consultation/liaison psychiatrist found a 25% death rate 6 months following diagnosis of Delirium.

An accurate estimate of the incidence of Delirium is difficult because of undetected episodes; lack of consistency of definition, terminology, and diagnostic criteria; lack of reliable tools to substantiate diagnosis; lack of epidemiological studies; and inaccurate diagnosis because of client lucidity at the time of evaluation. Actual frequency is influenced by specific client population and the clinical setting; there is a high prevalence in intensive care units, particularly during recovery from cardiovascular surgery. There has been an increased incidence resulting from increased life expectancy.

*References 2,4,15,23,24,29,30,32,34,36,47,52,53,56,57,59

- There is a reported incidence of 14% to 56% in hospitalized elderly with 11% to 42% of those among elderly medical-surgical inpatients.
- Reported incidence ranges from 5% to 57% in clients with burns.
- There is a range of 5% to 85% in clients with cancer, "depending on age, level of physical disability and stage of disease."[34, p. 371]
- Of the general hospital patients referred to a psychiatry consultation/liaison service for evaluation and treatment of depression, 41.8% were found to be delirious, not depressed.
- A recent report indicates that 16% of the clients admitted through an emergency room to a medical/surgical intensive care unit exhibited signs of Delirium (38 out of 323 consecutive admissions to the unit).

Dementia

- Over 70 types of dementia can occur in adults and the elderly.
- The 12-month prevalence rate of cognitive impairment in the population over the age of 17 years is 2.7%.
- Symptoms of dementias are reversible among 15% of population, but only 3% fully recover.
- A major risk factor is age: in persons over 65, 5% suffer from severe dementia and about 10% from mild dementia; at age 80, 20% have severe dementia; at age 90, 30% have severe dementia.

Dementia of the Alzheimer's Type

- There are 4 million Americans affected by Alzheimer's disease and related disorders, of which about 2.5 million are affected by Alzheimer's disease.
- It is the most common type of dementia in the elderly.
- It is the most common nonreversible type of dementia.
- It often starts insidiously in persons in their 50s, 60s, or older and leads to death in about 8 to 10 years from onset.
- It is the fourth leading cause of death in persons over 75.
- Depression occurs in 10% to 25% of clients with early-stage Alzheimer's disease.

Course*

Delirium

There is considerable variation depending on the specific cause. The fluctuation of symptoms, which may persist for weeks, and the overall clinical course may lead to vast differences in reported observations and can result in diagnostic confusion, as well as inappropriate management. Potential outcomes include full recovery; seizures; associated morbidity, e.g., fractures or subdural hematomas from falls; patients may progress "to stupor and/or coma with eventual recovery (with or without chronic brain damage), become chronically vegetative or die."[63, p. 321] Other possible outcomes include higher incidence of prolonged hospitalization, more frequent impairment of physical function, and increased rates of institutionalization. Rapid alleviation occurs, as a rule, with detection and appropriate treatment for the underlying condition; however, there is increasing evidence that the symptoms may often be persistent and not transient. The diagnosis may be indicative of future cognitive and functional decline.

Dementia

Dementia is manifested by cognitive symptoms such as alterations in memory (short term and long term) along with changes in the client's ability to reason; alterations in personality, ability to communicate, and ability to make sound judgments; alterations in abstract thinking, such as concept formation and logical reasoning; perceptual alterations, such as delusions and hallucinations; restlessness and agitation with extreme agitation at night (sundown syndrome); extremely agitated behavior (referred to as a catastrophic reaction), precipitated by change in cognitive status, medication side effects, changes in the environment, or psychosocial factors increasing demands on the client. The onset of Dementia is often insidious; early signs include subtle changes in personality, apathy, labile or shallow emotions, gradual loss of intellectual skills, more pronounced memory loss, and change in mood and personality. Eventually social skills are lost, psychotic symptoms

*References 2,5,23,50,52,53,57,63

arise, judgment is severely impaired, language impairments occur, and a regression to infantile behavior may occur. At the end stage, clients may become mute and unresponsive.

The causes of *reversible dementia* can be treated, e.g., Dementia related to Alcohol Abuse; Dementia related to depression; Dementia related to nutrition (pernicious anemia, pellagra), to metabolic and endocrine disorders (hypothyroidism, uremia, hyperparathyroidism), to toxicity (mercury), to infections (encephalitis, cryptococcal meningitis), to vascular conditions (MI, decreased cardiac output), and to mass effect (leukemia). The causes of *irreversible dementia*, such as Alzheimer's disease, cannot be treated.

Dementia of the Alzheimer's Type

Progressive irreversible deterioration in the cerebral cortex results in impaired social interaction, difficulty in handling stress, difficulty in making sound judgments, impaired memory, decreased ability to communicate, and impairment in performing activities of daily living. There is also a deterioration in language abilities, ranging from an inability to name an object to the inability to comprehend words to repetition of words. There is also a deterioration in behavior ranging from indifference to delusions to agitation. Gait/posture/movements deteriorate from normal to wandering to abnormal gait and flexed posture.

STAGES OF ALZHEIMER'S DISEASE

1. Forgetfulness—client manifests short-term memory loss; possible depression.
2. Confusion—client experiences declining short-term memory with long-term memory loss; may become disoriented to time, place, person; confabulation; depression common. Symptoms increase with fatigue, illness, stress, or in an unfamiliar environment. This results in difficulties in meeting instrumental activities of daily living independently, e.g., housekeeping, need for assistance when living home, need for day care.
3. Ambulatory dementia—client experiences declining ability to meet activities of daily living such as grooming and dressing; decline in reasoning ability, communica-

tion difficulties, is self absorbed; increasing memory loss with inability to retain or use past information for goal-directed behavior; increasing frustration with reduced stress threshold; decreasing depression; possible institutional care.

4. End stage—client unable to recognize significant others; inability to walk; mute or may scream and talk incessantly and repetitively; forgets how to eat and swallow with resulting weight loss; incontinence; seizures; institutionalization necessary.

The disease is progressive with stages merging into one another.

Alcohol-Induced Persisting Amnestic Disorder (Korsakoff's Syndrome)

Major memory impairment follows many years of heavy alcohol use; often exhibits an abrupt onset, although some persons develop deficits over many years with the occurrence of a final, more impairing episode; there is inability to learn and retain new information and lack of motivation. The condition can persist indefinitely; can result in severe impairment, often requiring lifelong care; and is preventable if treated early with thiamine repletion.

▌ Contributing Factors*

Delirium

1. Precipitating factors: intracranial and systemic infections; withdrawal syndromes, e.g., alcohol, sedatives; intoxication by drugs and poisons, e.g., prescribed medications, illicit drugs, industrial and animal poisons; metabolic encephalopathies, e.g., hypoxia, hypoglycemia, renal insufficiency; stroke; fluid and electrolyte disorders, hyperinsulinism, hyperthyroidism and hypothyroidism; head trauma, epilepsy; neoplasm; cerebrovascular or cardiovascular disorders; intracranial space-occupying lesions, e.g., abscess, neoplasm, subdural hematoma; disorders of the hematopoietic system, e.g., severe anemia; disorders

*References 1,2,13,36,53,56,61,63,64

due to hypersensitivity, e.g., serum sickness; injury by physical agents, e.g., heat stroke, radiation damage, electrocution.
2. Facilitating factors for onset, increased severity, and possible prolongation of course: bereavement and relocation to an unfamiliar environment; sleep deprivation; sensory deprivation and sensory overload; immobilization. However, these factors alone are not sufficient to *cause* Delirium.

Dementia

- Nonbiological facilitating factors are family history, psychosocial stressors, early life experiences.
- Physiological disruptions (e.g., CVA, trauma, metabolic imbalances, disease processes including brain tumors, toxins, medications, nutritional deficiencies) can lead to neuronal loss and cognitive disorder.
- Effects of substances such as drugs, toxins, medications
- Chemicals intrinsic to the body, e.g., neurotransmitters
- Environmental toxins such as pesticides
- Toxic effect of calcium in cells
- Medical condition
- Declining immune system in the aged may be a risk factor
- Systemic disorders possible related to brain cell destruction
- Nutritional deficiency
- Combination of substance abuse and medical condition
- Possible causes include a virus

Dementia of the Alzheimer's Type

- Autopsies reveal neurofibrillary tangles, senile plaques, Hirano bodies, neuronal granulovacuolar degeneration of nerve cell bodies.
- Heredity is indicated in about 10% of Alzheimer's disorders, e.g., genetic mutation on a chromosome (earlier onset).
- Abnormal protein structures; potential relationship between beta amyloid protein and Alzheimer's.
- Biopsies reveal high aluminum levels in the brain of Alzheimer's clients; role is unclear.

- Evidence of biochemical abnormality, e.g., reduced level of choline acetyltransferase, a catalyst for acetylcholine.
- Head trauma with loss of consciousness linked to Alzheimer's.
- Risk factors for Alzheimer's include age, history of head trauma, female gender (females live longer), low occupational and educational level, Down's syndrome, and first-degree relative diagnosed with Alzheimer's.

Alcohol-Induced Persisting Amnestic Disorder (Korsakoff's Syndrome)

Toxic and nutritional insults following heavy abuse of alcohol resulting in thiamine deficiency

▮ Laboratory and Physical Examination Findings[*]

- Assess for underlying psychiatric and medical condition.
- Review health history, physical exam, and mental status exam to determine presence of Delirium or Dementia.
- Assess for nature/onset of disorder, subsequent tempo of illness—gradual versus sudden, gradual versus stepwise progression.
- A neurological examination is extremely important in identifying the etiology of cognitive disorders.
- Neuropsychological testing is useful in detecting changes over time (Dementia).
- Obtain laboratory tests, e.g., blood chemistry profile, urinalysis, EKG, toxicology screen, liver and thyroid function tests, Lyme disease test, vitamin B_{12} levels, serological tests for HIV and syphilis, and chest X-ray.
- Obtain CT brain scan, EEG, magnetic resonance imaging (MRI).
- Other tests may be required: lumbar puncture, arterial blood gases, and cerebral blood flow (single photon emission computed tomography).
- "Diagnosis and Assessment Model [Demential]): (1) Case history interview; (2) neurologic and medical evaluation; (3) behavioral assessment (neuropsychological assessment; behavioral rating measures); (4) language and communication assessment (comprehensive language

[*]References 2,20,35,36,46,51,56

testing, pragmatics assessment, semantics assessment, syntax and phonology assessment, memory and language evaluation)." [51,p.188]

- Laboratory tests recommended to determine etiology of cognitive impairment: "Complete blood count, blood sugar, electrolytes, serum calcium, thyroid-stimulating hormone, blood urea nitrogen and creatinine, chest radiography, CT scan of the head, electrocardiogram, HIV titre, mammograms, plasma cortisol, serum vitamin B_{12}, serum folate, Venereal Disease Research Laboratory." [49,p.49]

▌Special Assessment Considerations[*]

Delirium

- Obtain information from all available resources, e.g., previous records, previous and current health care providers, client interview and family and friends, to determine if onset of cognitive-attentional disorder is sudden and abrupt (more indicative of Delirium) or insidious (indicative of Dementia). Compare baseline functional and behavioral information, if available, with client's current presentation.
- Consider the possibility of Delirium in hospitalized medically ill or postoperative clients who are labeled "difficult, obnoxious," who show poor impulse control, or make impulsive suicidal gestures or threats, or in clients who are reported to have a "sudden onset" of depression.
- Recognize that Delirium may be mistaken for uncooperative behavior in children, especially if familiar people are unable to soothe the child.
- Be alert for reports of the abrupt onset of "confusion" or "mental status changes" in the elderly; this is often the first indication of a urinary tract infection or pneumonia in this population or the first indication of sepsis in a postoperative client.
- Do not assume that abnormal vital signs are due to anxiety.
- Conduct routine cognitive assessments that take into consideration the client's cultural and educational background; names of presidents and dates of birth are not

[*]References 1,2,14,15,29,32,36,45,47,52,57

always useful indicators in some cultures. Try to ensure consistency of testing activities to obtain as accurate a profile as possible. Recognize that reports of intermittent and variable symptoms are indicative of the presence of Delirium. In assessing client, provide privacy to the extent possible and minimize distractions; individualize assessment based on client's physical status (in a cast, hemiplegic, aphasic, ventilator-dependent, ambulatory).

- Examples of components of a bedside cognitive mental status examination include:
  - ○ assessment of orientation to time, place, and person
  - ○ assessment of attention and concentration, e.g., subtracting 7s from 100, naming months of year backwards
  - ○ assessment of recent and remote memory and ability to retain new information, e.g., repeating and recalling three unrelated words, naming current and past presidents, providing home address and telephone number
  - ○ assessment of thought processes, e.g., coherence, presence of illusions, hallucinations
  - ○ assessment of ability to write a sentence and to name familiar objects
- Conduct a review of client's pharmacy profile of prescription and non-prescription medications.
- Recognize that use of the term "ICU psychosis" is often indicative of an inadequate search for the underlying cause of delirium.
- Recognize that "a delirium that is superimposed on a dementing condition may be difficult to distinguish from atypical dementia, progressive cognitive impairment, or a catastrophic reaction."[52,p.994]

Dementia

It is necessary to differentiate between Dementia and pseudodementia (i.e., "the dementia syndrome of depression," a condition in which a depressed person appears to have dementia).

Dementia of the Alzheimer's Type

- It is difficult to diagnose depression in clients with Alzheimer's disease because there is some overlap of symptoms, e.g., sleep disturbance, poor appetite, apathy, inefficiency of thought. The diagnosis is partly based on the presence of psychomotor retardation, thoughts of death, worthlessness, self-pity, and early morning awakening. Depressed elderly clients may be misdiagnosed as demented. When in doubt, a trial of antidepressant medications is warranted.

- Demented clients should be assessed for self-pity.
- Assess depressed Alzheimer's disease clients for more cognitive impairment, dependence in activities of daily living, and greater history of mental illness.

▌ Treatment*

Delirium

PROACTIVE INTERVENTIONS

- Identifying clients with significant risk factors for Delirium:
  - ○ age over 60
  - ○ clients with Dementia, preexisting brain damage
  - ○ post-cardiotomy clients
  - ○ clients with burns, clients with acquired immune deficiency syndrome
  - ○ clients with drug dependency who are in withdrawal.
- Avoiding polypharmacy
- Monitoring therapeutic doses and serum levels of prescribed drugs
- Being alert for potential drug interactions
- Recognizing agents that are associated with Delirium

When the diagnosis of Delirium is suspected or confirmed, the first step is to search for and treat the underlying cause(s), recognizing that Delirium is usually multifactorial in origin; the next step is to provide symptomatic and supportive measures.

NONPHARMACOLOGIC INTERVENTIONS

- Prevent self-harm by providing one-to-one staff for close surveillance; minimize the use of restraints. Restraints can increase paranoia and agitation and contribute to additional complications, e.g., pressure ulcers, pulmonary embolism, deep vein thrombosis, pneumonia.

- Enhance cognitive function through activities such as frequent reorientation; providing clock and visible calendar; ensuring sensory aids are available and in working order; and providing explanations based on ability of client to understand.
- Ensure client has adequate hydration and nutritional intake.
- Facilitate client's communication with caregivers by introducing self by name and calling client by preferred name; using simple, one-step commands, based on individual assessment; and individualizing communication devices if client is unable to speak (magic slate, letter board, hand signals, head nods).
- Facilitate communication with family and familiar friends and encourage them to remain with client if their presence helps to reduce client suspiciousness and paranoia.
- Eliminate unnecessary environmental stimulation, e.g., staff interaction, excessive use of TV, monitoring equipment and alarms; maintain semblance of day–night cycle via lighting and by providing routine care during daytime.
- Provide ongoing reassurance to client and the family that the symptoms will decrease and resolve as client's medical status improves.

PHARMACOLOGIC MANAGEMENT

- Review pharmacy profile for recently added drugs that may have precipitated onset of Delirium:
  - drugs with anticholinergic properties, e.g., antihistamines (diphenhydramine for sleep), tricyclic antidepressants, antispasmodics, antiparkinsonian agents
  - sedative-hypnotics, long-acting benzodiazepines, e.g., diazepam, prescribed for anxiety
- Neuroleptics remain the drugs of choice for management of agitation, e.g., haloperidol, droperidol. The advantages of neuroleptics over benzodiazepines, barbiturates, and opiates include no significant respiratory depression and less likelihood of further cognitive impairment. The IV route is preferable in intensive-care setting because it promotes quicker alleviation of signs and symptoms and results in more reliable blood levels

in clients who may have poor absorption with IM route due to poor muscle perfusion. Use of IV haloperidol, however, can cause severe hypotension.

- Haloperidol or droperidol are the neuroleptics of choice in the intensive care setting because of their minimal effects on cardiac function, blood pressure, and respiratory function, and their low incidence of hepatic or renal toxicity. Dosing is based on achievement of levels of sedation or calming. Factors that determine specific dosage include degree of agitation, the client's age, and presence of impaired metabolism. Initial IV dosage (haloperidol) varies from 0.5 to 2.0 mg to as high as 5.0 to 10 mg for a severely agitated client "previously exposed to psychotropic medications (especially neuroleptics)."[22,p.253] There is a rapid peak effect from the IV route; the dose can be repeated in 20 to 30 minutes if agitation continues, with a doubling of the dose every 20 to 30 minutes (up to 4 doses) until symptoms abate. The amount of medication required for the first 24 hours can be administered in divided doses, as needed; for the next 24 to 36 hours, supplemental doses may be used if needed. As symptoms subside and client becomes stable, medication is tapered by 25% daily and changed to an oral dose if possible.
- Droperidol (a butyrophenone, as is haloperidol), is used as a preanesthetic agent and for control of nausea and vomiting. It is also administered by IV for more rapid management of agitation. It "is more sedating than haloperidol and has a slight risk of hypotension."[64,p.440]
- Benzodiazepines are the drugs of choice for treating alcohol withdrawal or for clients who cannot tolerate neuroleptics because of additional medical conditions such as neuroleptic malignant syndrome and anticholinergic Delirium.
- Lorazepam is the benzodiazepine of choice in the ICU for treating agitation and Delirium because of its "relatively short half-life, absence of active metabolites, and elimination mechanisms that are not significantly affected by age or liver disease."[22,p.25]
- Effective treatment of Substance-Induced Delirium is based on the identification of the offending substance

and stopping or lowering the dose. Again, haloperidol is the drug of choice for most of these deliriums; exceptions include deliriums such as Alcohol Withdrawal Delirium and Benzodiazepine Withdrawal Delirium.

NURSING CARE CONSIDERATIONS FOR THE CLIENT ON HALOPERIDOL

Although the incidence of extrapyramidal symptoms is less with IV administration than with oral, the client should be observed for evidence of this group of side effects. Akathisia could be misinterpreted as increased agitation, with a subsequent inappropriate increase in haloperidol dosage.

Dementia

- Provide a therapeutic milieu that is safe and provides the appropriate level of routine, stimulation, and activity for the client's type and stage of Dementia.
- Use interventions to reduce or control problems demonstrated by clients with Dementia, e.g., balancing sleep, exercise, and activities in order to deal with sleep disturbances; medications to treat depression; use of cueing techniques or memory aides to cope with memory loss.
- Use remotivation therapy, a group technique to remotivate client by means of mental stimulation, involvement in the current world, and interpersonal interactions.
- Use validation therapy, a group technique in which the expression of feelings is encouraged, feelings are accepted as "the truth" and with empathy in order to help client resolve past conflicts and reach resolution instead of succumbing to a vegetative state.
- Use reminiscence therapy, an ego-supportive group technique, to reinforce life decisions and lifestyle without dwelling on current losses.
- Use reality orientation, a technique used to assist the client to remain oriented to time, place, and person.
- Other non-medical interventions include psychotherapy, resocialization, pet program, operant conditioning, memory retraining, direct cognitive stimulation, sensory

training, art therapy, music therapy, dance movement therapy, and behavioral contingency therapy.[9]
- Family interventions use education, problem solving, and support to aid the caregiver (informal and formal).
- Medications such as antipsychotics (thiothixene, haloperidol) and benzodiazepines (oxazepam, lorazepam) may be used to control symptoms of extreme anxiety and assaultiveness; anticonvulsants (valproate) and antidepressants (desipramine, fluoxetine, paroxetine) can be used to control depression; antimanic drugs (lithium) can be used to manage hyperactivity and agitation, with lower dosages used with debilitated clients; antioxidants vitamin E or L-Deprenyl may significantly slow down the progression of the disease that resulted in institutionalization.
- Sedatives/hypnotics may not be effective in all stages of Alzheimer's disease, particularly when there begins to be rapid deterioration in the sleep–wake cycle because of the destruction of a critical mass of cells in the suprachiasmatic nucleus (controls sleep–wake cycle).
- Trazodone can be very useful for sleep disorders in clients with Alzheimer's disease.

Dementia of the Alzheimer's Type

- Specialized care units for clients with Alzheimer's disease provide special environment.
- Tacrine is used to treat mild to moderate stages of the disease by improving cognition and the ability to perform tasks; may slow down but not otherwise alter course of Alzheimer's disease.

NURSING CARE CONSIDERATIONS FOR CLIENTS ON TACRINE

Administer drug between meals unless GI upset occurs; monitor hepatic transaminase levels carefully; note contraindications, particularly among clients who have previously developed treatment-related jaundice; observe for potential side effects such as vomiting, nausea, diarrhea, dyspepsia, bradycardia; monitor medications, especially for potential theophylline interaction.

Alcohol-Induced Persisting Amnestic Disorder (Korsakoff's Syndrome)

Thiamine is used for the emergency treatment of Wernicke-Korsakoff's syndrome; Korsakoff's psychosis is reversible in up to 50% of clients who abstain from alcohol and receive treatment with thiamine.

▎ Commonly Occurring Nursing Diagnoses[*]

Delirium

Acute confusion

Dementia

Altered family processes
Altered thought processes
Anxiety
Bowel incontinence
Caregiver role strain
Chronic confusion
Depression[†]
Fatigue
Fear
Impaired home maintenance management
Impaired memory
Impaired social interaction
Impaired verbal communication
Ineffective individual coping
Ineffective family coping: compromised
Ineffective family coping: disabling
Risk for fluid volume deficit
Risk for injury
Risk for violence
Self-care deficit, bathing/hygiene
Self-care deficit, dressing/grooming
Self-care deficit, feeding
Self-care deficit, toileting
Self esteem disturbance
Sensory/perceptual alterations

[*]References 16,33,41,48
[†]Non–NANDA-approved nursing diagnosis.

Sleep pattern disturbance
Social isolation

▌ Selected Nursing Diagnoses, Outcome Criteria, and Nursing Interventions With Rationale*

Client With Delirium

NURSING DIAGNOSIS #1:   *Acute Confusion, related to possible infection in a 70-year-old client transferred to rehabilitation unit following recent below-the-knee amputation*

EXPECTED CLIENT OUTCOME

- Client will experience no injury to self, will experience improved cognitive function, will participate in recommended rehabilitation activities.

NURSING INTERVENTIONS WITH RATIONALE

- Collaborate with client's treatment team in searching for the possible causes of acute confusion, *recognizing that client's mental status changes and concomitant behaviors are indicative of an underlying disease process that is usually reversible but can become life-threatening if left untreated and inappropriately managed.*
- Review client's current laboratory data for variations from normal limits, e.g., electrolytes, CBC, BUN, drug levels in terms of therapeutic/toxicology screen, *to determine possible sources for acute mental status changes.*
- Assess for presence of infection, including wound site, and collaborate with treatment team in obtaining additional information through diagnostic procedures, e.g., urinalysis, EKG, chest X-ray; *onset of Acute Confusion in the elderly is often indicative of an undetected urinary tract infection or pneumonia.*
- Conduct and record consistent ongoing assessments of client's cognitive status during periods of minimal environmental distraction *to monitor fluctuations in mental status and to determine when Acute Confusion is no longer present.*

*References 2–4,6,10,11,13,14,18,19,21–24,27,35,36,38,41–43,45,52–55,57,58, 60,61,64,65

- Explain the safety mechanisms in immediate environment, e.g., call light, availability of nurse, and remind the client to lock brakes on wheelchair *because the client is at risk for secondary complications, e.g., injury from falls. It may be necessary to repeat this information until Acute Confusion subsides.*
- Remove unnecessary clutter and objects from the client's bedside area *to prevent falls and to minimize client's potential for distortion of the environment until mentation clears.*
- Ensure adequate non-glare lighting in client's immediate environment, including a night light, *to facilitate reorientation to sensory cues and to reduce likelihood of visual distortions and misperceptions.*
- Be sure that client's eyeglasses and hearing aid are available.
- Remind client to wear dentures, *not only for adequate mastication of food but also to maximize his ability to communicate with others.*
- Reorient client to time, place, and person based on the findings of ongoing assessments.
- Ensure that all members of the client's treatment team use short, simple sentences when explaining procedures or planned therapies *because of client's decreased ability to attend to conversations.*
- Encourage client to participate as much as possible in self-care activities (hygiene, bathing, and grooming); provide a reasonable length of time for completion of these activities *based on the assessment of client's compromised mentation.*
- Defer providing specific educational information *until client experiences improvement in attention and concentration.*
- Encourage client participation in rehabilitation activities to the extent possible *based on the ongoing physical and psychological assessment findings.*
- Provide assurance to client and family that the complete disappearance of Acute Confusion may take several days or possibly a few weeks, *to reduce client and family anxiety associated with the recognition of the cognitive disturbance and uncertainty about its outcome.*

DSM-IV Disorder: Dementia of the Alzheimer's Type (Client at Stage of Confusion, Cared for in Home by Caregiver)

NURSING DIAGNOSIS #1:   *Impaired memory related to Dementia of the Alzheimer's Type*

EXPECTED CLIENT OUTCOME

• Client will participate in environmental routine and maintain optimal cognitive functioning.

NURSING INTERVENTIONS WITH RATIONALE

• Teach the caregiver to maintain a safe home environment, yet one that does not unnecessarily restrict the activities of client.
• Teach the caregiver to permit the client to live as independently as possible.
• Involve client, family, and significant others in identifying previous strengths, skills, organizational styles, and most appropriate therapeutic approaches. *Information is more easily learned and retained if it is linked to knowledge previously possessed by client.*
• Assist client, family, and/or significant other to select the most useful memory aides such as large calendars, note pads, or a memory book. *Such memory aides can assist the client to compensate for the initial memory loss experienced in the course of Alzheimer's disease.*
• Discuss with family why it may be difficult for the client to learn new material.
• Use symbols on signs to indicate location of bathroom, etc.
• Have the client wear an identification bracelet or necklace and print client's name on room in large letters.
• Assist caregiver in providing milieu that incorporates appropriate level of routine and consistency that client can follow every day, e.g., keep a regular daily schedule, provide reality orientation when needed *in order to compensate for client's difficulty in dealing with change and overstimulation.*
• Approach in calm, warm, reassuring, and consistent manner, e.g., keep voice calm; talk in an encouraging way; repeat answers to questions in a warm, calm way; use touch when appropriate; stand or sit to face client;

maintain eye contact. *Clients with a loss in mental competence become more sensitive to the moods and feelings of others.*

NURSING DIAGNOSIS #2:   *Chronic confusion related to Dementia of the Alzheimer's Type*

EXPECTED CLIENT OUTCOMES

- Client will experience the least amount of anxiety and stress and remain at optimal level of functioning for the stage of the condition.

NURSING INTERVENTIONS WITH RATIONALE

- Monitor any physiological changes that might contribute to increased confusion.
- Identify client's current level of functioning given the stage of illness present.
- Provide a safe environment by assessing the appropriate level of safety precautions that need to be implemented based on the stage of the client's condition.
- Monitor client's tendency to wander, and intervene as needed, e.g., provide a safe area in which client can wander, use appropriate identification, engage in appropriate activities for outlet of energy, use Med-Alert bracelets. *Wandering can result from such factors as boredom, restlessness, confusion, or the need for exercise.*
- Teach and work with caregivers to control selected factors and stressors that can contribute to increased anxiety, stress, and dysfunctional behavior. *Factors and stressors such as unreasonable expectations, fatigue, too much stimuli, physiological problems, and too much change can lead to an increase in stress, anxiety, and dysfunctional behaviors.*
- Determine client's usual patterns of behavior and level of stress. *Stress can lead to anxiety and dysfunctional behaviors.*
- Maintain as much stability and consistency in environment as possible by avoiding abrupt changes in caregivers, routine, and environmental surroundings; post daily routine and schedule in client's room; minimize situations that are unfamiliar; provide one simple instruc-

tion at a time. *Changes in cognitive abilities affect client's ability to cope with change. Difficulty in interpreting sensory input can lead to feelings of being overwhelmed. Consistency reduces fear, anxiety, and stress and permits client to focus on goal-directed behavior and the necessary activities of daily living. Consistency in routine can reduce confusion and agitation.*

- Carefully assess expectations of client *so that capabilities are not overextended.*
- Space personal care and activities to minimize client fatigue; provide regular periods for rest during the day in a comfortable recliner. *Fatigue can easily develop while performing the essential activities of daily living.*
- Help client keep active and involved in activities that are within client's level of capability. *Demands that exceed functional capacity increase stress and the potential for dysfunctional behavior.*
- Keep stimuli within tolerance; avoid subjecting client to competing stimuli, e.g., decrease noise level or crowds of people as much as possible. *Competing stimuli increase frustration, stress, and misinterpretations and reduce client's ability to engage in the task at hand and the necessary activities of daily living. Sensory deprivation or overload can lead to dysfunctional responses.*
- Monitor health status and avoid complications such as infections and electrolyte imbalances; relieve pain; treat constipation; encourage good nutritional and fluid intake; avoid use of caffeine.
- Teach caregiver to avoid probing questions to determine orientation that client cannot answer; use praise and encouragement when assessing for orientation.
- Teach caregivers to set reasonable expectations for behavior and to communicate to client in ways that can be understood; monitor and modify these expectations with changes in condition.
- Point out to caregiver selected diversional activities that are based on client's interest, tolerance, and cognitive abilities, e.g., favorite TV programs, music.
- Provide frequent, positive feedback.
- Limit visitors to a number that the client can tolerate, and encourage visitors to discuss topics that might be of interest to client.

- Orient client as much as and when needed. *Reality orientation may be useful with clients with mild cognitive impairment.*
- Have family member write names of persons in familiar photos.
- Teach caregivers how to manage problem behaviors:
  ○ Demanding or abusive behavior: Listen and observe for the information that client is trying to communicate. Attempt to eliminate the cause of behavior; use distracters to manage behavior.
  ○ Refusal to eat: Offer extra treats or special desserts when client has eaten some of main meal.
  ○ Refusal to bathe: Try a different method; substitute a shower for a tub bath. Offer rewards after bathing is completed.
  ○ Agitation when trying to communicate: Listen actively and convey acceptance of the communication. Attempt to rephrase message that was heard. Speak naturally but use simple sentences. Involve the client to ensure an understanding of the client's response.
- Discuss with caregiver the necessity of accepting the client's confusion *to minimize unrealistic caregiver expectations of self and client.*

NURSING DIAGNOSIS #3: *Caregiver role strain related to health care demands of client with Alzheimer's disease*

EXPECTED CAREGIVER OUTCOMES

- Caregiver will participate in managing environmental routine, assist client in maintaining optimal cognitive functioning, and provide optimal care to client.
- Caregiver will avoid reaching physical and emotional exhaustion and caregiver role strain from caregiver activities.

NURSING INTERVENTIONS WITH RATIONALE

- Teach caregiver about Alzheimer's disease, e.g., can use Caregivers–Alzheimer's Disease Assessment Tool (C-ADAT).
- Assist caregiver in understanding the caregiving process:

- ○ anticipatory behaviors (caregiver actions influenced by external events)
- ○ preventive care (caregiver actions taken to assure maximum health of client)
- ○ supervisory and instrumental (actions surrounding the caregiving act, including the hands-on actions to maintain health of client)
- ○ protective (protecting client from consequences that are not preventable)
- Assist caregiver in identifying the availability of interdisciplinary team resources that can be contacted for assistance, e.g., home health nurse, occupational therapist, social worker, home health aides, and counselors.
- Assist caregiver in identifying and using other community resources as necessary, e.g., adult day care, day programs, respite care, partial hospitalization, case management, homemaker services, transportation, home delivered meals, agencies supplying daily telephone reassurance, medical equipment to *reduce the burden of care. Adult day care may be an appropriate placement for clients who remain oriented, comprehend communication, are cooperative, and can remain out of bed in the daytime.*
- Encourage participation in Alzheimer's support group.
- Encourage discussion of perception of one's own role as caregiver versus previous role in family and community.
- Teach caregiver the importance of maintaining balance between caregiver role and individual needs, e.g., teach importance of identifying needs such as getting enough rest and sleep.
- Offer emotional support and assist caregiver to work through issues such as emotional grief.
- Teach caregiver about client's condition and potential problematic behaviors.
- Encourage solution of one problem at a time. *Identifying one problem to focus on at a time can make an overall insurmountable task more manageable.*
- Teach caregiver to involve client in planning care as much as the stage of client's condition will allow.
- Teach caregiver communication skills useful in working with client.

- Teach caregiver to problem solve when faced with problematic behavior in client.
- Identify when the problem behavior occurs and what happened prior to the onset of the behavior or who was involved. Determine emotional response of client, caregiver, and others involved.
- Identify potential factors contributing to the occurrence of the problem behavior, such as client fatigue, difficulties in communication, nature of the task challenging the client, and client's physical health.
- Assess approaches that have been used. What have been the results? Are there other interpersonal approaches that could be used?
- Encourage creativity and adaptation in developing strategies that are successful.
- Teach caregiver use of effective interpersonal responses to manage problem behaviors.
- Encourage the use of distraction, such as changing the tone of voice, giving food, changing the subject.
- Allow for pacing in a safe environment, e.g., an enclosed backyard. *It is important to allow as much freedom for the client as possible while providing the safety and structure that are needed for the client's current condition.*
- Permit wandering within safe, restricted environment; prevent leaving the safety of home.
- Permit rummaging; ask client what is being sought; use distraction to limit rummaging behavior.
- Reduce effects of sundowning (increased restlessness in late afternoon or early evening) by encouraging early afternoon exercise.
- Reduce sleep disturbances by setting a regular schedule for sleep and creating an atmosphere conducive to sleep.
- Encourage caregiver to participate in support groups. To determine which support group to select, have the caregiver ask such questions as: What is the goal of the group? What will it accomplish? Do the persons attending the group gain something positive from attending the group?
- Encourage family member and client to engage in early financial and legal planning *in order to reduce the severe*

potential negative impact on the family of this devastating illness.

- Be aware of signs of elder abuse or neglect, e.g., weight loss, dehydration, sunken eyes, pallor, inappropriate fractures, lacerations, bruises, burns, rope burns, and head injuries. (See also Abuse Protection in Chapter 5.)

CHAPTER 7

Mental Disorders Due to a General Medical Condition

Definition/Major Symptoms[*]

Mental Disorders Due to a General Medical Condition are a group of conditions in which the mental symptoms are caused by general medical problems. These symptoms are severe, significant, and problematic enough to cause clinicians working with the client to label and treat the conditions/syndromes. Many medical conditions exhibit mental symptoms. The category "mental disorders due to a general medical condition" facilitates the diagnostic and treatment process.

The most common psychiatric symptoms related to medical conditions are:

- Anxiety: irritability, feelings of tension and apprehension, distractibility.
- Depression: feeling blue, loss of interest, hopelessness, worthlessness, inability to concentrate, tiredness, sleeplessness, irritable, somatic complaints.
- Confusion and memory loss, particularly recent memory.
- Psychotic symptoms: hallucinations, delusions, bizarre behavior.
- Delirium: confusion, restlessness, disorientation related to hallucinations and fear.

[*]References 1,7,10,13,14

▌ Definition/Major Symptoms of Selected Major Categories[*]

The DSM-IV has a general category for Mental Disorders Due to a General Medical Condition. Each disorder is found under the specific DSM-IV category according to the major mental symptoms that the medical condition exhibits. The categories are listed below with examples. (Refer to the chapters that discuss particular disorder categories for further identification of symptoms.)

Delirium—e.g., Delirium due to third degree burns on 10% of body

Dementia—e.g., Dementia due to HIV

Amnestic disorders—e.g., Amnestic Disorder due to alcohol abuse

Schizophrenia and other psychotic disorders—e.g., Psychotic Disorder due to renal failure

Mood disorders—e.g., Mood Disorder due to frontal lobe tumor

Anxiety disorders—e.g., Anxiety Disorder due to hypoxia from COPD

Sexual disorders—e.g., Male Erectile Disorder due to atherosclerosis

Sleep disorders—e.g., Sleep Disorder, Insomnia Type due to sleep apnea

In addition there are:

Catatonia disorder due to a medical condition—e.g., Catatonia Disorder due to hepatic encephalopathy

Personality change due to a general medical condition—e.g., Personality Change due to seizure disorder

▌ Incidence[†]

- Unknown
- 25%–30% of medical outpatients and 40%–50% of medical inpatients have a psychiatric disorder.

[*]References 1,7,10,13,14
[†]References 1,7,10,13,14

Course

The course of the disorder is related primarily to the treatment of the medical condition.

Contributing Factors*

- Trauma—e.g., head trauma
- Infectious disease—e.g., encephalitis, syphilis
- Cardiovascular conditions—e.g., arrhythmias
- Pulmonary conditions—e.g., COPD
- Drug intoxication—e.g., alcohol
- Drug withdrawal—e.g., caffeine
- Tumors—e.g., cancer, brain tumor
- Degenerative disease—e.g., Parkinson's disease, Huntington's disease
- Demyelinating disorders—e.g., multiple sclerosis
- Metabolic diseases—e.g., diabetes, hepatic failure, renal failure
- Endocrine disorders—e.g., thyroid dysfunction, adrenal disease
- Immune disorders—e.g., AIDS, lupus
- Vitamin deficiency—e.g., pernicious anemia, pellagra
- Medications—e.g., cardiac drugs, diuretics
- Malformations

Laboratory and Physical Findings†

The usual psychiatric screening includes complete blood count (CBC), blood chemistry screening, thyroid function tests (TSH, T_4), chest X-ray, and urinalysis. Additional screens commonly include vitamin B_{12}, drug levels, CT scan, and EEG. Differential diagnosis continues until the clinical presentation clarifies the diagnosis as a medical condition, a mental disorder, or a mental disorder due to a medical condition.

*References 1,7,10,13,14
†References 7,10,13,14

▌ Special Assessment Considerations*

Since approximately 60% of psychiatric patients are treated by medical physicians, the diagnostic category "mental disorders due to ..." provides a mechanism for considering a psychiatric diagnosis and acknowledging the presence of mental symptoms; highlights the importance of the recognition and identification of symptoms in the diagnostic process; and guides the treatment of the mental disorder and/or symptoms when they appear.

Problems related to death and dying frequently emerge in clients experiencing serious medical conditions. Symptoms may include suicidal thoughts and acts. Careful assessment of the client's overall condition is required; compassion and support need to be provided.

▌ Treatment†

- Treatment of the underlying etiology of the specific medical condition is *very important*, e.g., renal dialysis for renal failure, antibiotics for infectious disease, or thyroid replacement for hypothyroidism. The first step is to remove or minimize the medical condition causing the psychiatric disorder.
- Psychopharmacology.
  ○ Antidepressants or ECT for Mood Disorder
  ○ Antipsychotics, if not contraindicated by medical condition, for psychotic disorders
  ○ Anxiolytics, benzodiazepines for anxiety disorders
- Teaching of good health habits/routines (i.e., fluid intake, diet, exercise, sleep, hygiene).
- Supportive psychotherapy focusing of relief of anxiety and fears.
- Engagement of support system in treatment process.

▌ Commonly Occurring Nursing Diagnoses

- Adjustment, impaired
- Anxiety
- Breathing pattern, ineffective

*References 1,7,10,13,14
†References 7,10,13,14

- Confusion, acute or chronic
- Coping, defensive
- Coping, ineffective, individual
- Denial, ineffective
- Gas exchange, impaired
- Grieving, anticipatory
- Grieving, dysfunctional
- Hopelessness
- Memory, impaired
- Mobility, impaired physical
- Pain
- Pain, chronic
- Sexual dysfunction
- Sleep pattern disturbance
- Thought processes, altered

■ Selected Nursing Diagnoses, Outcome Criteria, and Nursing Interventions with Rationale*

Example: Client With Mood Disorder due to HIV Associated With Dementia in an Outpatient Setting

NURSING DIAGNOSIS #1:   *Hopelessness related to deteriorating physiological condition, to little belief in a future, and no hope for change.*

EXPECTED CLIENT OUTCOME

- Client will identify which of his abilities have not changed, which have altered somewhat, and how he will manage.

NURSING INTERVENTIONS WITH RATIONALE

- Provide self-awareness enhancement *to assist the client in identifying and valuing his positive attributes that contribute to lessening of anxiety and/or depression associated with physical losses.*
  - Provide opportunity to vent feelings of anger and frustration being experienced as he alters his goals.
  - Identify changes he has made in his life routines to make activities easier, *thus providing feedback about ability to cope.*

*References 2–6,8,9,11,12,15

- Provide coping enhancement *because the client is experiencing problems in processing information and making decisions.*
  - Focus on simplifying his tasks/routines during the day.
  - Give explanations in concrete manner and use several illustrations *to make directions and/or information clear, since he is processing information at a slower rate.*
  - Write down directions for taking medications.

EXPECTED CLIENT OUTCOME

- Client will identify a goal for a month and for six months from now.

NURSING INTERVENTIONS WITH RATIONALE

- Enhance the instillation of hope *to promote change in the outlook he has about the future.*
  - Review goals he has achieved and those he wants to accomplish; give feedback as he begins to alter them.
  - Emphasize caring for self rather than searching for a cure; focus on present and not past, *because this enables a person to take some actions for the self rather than feeling that all is useless, because there is no cure.*
  - Identify next appointment date and other significant dates in future *as another way of supporting a look forward, even if only for a few days or months.*
- Provide presence *to allay fears and anxiety as one communicates empathy to the client.*
  - Set specific appointment time every two weeks.
  - Develop plan for communicating with client at other times, e.g., taking phone calls at certain times or having access to voicemail.

NURSING DIAGNOSIS #2: *Knowledge deficit of good health habits or habits that will tend to maximize one's resistance to opportunistic infections.*

EXPECTED CLIENT OUTCOME

- Client will demonstrate one or two changes in diet, exercise, sleep, and sexual habits.

NURSING INTERVENTIONS WITH RATIONALE

- Provide teaching of basic healthful living practices *to improve overall health routines and ways of coping with these areas of one's life.*

○ Discuss and set priorities with client for review of basic health routines, i.e., food, exercise, fluid intake, sleep, sex.

○ Teach ways to keep self oriented, less forgetful, and feeling less overwhelmed or confused.

○ Identify ways to deal with tiredness, occasional unsteadiness, stumbling.

○ Discuss importance of contact with others and techniques to help others feel comfortable when in their presence. Encourage attendance at support group.

EXPECTED CLIENT OUTCOME

• Client will identify undesirable health practices and will make appropriate change with assistance from variety of resouces.

NURSING INTERVENTIONS WITH RATIONALE

• Review poor practices that increase one's risk for infection and disease or weaken the response of immune system, *so the client is knowledgeable and can make informed decisions and action plans in his own behalf.*

• Teach client to change poor habits such as:

○ Injecting recreational drugs. If client still is injecting, then teach to sterilize needles with 1-to-5 ratio of bleach to water *to sterilize needles and thus prevent infection.*

○ Sexual contact without practicing safe sex.

○ Use of alcohol, tobacco.

○ Not taking HIV medicines because of side effects, e.g., zidovudine (Retrovir, AZT) may cause headache, nausea.

○ Not avoiding situations where possibility of infection exists, e.g., caring for cat litter box, attending school function in height of flu season.

○ Not preparing/keeping food in safe manner; not cooking meat and fish thoroughly; not eating from clean dishes.

○ Not seeking help for discomfort/pain.

○ Isolating self from others.

• Provide cognitive restructuring *to manage the depressive symptoms and other sources of stress.*

○ Assist the client in making positive self statements.

○ Assist the client in separating the fears and anxieties of others from fears/anxiety he is experiencing.

○ Review ways to manage stress (see Chapter 4).
• Emphasize importance of notifying physician when signs of infection occur, e.g., fever, rash, cough, *so that preventive action can be taken or early treatment begun.*

CHAPTER 8

Substance-Related Disorders

▎ Definition*

Substance-Related Disorders are clinical conditions resulting from using a drug of abuse, e.g., alcohol, to alter one's mood or behavior, as well as clinical conditions that are induced as the result of side effects from a prescribed medication or from an individual's unintentional exposure to toxic substances. These disorders are divided into two major groups: Substance Use Disorders (Substance Dependence and Substance Abuse) and Substance-Induced Disorders.

▎ Definition/Major Symptoms for Substance Dependence†

Substance Dependence is a pattern of repeated self-administration of a substance that causes cognitive, behavioral, and physiological symptoms that are associated with significant substance-related problems. Signs and symptoms in the elderly may be overlooked because they are subtle and resemble symptoms of other geriatric medical conditions; memory loss and feeling of shame that substance abuse is immoral contribute to inadequate reporting. The

*References 1,17
†References 1,3,17

symptoms of Substance Dependence span all categories of substances. Specific symptoms include:

1. *Tolerance*, the need for increased amounts of substance to achieve intoxication or the desired effect, or experiencing less effect when continuing to use same amount of substance; person may be unaware of tolerance.
2. *Withdrawal* following decreased blood or tissue concentrations of the substance after prolonged or heavy use of the substance with increased use of substance to relieve or avoid recurrence of withdrawal.
3. *Compulsive substance use* evidenced by increased amount or longer duration than originally intended; persistent desire or unsuccessful efforts to reduce or control substance use; time-consuming efforts for obtaining, using, or recovering from effects of substance; relinquishment or decreased participation in important social, occupational, or recreational activities or withdrawal from social and leisure activities to engage in private substance use or to be with others with similar problems; inability to abstain from substance use despite recognition of persistent or recurrent physical or psychological problems from substance use.

▌ Definition/Symptoms for Substance Abuse*

Substance Abuse is "a maladaptive pattern of substance use manifested by recurrent and significant adverse consequences related to the repeated use of substances."[1,p.182] Symptoms include failure to perform role responsibilities, e.g., absence, poor performance; neglect of children or household during times of intoxication; repeated intoxication in physically hazardous situations, e.g., driving an automobile, operating machinery; recurrent legal problems, e.g., arrests, related to substance use; and ongoing substance use despite persistent or repeated social or interpersonal problems associated with substance use, e.g., verbal and physical altercations with family.

Serious, nonspecific symptoms of Substance Abuse in the elderly overlap with problems commonly seen in this population and may erroneously be attributed to other

*References 1,3,17,33

causes. These symptoms include poor grooming, depression, malnutrition, bladder and bowel incontinence, muscle weakness, gait disorder, recurring falls, burns, or head trauma. The category of Substance Abuse does not apply to caffeine and nicotine.

▌ Definition/Symptoms for Substance-Induced Disorder, Substance Intoxication[*]

This is "the development of a reversible substance-specific syndrome due to recent ingestion of (or exposure to) a substance. Different substances may produce similar or identical syndromes."[1,p.184] Maladaptive behavioral or psychological changes occur during or shortly after substance use, e.g., euphoria, belligerence, mood lability, cognitive impairment, impaired judgment, and impaired interpersonal functioning and psychomotor disturbances. Symptoms vary according to the specific substance, dose, person's tolerance, length of time since last dose, and the environmental or social context in which substance is taken. Symptoms may persist for hours or days after the substance can be detected in body fluids.

▌ Definition/Symptoms for Substance-Induced Disorder, Substance Withdrawal[†]

This is "the development of a substance-specific syndrome due to the cessation of (or reduction in) substance use that has been heavy and prolonged."[1,p.185] Substance Withdrawal often, but not always, occurs with Substance Dependence. Symptoms, which begin when the dose is decreased or stopped, include a craving for the substance to decrease the symptoms and may include autonomic or physiological symptoms such as tremor, tachycardia, hypertension, insomnia, sweating, or seizures. Symptoms are influenced by the type of substance, dose, length of use, and the presence or absence of other illnesses.

[*]Reference 1
[†]Reference 1

▮ Definition/Symptoms of Selected Major Categories: Alcohol-Related Disorders*

Alcohol Use Disorder, Alcohol Dependence

Symptoms include physiological dependence on alcohol as evidenced by tolerance or symptoms of alcohol withdrawal, which develop approximately 12 hours after a decrease in prolonged or heavy alcohol intake. A pattern of compulsive use includes devoting significant amounts of time to obtaining and consuming alcoholic beverage and continuing to drink while recognizing potential adverse physiological or psychological consequences, e.g., depression, blackouts, cardiac or liver disease/failure. (See also previous Definition/Symptoms for Substance Dependence and subsequent Definition/Symptoms for Alcohol Withdrawal.)

Alcohol Use Disorder, Alcohol Abuse

This is a maladaptive pattern of alcohol use. (See also previous Definition/Symptoms for Substance Abuse.)

Alcohol-Induced Disorder, Alcohol Intoxication

This consists of "...maladaptive behavioral or psychological changes...that develop during or shortly after the ingestion of alcohol."[1, p. 196]

   Symptoms include odor of alcohol on person's breath; alterations in mood; inappropriate sexual or aggressive behavior; slurred speech; incoordination, which can impede driving ability; unsteady gait, which may result in falls; nystagmus; impaired attention or concentration; and stupor or coma. (See also previous Definitions/Symptoms for Substance Intoxication.)

Alcohol-Induced Disorder, Alcohol Withdrawal

This is a withdrawal syndrome that develops in close proximity (several hours to a few days) after person abruptly stops or decreases heavy and prolonged alcohol consumption. Symptoms include autonomic hyperactivity,

*References 1,5,6,17

e.g., profuse sweating, increased blood pressure, piloerection, pulse rate over 100, as well as malaise, nausea or vomiting, increased hand tremor, sleep disturbance, tactile illusions or hallucinations, visual or auditory hallucinations or illusions, psychomotor agitation, anxiety, and generalized tonic-clonic seizures. (See also previous Definition/Symptoms for Substance Withdrawal.)

▌ Definition/Symptoms of Selected Major Categories of Amphetamine (or Amphetamine-Like) Related Disorders*

Amphetamine Use Disorder, Amphetamine Dependence and Amphetamine Use Disorder, Amphetamine Abuse

Specific substances within these categories include amphetamine, dextroamphetamine, methamphetamine ("ice" or "speed"), crystal methedrine ("crank"), as well as substances that have amphetamine action, e.g., methylphenidate and appetite suppressants. Psychic and physical dependence develops with only a few months between first drug use and chronic use. (See previous Definition/ Symptoms for Substance Dependence and Substance Abuse.)

Amphetamine-Induced Disorder, Amphetamine Intoxication

After an initial "high" feeling, person develops maladaptive behavioral or psychological changes, e.g., hypervigilance; interpersonal sensitivity; anxiety, anger, fighting; grandiosity; impaired judgment; and psychotic symptoms. Additional signs and symptoms may include "tachycardia or bradycardia; pupillary dilation; elevated or lowered blood pressure; perspiration or chills; nausea or vomiting; evidence of weight loss; psychomotor agitation or retardation; muscular weakness, respiratory depression, chest pain, or cardiac arrhythmias; and confusion, seizures, dyskinesia, dystonia, or coma."[1,p.207] (See also previous Definition/Symptoms for Substance Abuse.)

*References 1,7,48,52

Amphetamine-Induced Disorder, Amphetamine Withdrawal

Symptoms include dysphoric mood, suicidal ideation, fatigue, vivid and unpleasant dreams, sleep disturbance, increased appetite, psychomotor agitation or retardation, lassitude, and weight loss. Although withdrawal symptoms are not life threatening, depression and suicidal symptoms may continue for weeks and craving can continue for months. (See also previous Definition/Symptoms for Substance Withdrawal.)

▐ Definition/Symptoms of Major Categories of Selected Caffeine-Related Disorders

Caffeine-Induced Disorder, Caffeine Intoxication[*]

Symptoms include nervousness, anxiety, excitement, insomnia, flushed face, diuresis, gastrointestinal complaints, muscle twitching, rambling flow of thoughts and speech, tachycardia, premature ventricular contractions, periods of inexhaustibility, and psychomotor agitation. Symptoms of toxicity include agitation, tinnitus, dyskinesias, and cardiac arrhythmia. Sources for caffeine, in addition to coffee, include caffeinated soft drinks, cocoa, milk chocolate, prescription medications (e.g., Cafergot, Fiorinal), over-the-counter analgesics and cold preparations (e.g., Anacin, Midol, Dristan), and weight-loss products. (See also previous Definition/Symptoms for Substance Intoxication.)

▐ Definition/Symptoms of Selected Major Categories of Cannabis-Related Disorders

Cannabis Use Disorder, Cannabis Dependence and Cannabis Use Disorder, Cannabis Abuse[†]

This category includes various forms, commonly referred to as marijuana, pot, hashish, reefer, weed. Physical dependence is controversial; compulsive use is common. (See previous Definition/Symptoms for Substance Dependence and Substance Abuse.)

[*]References 1,7,12,58
[†]References 1,7,12

◼ Definition/Symptoms of Selected Major Categories of Cocaine-Related Disorders[*]

Cocaine Dependence

Cocaine is the most behaviorally reinforcing of all drugs. There are various preparations, e.g., cocaine hydrochloride powder that is "snorted" through the nostrils or dissolved in water for intravenous use, and "crack," a cocaine alkaloid that is a prepackaged, freebased derivative ready for smoking. Slang terms include "coke," "snow," "girl," and "nose candy." Early indication of dependence is difficulty refusing opportunity to use it. Dependence is often associated with illegal activities to obtain money to pay for the drug. Mental complications include hallucinations, paranoia, mood disturbances, and repetitive and aggressive behaviors; physical complications include weight loss. (Refer to definition, criteria/symptoms for Substance Dependence.)

◼ Definition/Symptoms of Selected Nicotine-Related Disorders[†]

Nicotine Use Disorder, Nicotine Dependence

Dependence can occur with all forms of tobacco as well as nicotine gum and nicotine patches. (Refer to definition and criteria/symptoms for Substance Dependence.)

Nicotine Use Disorder, Nicotine Withdrawal

Withdrawal, which begins within 24 hours in person with several weeks' history of daily use, is more commonly associated with cigarette use. Symptoms include headache, anxiety, gastrointestinal disturbance, irritability, problems with concentration, restlessness, and weight gain (more common in women). (Refer to definition and criteria/symptoms for Substance Withdrawal.)

[*]References 1,12,17,48,58
[†]References 1,7,12,47,58

▌ Definition/Symptoms of Selected Opioid-Related Disorders[*]

Opioid-Related Disorder, Opioid Dependence

The opioids include morphine (a natural opioid), heroin (semisynthetic); and codeine, hydromorphone, methadone, oxycodone, meperidine, and fentanyl (synthetics with action similar to morphine). Drugs may be prescribed, e.g., analgesics, cough suppressants, or obtained through street use. Signs and symptoms of dependence include self-administration for no legitimate medical condition, requirement for dose that is in excess of usual amount, daily activities that are based on obtaining and administering the drug, purchasing of drug through illegal market, forging prescriptions, and obtaining prescription for same drug from numerous providers. A health care professional with opioid dependence may write own prescription, take drugs that have been prescribed for a client, or steal from pharmacy supplies. (Refer to definition and criteria/symptoms for Substance Dependence.)

▌ Incidence[†]

The number one health problem in the United States is Substance Abuse.

Alcohol is the most commonly used recreational drug in the United States. Alcoholism affects approximately 14% of the population at some point in time. "Approximately 48% of youths (age 12 to 17 years) have tried alcohol and about 15% have tried marijuana...illicit drug use among females aged 15 to 44...is 25% greater than general population."[11,p.1001] Caffeine use varies according to culture. Cannabis is the most commonly used illicit substance in the world. There is an epidemic of Cocaine Abuse in the United States, with an estimated 3 million current cocaine users in 1991. Approximately 50 to 60 million Americans smoke tobacco, the second most commonly used recreational drug in the United States. Prevalence of nicotine use decreases with amount of education. Opioid incidence

[*]References 1,12,58
[†]References 1,7,11,13,17,33,51

varies according to specific drug. Approximately 500,000 persons are heroin dependent, and an even greater number use other opiates.

▌ Course[*]

- There may be fluctuations in drinking patterns, with intervals of sobriety of 10 years or longer. The interval from initial onset of alcohol problems until entry into treatment can be as long as 50 years; high mortality rates occur with active drinking after presence of dementia.
- Amphetamine Abuse often begins through weight control attempts; there is a rapid tolerance to effects; occlusive and hemorrhagic stroke are a frequent complication; intracranial hemorrhage has been reported in clients 16 to 60 years of age after amphetamine use.
- Caffeine half-life is 2 to 6 hours; development of tolerance to behavioral effects of caffeine reduces occurrence of Caffeine Intoxication; intoxication occurs in infrequent users or persons who have substantially increased their intake.
- Cannabis Dependence and Abuse develop over time; chronic use can result in same problems as tobacco use, as well as what is referred to "amotivational syndrome," with behavioral patterns such as "apathy, dullness, impaired judgment, decreased concentration and memory, loss of interest in personal hygiene and a general reduction of goal-directed behavior."[11,p.1009]
- Cocaine use may be daily or episodic, i.e., "binges" that end when supply is no longer available; there is a rapid progression from use to Abuse or Dependence with decrease in pleasurable effects and increase in dysphoria. Intravenous use with impurities is associated with complications such as endocarditis, septicemia, HIV, hepatitis B, pulmonary emboli, and death.
- Tobacco use accounts for 85% of deaths from lung cancer in the U.S. and also contributes to numerous other cancers (e.g., oropharyngeal, esophageal, pancreatic, kidney and bladder), COPD, and coronary and peripheral vascular disease.

[*]References 1,2,3,7,12,47,58

- Opioid Abuse and Dependence are also associated with frequent use of medical and surgical services, e.g., life-threatening infections, accidents, injuries, general medical complications, and very high rate of death.

▌ Culture, Age, and Gender*

- Substance Abuse (both alcohol and drug) has been identified as a problem of older women.
- First episode of intoxication from alcohol (male and female) is most likely to occur during the mid-teens, with dependence peaking in the 20s to mid-30s.
- Ethnic variation exists on perspectives and values regarding definition, nature, and treatment of Substance Abuse, e.g., alcohol is a part of communion in some Christian churches or ceremonies of the Native American church; some groups see overindulgence as normal; drugs may serve occupational as well as recreational need in some urban African-American communities.
- IV drug use is more common in lower socioeconomic groups with a male-to-female ratio of 3/4:1.
- Use patterns of caffeine, the most widely used psychoactive drug in the world, indicate greater use among males, smokers, and Caucasians; consumption increases in the 20s with a decrease after 65 years of age.
- Cocaine use is most commonly found in people 18 to 30 years of age and spans all races, socioeconomic, age, and gender groups in the U.S., with an equal distribution between males and females.
- Use of "smokeless tobacco," chewing tobacco or snuff, has increased among high school seniors. Although cigarette use has decreased in men, it has increased in women and teenagers.
- More men than women are affected with Opioid Dependence (ratio of 3/4:1); opioid dependency is known to last as long as 50 years; health care providers have an increased risk for Opioid Abuse and Dependence because of their ready access to drugs.

*References 1,2,3,7,8,16,59

▌ Contributing Factors to Substance-Related Disorders[*]

Neurobiological/Genetic

"...[T]he etiology of substance abuse remains obscure and controversial"[43,p.179]; there are possible differences in etiological factors for men and women. Biological theories propose predisposition to alcoholism in some persons; children of alcoholics have increased risk for developing alcohol problems, even when they grow up in a non-alcoholic home. Genetic factors offer only a partial explanation, with additional factors such as environmental and interpersonal factors playing a role in increased risk for alcohol dependence. Studies of families, twins, and adoption demonstrate genetic influences on tobacco addiction. A lack of endogenous opioid peptide homeostasis is one hypothesis for the fact that some persons are more prone to opioid addiction; other models link opioid tolerance and dependence to an imbalance between endogenous opioids and adrenocorticotropic hormone (ACTH).

Psychological Model

The inability of addicted people to outwardly manifest feelings and emotions when they experience psychic trauma can result in substance use as a protection from recognizing and expressing overwhelming feelings or emotions. Pathological shame that influences the person's core sense of self has been linked to Substance Abuse. There may be pathological identification with destructive or psychotic parents. Insufficient data exist to substantiate psychological explanations for "alcoholic personality." Severe stress, associated with war-related assignments and activities in conjunction with substance availability, is a possible factor in some opioid use, as well as social stressors experienced by disadvantaged communities who have high unemployment, family instability, and increased tolerance of criminal activity.

[*]References 1,7,18,39,43,50,51

▌ Laboratory Findings*

Tests for detection of adverse medical consequences from alcohol and drug use include urinalysis, CBC, blood chemistry, liver enzymes, serology, and testing for tuberculosis. HIV testing, with the client's permission, is also important because of high rates of infection in intravenous drug users, freebase and crack cocaine users, and alcohol abusers. *Serum and urine toxicologic samples for screening for assessment and treatment of substance use disorders should be obtained under direct observation to minimize collection errors; it is important to take into consideration that compounds in some foods or medications can mimic illicit drugs in analysis of these tests; positive test results indicate probable past use of substance but do not indicate extent of use or when use occurred.*

Elevations in liver function tests and mean corpuscular volume (MCV), adjunctive tests, are not always reliable and specific for confirming diagnosis of Substance Abuse because findings may be similar to other medical conditions, e.g., liver disease and nutritional deficiencies not associated with Substance Abuse.

Use of a breathalizer is preferable to urine drug testing for alcohol because of its convenience, reliability, and low cost.

Findings in Nicotine Withdrawal include the following: EEG shows slower frequencies during abstinence from smoking; decrease in catecholamine and cortisol levels; REM changes; diminished pulmonary function tests; increased MCV; decreased metabolic rate; and increased metabolism of certain medications prescribed for treatment of mental disorders or other substances.

▌ Physical Examination Findings†

- Indications of possible Substance Abuse include:
  - repeated trauma to head from injuries while intoxicated
  - elderly client with history of accidents or falls, bruises on legs or arms from bumping into furniture (possible Alcohol Abuse)
  - elderly client with bladder and bowel incontinence, muscle weakness, gait disorders, tremulousness that

*References 1,9,17,53,58
†References 1,3,7,9,17,33,44,47,50,53,54,58

affects ability to bathe, brush teeth (possible Alcohol Abuse/Withdrawal).
- Indicators of Alcohol Abuse include:
  - peripheral neuropathy
  - gynecomastia
  - cardiovascular disease (e.g., cardiomyopathy, essential hypertension)
  - digestive disease (e.g.,alcoholic fatty liver, cirrhosis).
- Cocaine Abuse is associated with acute and chronic medical complications that include sudden death from ventricular arrhythmias, septal necrosis from chronic intranasal use; dental neglect because of anesthetic properties; and malnutrition, severe weight loss, and dehydration from binges. Perinatal and neonatal cocaine-exposed infants are at risk for strokes; babies born to cocaine-using mothers have five times as many birth defects compared with non-using mothers.
- Tobacco: morning cough, sputum production, hoarseness, nicotine stains on teeth and hands, fatigue.
- Cellulitis, abscesses, sclerosing of veins, and track marks from intravenous drug abuse are noted in clients with Opioid Dependence.
- Signs and symptoms of HIV, AIDS, tuberculosis, liver disease, bacterial endocarditis (IV opioid use), gastrointestinal bleeding, chronic diarrhea, and malabsorption are suggestive of Substance Abuse with medical complications.
- Depressed respiration and marked somnolence may be indicative of an impending drug overdose.

▌ Special Assessment Considerations[*]

- Use client and (based on client consent) family, peers, employers, and past and current health providers to determine nature and extent of Substance Abuse by obtaining information such as all substances used by client; the degree of physical and psychological dependence; extent to which substances interfere with daily life; severity of past withdrawal patterns; time since most recent dose; method of use, e.g., smoking, injecting, quantity, frequency, duration, source of supply

[*]References 1,2,4,8,10,15,30,33,35,44,50,53–55,57,60

(drugs); history of previous treatment as well as attempts by client to stop outside formal treatment; family history of Substance Abuse, substance and psychiatric disorders; financial, legal problems.

- Recognize tendency for client to minimize, deny, lie about substance use and concomitant problems; avoid use of "Why did you..." and focus on "How did that affect you?" to minimize client's defensiveness and perception of questions as judgmental.

- Assess for psychosocial problems associated with Substance Abuse that could be related to culture, e.g., alienation from client's cultural group, being forced out of religious or ethnic association, failing to meet reciprocal obligations to his or her cultural group, failure to adhere to cultural norms with loss of social status and loss of self-esteem.

- In non-emergency situations begin assessment by asking client to review successes as well as problems in work, school, family, friends, and medical, legal and psychological problems without attempting to make a direct connection to substance use; then focus on specific questions that address history of substance and associated problems.

- Assess for presence of risk factors associated with suicide in client with alcohol problems, e.g., ongoing Alcohol Abuse, living alone, inadequate social support, unemployment, suicidal ideation, coexisting Major Depressive Disorder, serious medical condition(s).

- Assess client's motivation for treatment. For example, is spouse threatening to end relationship? Is employer mandating treatment? Is client attempting to obtain leniency in pending court case, such as DWI? Many clients with Substance Abuse problems do not enter treatment voluntarily.

- How has client obtained money for alcohol or drugs? To what extent did client engage in risk-taking activities to obtain substance?

- Inquire what client is like when on drugs or using alcohol; what are effects on family, friendships, employment?

- Conduct mental status examination that includes assessment of cognitive functioning (see also Chapter 3) to facilitate accurate recognition of Substance Dependence, comorbid psychiatric disorders, and medical conditions; comorbid disorders (dual diagnosis) are common and affect the client's prognosis and implications for treatment.

- Use short, self-report questionnaires for routine assessment of Alcohol Abuse and Dependence, such as:
  ○ CAGE: four questions that inquire about attempts to *C*ut back on alcohol, being *A*nnoyed by comments about drinking, *G*uilt about drinking, having an *E*ye-opener first thing in the morning to steady nerves[15]
  ○ Short Michigan Alcoholism Screening Test (SMAST): 13 items for assessment of lifetime problems associated with drinking[55]
  ○ Beck Depression Inventory,[4] which may help to detect comorbid depressive disorders
- Recognize that the following symptoms in an older client are indicative of need for careful assessment for history of alcohol use: difficulty with performing activities of daily living, self-care deficits in area of personal hygiene and appearance, incontinence and/or diarrhea, short-term memory loss, symptoms of depression with suicidal ideation, and anxiety and insomnia.
- Explore issues of religiosity or spirituality to determine role that they may have in client's attempt to rebuild a life free of substance-related problems.
- Assess stability of client's current living situation; approximately 50% of all homeless adults suffer from Substance Abuse—predominantly alcohol.

▊ Treatment

Psychopharmacologic*

SPECIFIC DISORDERS AND DRUG TREATMENT

- Mild to moderate symptoms of Alcohol Withdrawal in outpatient setting: Short-acting benzodiazepines (BZs), e.g., oxazepam (30 mg qid) or lorazepam (1 mg tid or qid); BZ use is typically PRN and guided by signs of autonomic instability, e.g., tachycardia, sweating, increased blood pressure, piloerection, agitation; thiamine (50 to 100 mg per day) and multivitamins are also prescribed to reduce risk for CNS damage from Wernicke's encephalopathy.

*References 2,7,11,17,21,22,25,27,31,32,47,48,51,60,

- Severe Alcohol Withdrawal, Alcohol Withdrawal Delirium (requires immediate hospitalization): BZs are used
  for clients with recent history of alcohol withdrawal convulsions; diazepam, chlordiazepoxide, oxazepam, or
  lorazepam are appropriate for client with moderate liver
  damage because they do not require metabolism in the
  liver and do not accumulate; specific dosage takes into
  consideration the client's alcohol consumption before
  withdrawal, previous history of withdrawal, weight, and
  severity of withdrawal symptoms; severe Alcohol Withdrawal Delirium may require higher doses of oxazepam
  (60 mg qid) or diazepam (20 mg qid); caution should be
  used to avoid "overtreating," which could result in BZ-
  induced delirium; intramuscular preparations of BZ, e.g.,
  lorazepam absorbs readily after administration and is
  indicated for clients whose vomiting precludes ability to
  take oral preparations; *intramuscular forms of chlordiazepoxide and diazepam are poorly absorbed*; pro-
  chlorperazine suppository (25 mg) can be used for emesis; glucose for clients whose excessive vomiting and
  diarrhea have resulted in dehydration; infusion should
  be administered in conjunction with parenteral thiamine
  to reduce the risk of Wernicke's encephalopathy in client
  who may be thiamine deficient.
- Alcohol abstinence phase: Disulfiram (Antabuse) is an
  aversive agent for alcohol ingestion that also symbolizes
  the client's commitment to remain in a state of enforced
  sobriety; more effective and has greater therapeutic
  gains when administered by spouse or cohabitant who
  has received positive reinforcement therapy with social
  skills training for administering this drug; 250 to 500 mg
  per day, preferably in the morning when urge to drink is
  least; Native Americans whose refusal to drink may be
  taken as a personal cultural affront have benefited from
  having this drug prescribed because it gives them a valid
  reason for not drinking. Disulfiram, which is rarely associated with serious side effects, blocks the oxidation of
  acetaldehyde; adverse effects from alcohol begin within
  5 to 10 minutes after alcohol ingestion, e.g., warmth and
  flushing of face and chest, throbbing headache, respiratory difficulty, hyperventilation, dyspnea, nausea, copi-
  ous vomiting, sweating, thirst, chest pain, palpitations,

hypotension, anxiety, confusion, weakness, vertigo, and blurred vision; severe reactions, e.g., cardiovascular collapse, myocardial infarction, convulsions, are potentially fatal; client can experience reactions for as long as 1 week following the last dose; drug should be used with caution in clients with comorbid diagnosis of schizophrenia (small doses, 125 mg) as well as those with severe myocardial disease or coronary occlusion, diabetes mellitus, hypothyroidism, epilepsy, cerebral damage, chronic and acute nephritis, hepatic cirrhosis or dysfunction; use caution in clients with current or recent treatment with alcohol or alcohol-containing preparations.

- Alcohol or Opioid Dependence: Naltrexone (ReVia), an opioid antagonist, is used as an adjunct to comprehensive treatment program to reduce craving and to block the reinforcing effects of alcohol or opioid by blocking opioid receptors. Drug has had good effect, from a cultural perspective, when prescribed for Southeast Asian opium smokers because it provides these clients with a valid reason for abstinence. Contraindications and cautions are indicated for client with opioid addiction (because of potential for producing withdrawal symptoms) as well as for conditions such as opioid withdrawal, acute hepatitis, liver failure, lactation, depression, and client with suicidal tendencies. Client should be opioid free from 7 to 10 days before medication is administered. Actual maintenance dose is preceded by an IV or subcutaneous test dose of naltrexone to assess the degree of opioid dependence; the test dose may be repeated in 24 hours to observe for signs and symptoms of withdrawal and repeated again until there are no indications of withdrawal. Maintenance dosage (oral) for alcoholism is 50 mg per day. Dosage for Opioid Dependence begins with 25 mg (oral) with observation for 1 hour for signs or symptoms of withdrawal before completing dose with 25 additional mg. Because of its long duration, maintenance dosage may vary from 50 mg every 24 hours to flexible dosing schedule of 100 mg every other day or 150 mg every third day. This drug has no abuse potential. Common adverse effects may include dysphoria, sleep disturbance, anxiety, nervousness, headache, low energy, abdominal pain or cramps, nausea, vomiting, delayed ejaculation, decreased sexual potency, skin rash, chills, increased thirst, and joint and muscle pain. This medication should be prescribed in conjunction with a strong psychosocial rehabilitation program, e.g., family involvement, behavioral contingencies (reinforcement or punishment), to be most effective. Improved compliance is seen when client is directly observed and supervised by a designated health care professional, responsible family member, or work supervisor. Higher rates of success are reported when used as court-mandated treatment and for health professionals who risk losing their license if they do not adhere to designated treatment regimen.

- Mixed results of improved mood and reduced alcohol intake with desipramine and decrease in problem drinking in non-depressed social drinkers who were prescribed selective serotonin reuptake inhibitors (SSRIs) have been reported.

- Cocaine Dependency: No clearly identified effective pharmacotherapy, although desipramine has been moderately effective at influencing abstinence.

- Nicotine addiction: No effective treatment exists. Clonidine and alprazolam decease anxiety and irritability during withdrawal; mixed findings in clonidine's effectiveness for inducing abstinence. Nicotine-containing gum (Nicorette) is sometimes effective for cessation when used in conjunction with behavioral treatment, permitting smoker to regulate nicotine intake; dosage is one piece of gum to be chewed slowly when client experiences urge to smoke; dosage should not exceed 30 pieces (2 mg) or 20 pieces (4 mg) per day; 10 pieces per day is common during first month of use; should not be used longer than 6 months. Nicotine transdermal patch is a useful adjunct for treatment of nicotine withdrawal and for encouraging abstinence when used in conjunction with behavioral treatment; provides steady state of nicotine; dosage is based client's response, stage of withdrawal, specific brand/formulation of drug; drug is administered over an 8- to 10-week period with tapering of dosage at specified intervals. Contraindications for both gum and patch include recent myocardial infarction, increasing angina, pregnancy, and lactation. Gum is contraindicated in patients with tempromandibular joint disease (TMJ).

- Chronic Opioid Dependence: Methadone, an opioid agonist analgesic, is used to reduce opioid craving and illicit use and to prevent dependence on or abuse of other substances. Contraindications include hypersensitivity to opioids, bronchial asthma, chronic obstructive pulmonary disease, respiratory depression, and acute alcoholism. No optimal single dose exists for all clients; maintenance varies from low doses of 10 to 20 mg per day to more than 100 mg per day to block craving for opiates and associated drug use. Common adverse effects include lightheadedness, dizziness, sedation, nausea, vomiting; major adverse effects include respiratory depression, apnea, circulatory depression, respiratory arrest, shock, and cardiac arrest. Methadone is less effective if taken in conjunction with hydantoins, rifampin, urinary acidifiers; increased effects and risk for methadone toxicity if taken in conjunction with cimetidine or ranitidine. The decision to withdraw client from long-term maintenance is based upon successful treatment that results in client's progress toward a drug-free lifestyle, as well as personal and occupational adjustment and stability and the absence of other Substance Use Disorders or comorbid psychiatric disorder(s). Relapse rate increases with abrupt discharge from maintenance programs and voluntary termination by client; supportive treatment during detoxification and provision of after-care services increases potential for abstinence; clients with repeated relapse even with support benefit from option of voluntary lifetime maintenance on methadone. L-Alphacetylmethadol (LAAM), an opioid agonist, is used for same purposes as methadone; longer-acting preparation administered less frequently than methadone; suppresses withdrawal symptoms for 72 to 96 hours; usual dosage of 20 to 140 mg with an average dose of 60 mg; dosing can be three times per week. Criteria for withdrawal from maintenance are similar to those for methadone.

CLIENT EDUCATION: PHARMACOLOGIC
MANAGEMENT[*]

- Disulfiram: Client should not take medication until at
  least 12 hours after last alcohol use; reaction can occur
  up to 2 weeks after last disulfiram use; abstain from all
  forms of alcohol, including wine, liquor, vinegars, cough
  medication, aftershave lotions; emphasize importance of
  client's knowing that use of alcohol while taking disulfiram can cause a variety of unpleasant reactions, e.g.,
  vomiting, headache, breathing difficulty, and even death;
  teach recognition of medication side effects and to
  report unusual bleeding or bruising, yellowing of skin or
  eyes, chest pain, breathing difficulties, or use of alcohol
  in any form; periodic blood tests are necessary to monitor effects on liver; client should wear Medic Alert identification while taking medication.
- Naltrexone: Teach client to recognize side effects such as
  drowsiness, dizziness, blurred vision, and anxiety and to
  avoid driving or operating heavy equipment if these
  occur; client should report unusual bleeding or bruising,
  presence of dark or tarry stools, yellowing of eyes or skin,
  running nose, tearing, sweating, chills, joint or muscle
  pain; ensure that client is aware that because medication
  blocks effects of opioids, client should avoid opioid-con-
  taining preparations, e.g., cough medications with
  codeine or antidiarrheal preparations such as paregoric;
  emphasize that self-administration of large doses of
  heroin or other opioids may cause serious injury, coma,
  or death; periodic monitoring of liver function tests is necessary; client should wear Medic Alert tag.
- Nicotine gum: For maximum absorption, client must
  chew gum slowly and not let it sit between teeth; important for client to chew sufficient number of pieces per
  day and to use gum for adequate length of time to be
  effective; gum that has been chewed should be wrapped
  before being discarded to minimize accidental ingestion
  by children or pets; side effects include dizziness and
  lightheadedness as well as nausea and vomiting.
- Nicotine transdermal patch: New patch is applied every
  24 hours with 1-week interval before reapplication in
  previous site; wash hands thoroughly after application,

[*]References 7,32,47

avoiding contact to eyes; discontinue if client is unable to stop smoking after 4 weeks of application; safety precautions for discarding are same as for nicotine gum; side effects include dizziness, lightheadedness, GI problems (nausea, vomiting, constipation, diarrhea), and redness and swelling at site where patch is applied.

- Methadone: Client should avoid alcohol while taking drug. Teach management of side effects, e.g., nausea and lack of appetite may be minimized by taking drug with food, lying down, eating small frequent meals; use laxative for management of constipation; avoid tasks that require alertness (including driving) if dizziness, sedation, drowsiness, blurred vision occur; no one else should use prescription; problems such as severe nausea, vomiting, constipation, shortness of breath, or difficulty breathing should be reported at once.

Psychosocial Treatments[*]

- Develop an oral or written contract following end of initial evaluation or after detoxification; client and family are included in developing and agreeing to specific aspects of contract, which may include agreement on method for maintaining abstinence, therapy for comorbid psychiatric disorder(s) or medical conditions, family participation in educational aspects of treatment, beginning commitment to client's living in a drug- and alcohol-free environment by removing all abusable substances from house, avoiding known substance abusers and providers, and avoiding geographical locations where past Substance Abuse occurred. (See also Contracting in Chapter 5.)
- Cognitive behavior therapies focus on identification and modification of maladaptive thinking patterns so that client can decrease or eliminate negative feelings and behavior; includes self-control strategies for relapse prevention, e.g., goal setting, self monitoring, analyzing antecedents of substance use.
- Behavioral therapies include operant rewarding for treatment compliance or punishment for undesirable behaviors; contingency management is based on predetermined positive or negative consequences, e.g., notification of

[*]References 2,13,14,25,28,34,35,37,50,54,56,60,64

court or employer if client resumes Substance Abuse (this approach requires written permission from client).

- Individual psychodynamic/interpersonal psychotherapy, supportive-expressive therapy, and individual interpersonal therapy are more effective for clients who do not have comorbid antisocial personality disorder or high levels of sociopathy and for those who do not have cognitive deficits.

- Group therapy, e.g., modified psychodynamic, interpersonal, interactive, rational emotive, Gestalt, psychodrama, can be a supportive, therapeutic, and educational experience that can motivate clients and help them to successfully cope with life stresses and substance craving without the use of drugs or alcohol. Focus is on group confrontation of client's denial, dealing with interpersonal conflict or closeness, and experiencing painful emotions. Female clients with chemical dependence may benefit from a women-only treatment group. Group participation provides opportunity for therapist and members to recognize early warning signs of relapse so that they can take constructive action for members.

- Family therapy, with structural, strategic, psychodynamic, systems or behavioral approaches, is a modality that encourages family support for the client's abstinence and provides relevant information about his or her current attitudes toward substance use, treatment participation, and compliance; family therapy also contributes to maintaining marital relationships and improving treatment compliance and long-term outcome.

- Social Skills Training includes learning how to form and maintain constructive interpersonal relationships and refusing substance use. (See also Social Skills Training in Chapter 5.)

- Stress Management includes relaxation training. (See also Stress Management in Chapter 5.)

- Self-help groups and 12-step groups, e.g., Alcoholics Anonymous, Cocaine Anonymous, and Narcotics Anonymous for identified client and Al-Anon, Ala-Teen, and Nar-Anon for client's family and friends, are effective for many, although not always helpful to other clients; preferable to encourage but not require participation;

refusal to attend should not be equated with treatment resistance; focus is on group support with ongoing reminders of disastrous consequences if client reverts to alcohol or drug use; emphasis on benefits of abstinence and sobriety; mutual support and advice with personalized support of a recovering sponsor.

- Treatment for clients with dual diagnosis or comorbid psychiatric disorders requires an integrated approach that focuses on both the Substance Abuse or Dependence and the mental disorder. Treatment may be offered in a variety of settings, e.g., inpatient psychiatric units, chemical dependency units, mental health clinics, shelters for the homeless. Treatment modalities include any of the previously described.

▌ Commonly Occurring Nursing Diagnoses[*]

Adjustment, impaired
Anxiety
Confusion, acute
Confusion, chronic
Coping, ineffective individual
Denial, ineffective
Family Process, altered: alcoholism
Fear
Grieving, anticipatory
Grieving, dysfunctional
Hopelessness
Impaired environmental interpretation syndrome
Impaired memory
Impaired social interaction
Infection, risk for
Injury, risk for
Knowledge deficit
Loneliness, risk for
Noncompliance
Nutrition, alteration in: less than body requirements
Oral mucous membrane, altered
Pain, chronic
Parenting, altered
Poisoning, risk for

[*]References 9,16,19,20,33,35–37,45,46,52,61,62

Powerlessness
Self-care deficit
Self-esteem disturbance
Self-esteem chronic low
Self-esteem, situational low
Sensory/perceptual alterations (visual, auditory, tactile)
Sexual dysfunction
Sleep pattern disturbance
Social interaction, impaired
Social isolation
Spiritual distress
Thought processes, altered
Violence, risk for, self-directed or directed at others

▌ Selected Nursing Diagnoses, Outcome Criteria, and Nursing Interventions with Rationale

Client With Alcohol-Induced Disorder, Alcohol Withdrawal

NURSING DIAGNOSIS #1:* *Risk for injury related to Alcohol Withdrawal*

EXPECTED CLIENT OUTCOME

• The client will experience a decrease in symptoms indicative of Alcohol Withdrawal with no physical harm to self.

NURSING INTERVENTIONS WITH RATIONALE

• Provide a safe and monitored environment that has minimal external stimulation, "*to decrease possibility of agitation, anxiety, and belligerence caused by central nervous system (CNS) stimulation during withdrawal.*"[42,p.1307]
• Initiate close monitoring and necessary restrictions, e.g., side rails, based on individual assessment of client's safety needs; *close supervision is necessary because client who is intoxicated is likely to become disoriented, experience motor instability, and be impulsive.*
• Monitor for initial symptoms of Alcohol Withdrawal, e.g., vital signs, ability to perform "serial sevens" (see Chapter 3), anxiety, mild tremor, diaphoresis, headache, mild

---

*References 2,5,6,12,22,,42,44,46,51,58

hypertension, *recognizing that early or mild withdrawal can begin within 6 to 8 hours after client's last drink.*

- To the extent possible, obtain information from family, friends, records, and health care providers about client's alcohol history, e.g., last drink, past history of withdrawal, whether current intoxication is waxing or waning; *factors such as a history of previous withdrawal episodes and severity of Alcohol Dependence increase the risk and severity of client's withdrawal in the current situation.*
- Collaborate with health care providers in assessing for the possible presence of other substances in addition to alcohol, e.g., laboratory tests to detect presence of other drugs.
- Conduct mental status examination that includes assessment for presence of suicidal ideation, intent; *continued drinking is a risk factor for suicide in alcoholics.* Continue to monitor mental status and provide ongoing orientation and reality testing, based on findings.
- Monitor physical status, including vital signs, at scheduled intervals. *Alcohol Withdrawal increases the risk for temperature elevation and tachycardia. Temperature of 100°F or above and pulse rate over 100 beats per minute are indicators of delirium tremens.*
- Ensure adequate food and oral fluid intake *because of requirements for high caloric intake and risk for client being dehydrated;* monitor intake and output *to reduce possibility of overhydration or electrolyte imbalance.*
- Collaborate with health care provider in administration of medications (usually benzodiazepines) to reduce agitation and to prevent seizures, recognizing that dosages may be higher than for nonalcoholic client; *do not undermedicate because early intervention reduces the severity of the withdrawal syndrome; inadequate treatment of withdrawal may increase potential for future withdrawal of increased severity; it is important, however, not to overmedicate the elderly client.*
- Collaborate with health care provider in administration of additional pharmacologic measures *to prevent development of Wernicke-Korsakoff syndrome (IM thiamine immediately and other B vitamin supplements) or magnesium for electrolyte replacement to reduce risk for seizures.*

- Notify appropriate health care provider(s) when with-drawal symptoms are out of specified parameters *to ensure appropriate management for reducing risk for additional complications, e.g., seizures, delirium tremens, and death.*
- Ensure that client has quiet night-time environment *to promote relaxation and sleep*; use night light *to minimize misinterpretation and distortions of environmental stimuli.*

For Family of Client With Alcohol Use Disorder, Alcohol Dependence or Alcohol Abuse or Alcohol-Induced Disorder, Alcohol Withdrawal

NURSING DIAGNOSIS #2:* *Altered family processes, alcoholism, related to family history of alcoholism, resistance to treatment, lack of problem-solving skills*

EXPECTED FAMILY OUTCOME

- The family will acknowledge recognition of effects of alcoholism on family unit, will participate in alcohol treatment, and will engage in constructive problem-solving resolution.

NURSING INTERVENTIONS WITH RATIONALE

- Encourage members to verbalize their recognition of effects of alcohol on individual members, e.g., husband–wife, parent–child, and family as a unit *because of common pattern of family unwillingness to acknowledge that a problem with alcohol exists.*
- Determine individual members' knowledge about client's alcoholism.
- Encourage description of specific areas of need for emotional and/or social support, e.g., ability to trust, need for and fear of intimacy, need for sense of internal locus of control *(common characteristics in substance-abusing families)*, and help family begin to resolve some of these problem areas *to improve their relationships with one another and to develop realistic expectations of one another.*
- Observe for behaviors indicative of detrimental denial in individual family members or in family as a unit, e.g., fabrication of information, attempts to manipulate others

*References 9,19,26,29,33,36,40–42,46,54,57,61–63

into empathizing with stories of what was done to individual.

- Confront individual member and/or family when denial is evident, e.g., redirect the focus to "What was your role in allowing this to happen?" *to increase family member's objective recognition of reality.*
- Provide family with educational information about alcoholism, e.g., it is a disease that, if not treated, results in severe physical, psychological, and social consequences.
- Observe for presence of enabling or co-dependent behaviors, e.g., spouse or child feeling guilty when client experiences problems, individual member(s) accepting responsibility for maintaining smooth relationships in family, feeling powerless to change own life. *Recognize cultural variations in this area to avoid "imposing unfamiliar values on clients and their families..."*[29,p.247] *For example, one integral Hispanic cultural norm for family membership is "[p]rotecting other family members, advising them, and assuming responsibility for them..."*[29,p.251]
- Determine family's willingness to engage in treatment, e.g., family therapy; inquire about past treatment experiences, what helped, what did not help, *to capitalize on family motivation and to minimize treatment resistance.*
- Evaluate need for referral to family therapist or alcoholism counselor.
- Provide additional appropriate referrals to self-help groups, e.g., Al-Anon for spouse, Ala-Teen for children, ACOA (Adult Children of Alcoholics); *participation in these groups provides opportunity for family members to obtain support from others in similar situations, to examine their role in "enabling" behaviors, to share constructive coping strategies, and to learn to accept responsibility only for their own behavior.*
- Assist family in problem-solving activities by helping them to recognize that sobriety does not necessarily result in disappearance of pre-existing or current stressors and that achievement of sobriety will likely affect familiar established roles and behavioral patterns of individual members.
- Provide information about medical, social, and child care services *to maximize opportunity for client and family to participate in appropriate treatment regimen.*

- Based on assessment of factors such as ongoing family conflicts, employment status, and financial difficulties, provide referrals to additional resources, e.g., marriage counselors, career counselors, financial planners *to assist with achievement of life-planning goals.*
- Help family to recognize that client's recovery from alcoholism is a continuous process *so that they will not underestimate the potential threat of relapse for the client and so that they and the client will continue to engage in appropriate maintenance programs or after-care to ensure continuation of recovery.*

Client Unable to Cope With Anxiety Related to Drug Use

NURSING DIAGNOSIS #3:[*]   *Ineffective coping related to substance use (drugs) for coping with anxiety and stressors*

EXPECTED CLIENT OUTCOME

- The client will participate in Substance Abuse/Dependence treatment and will develop adaptive coping strategies and constructive behaviors for coping with anxiety and stressors.

NURSING INTERVENTIONS WITH RATIONALE

- Assess client's motivation for seeking treatment to change behaviors.
- Collaborate with mental health team and client to determine appropriate treatment setting.
- Establish and maintain a therapeutic alliance with the client; *this is a significant predictor of successful outcome, e.g., less drug use and better psychological functioning during follow-up.*
- Suggest that client keep a drug diary *to obtain a clearer picture of precipitant and how it connects to client's responses to anxiety and stressors*; emphasize importance of abstaining from drug use; however, if client is unsuccessful in abstinence, he or she should still record drug use.
- Assist client in recognizing current health coping strategies *that can be used to reinforce strengths for drug abstinence.*

[*]References 2,9,13,17,27,33,40,42,49,52,54,57

- Evaluate the need for client to participate in assertiveness training or social skills training *to strengthen self-esteem and to increase client's sense of control in anxiety- and stress-producing situations, e.g., social and/or work.* (See also Assertiveness Training and Social Skills Training in Chapter 5.)
- Ensure that client's discharge plan devotes time for him or her to focus on anticipation of post-discharge stressors *so that client can begin to develop and practice strategies for managing without resorting to use of drugs.*
- Encourage client to develop alternative strategies for coping with anxiety that do not involve the use of drugs, e.g., relaxation techniques, recreational activity, and exercise. (See also Stress Management in Chapter 5.)
- Use role-playing in individual or small group setting *to prepare client for dealing with potential pressures to resume drug use.* Emphasize importance of avoiding situations in which drugs are available.
- Help client to develop plans for management of non–drug-related activities *to reduce potential feelings of emptiness and anxiety related to free time.*
- Evaluate need for referral for psychotherapy, Narcotics Anonymous, or therapeutic communities. *For example, professional psychotherapy has been found to be more effective than drug counseling alone. Narcotics Anonymous provides group support and ongoing reminders of negative consequences of drug use as well as benefits of abstinence. Therapeutic communities provide a drug-free environment for peer confrontation, with an emphasis on client's assuming personal responsibility for drug abstinence.*
- Teach client to be aware that long-term treatment for drug abuse and dependence lasts a lifetime. *Client will always be at risk for relapse; therefore, total, long-term abstinence is essential.*

Client With Nicotine Use Disorder, Nicotine Dependence

NURSING DIAGNOSIS #4:* *Impaired adjustment, related to disability requiring a change in life style; 45-year-old male with second MI and history of inability to stop smoking*

*References 7,23,24,46,47,52

EXPECTED CLIENT OUTCOME

- The client will involve himself in goal setting for plans to stop smoking and will demonstrate self-care practices that are within his prescribed cardiac regimen.

NURSING INTERVENTIONS WITH RATIONALE

- Encourage client to discuss thoughts and feelings associated with recurrence of cardiac problems and perception of ability to modify changes in lifestyle, including smoking cessation.
- Assess for presence of depression; *there is a link between smoking and depression.*
- Obtain a smoking history that examines client's past attempts to quit, resources that helped, factors that hindered, and factors that client believes contributed to inability to quit or to relapse.
- Encourage client to reframe past periods of smoking cessation as successes and not failures *to increase client's self-confidence.*
- Assess client's desire and motivation to stop smoking through use of behavioral self-monitoring: client prepares for monitoring by wrapping a piece of paper around cigarette pack for recording specific information each time a cigarette is smoked, e.g., time, place, mood, and thoughts; pattern can be graphed after first week, giving nurse and client a better understanding of behaviors, thoughts, and environmental factors that influenced client's smoking.[47] *This approach also engages the client as an active participant in treatment for Nicotine Dependence and can assist him in cutting back on cigarettes, especially automatic smoking.*
- Encourage discussion of smoking cessation with focus on *benefits* of stopping smoking, e.g., longer life expectancy, decreased risk for further cardiac problems, instead of emphasizing potential serious consequences.
- Provide client with information about health risks associated with smoking. *It is important to present this information in a way that does not unnecessarily frighten the client and cause increased denial or resistance; a high rate of success in helping clients stop smoking has been experienced with the skillful presentation of health risks.*

- Assist client to examine alternatives, e.g., making no immediate changes in cigarette use, reducing the number of cigarettes smoked, or quitting entirely.
- Inform client of available resources for smoking cessation, e.g., nicotine gum and transdermal patch, relaxation training, group treatment, hypnosis, acupuncture.
- Encourage client's use of problem-focused strategies for smoking cessation *to increase perception of self-control and to maximize psychosocial coping with post-MI adjustment and smoking cessation.* Examples of stop-smoking strategies include: determining a specific day for stopping smoking after tapering to 5 to 10 cigarettes per day *to minimize "cold turkey," withdrawal distress;* using chewing gum or chewy candy to manage potential craving for cigarettes; avoiding situations that trigger desire to smoke, including social contacts with smokers; monitoring caffeine intake if feeling anxious, and avoiding or decreasing caffeine during these times; avoiding usual cues to smoke, e.g., cup of coffee after breakfast; and developing incompatible alternative behaviors when feeling urge to smoke, e.g., low-calorie snacking.[47,52]
- Promote development of a behavioral contract that specifies mutually agreed-upon plan, process, and strategies for smoking cessation. (See also Contracting in Chapter 5.)
- Use cognitive restructuring, e.g., learning to direct thoughts to other choices that do not result in smoking, visualizing unpleasant aspects of smoking, visualizing benefits from smoking cessation, diverting focus from smoking to pleasant, enjoyable thoughts (e.g., favorite fishing hole, favorite vacation spot), *to help client reduce positive associations with smoking.*
- Help client to develop an overall plan for stress management *to reduce feelings of anxiety that may be associated with smoking cessation and other lifestyle changes for management of recovery from MI.* (See also Stress Management in Chapter 5.)
- Encourage client to plan rewards, e.g., dinner with friends, weekend outing, for progress in modifying lifestyle *to maintain motivation.*
- Encourage client to use family, friends, and coworkers *for social support to strengthen commitment to improved lifestyle.*

- Collaborate with client in the development of an individualized health care regimen that can be incorporated in the work setting as well as at home; have client identify possible factors that could interfere with following this regimen and to identify and practice responses he or she can use to avoid pitfalls. *Coping rehearsal helps client prepare for alternatives to reduce risk for relapse and resuming "old behaviors" that are incompatible with current goals.*
- Help client to evaluate extent to which his or her choice of health care practices influences recovery from MI and ability to engage in a maximally independent and constructive lifestyle.

CHAPTER 9

Schizophrenia and Other Psychotic Disorders

▌ Definition/Major Symptoms*

Schizophrenia and Other Psychotic Disorders are a group of mental disorders with marked impairment in thinking, perception of reality, and emotions affecting motor behavior and the ability to choose, act, and relate to others.

Behavior or symptoms may be labeled "psychotic" because of their seriousness, severity, and impact on the total functioning of the person.

Psychotic symptoms are generally considered to be hallucinations, delusions, disorganized speech, disorganized behavior, and negative symptoms.

1. Thought form dysfunction in which the client's thoughts can be described by the following:

   Derailment or loose association: when the relationship between one idea and the next is lost or only obliquely related, or when two ideas are expressed that are completely unrelated

   Tangentiality: when the main idea of the discussion is lost

   Circumstantiality: when an unnecessary amount of detail or a lengthy explanation is added so that the main idea is almost lost

   Incoherence: when speech cannot be understood

*References 2,10,12,27,28,46,58,59,66,70

Neologisms: when new words are created

Clanging: when rhyming speech is used

Concreteness: when there is a literal focus on content with an inability to abstract or generalize

Alogia: when there is a poverty of speech, that is, speech provides little information, or there is poverty of speech content, that is, speaking only a few words

2. Thought content dysfunction in which the client's thoughts can be described by the following:

Delusions: false beliefs that are not altered by reason; they are incongruent with the person's education, social class, and culture. The classic delusion is of passivity, i.e., being controlled by an outside force. There are delusions of persecution, influence, reference, thought broadcasting, thought insertion, and guilt. Delusions can be described as grandiose, somatic, sexual, and religious.

It is important for the clinician to determine if the "delusion" reflects the client's view of situation or describes the client's belief in the reality of the situation. The "delusion" may be an attempt to communicate how a situation is understood and not its actual existence.

3. Perceptual dysfunction in which the client's perceptions can be described by the following:

Hallucination: an experience of sensory perception without a stimuli.

Auditory hallucinations: the most common type. They may be a first sign of schizophrenia; some persons never hear voices or it happens once, or the voices are always present. Comments about the environment, obscure remarks, or threats may be heard as coming from outside or inside one's head; most of them are derogatory or threatening.

A command hallucination may cause the client to engage in violent acts.

Visual hallucinations are rare and described as light, spots, different colors, or shadings, or they may be small human figure(s) or animals; they may be due to general medical conditions, alcohol or drug use.

Olfactory hallucinations are rare and generally associated with seizure disorders.

4. Emotional dysfunction: Emotional states that are varied and may change from ones of intense expression to ones of unresponsiveness

   Affect: The expression of feeling may be described as *flat or blunted* when the client is expressionless or seemingly unresponsive or less responsive than is generally expected. At times affect may be *inappropriate* because it is not related to the content the client is expressing. Affect may also be described as *labile* when there is a frequent changing of the person's emotional state with little or no apparent cause.

   Mood: The expression of the state of mind and other emotions being experienced. Common moods expressed are anxiousness, agitation (increased motor activity and anxiety), depression, ambivalence, hostility, etc. Anhedonia is the lack of the ability to experience pleasure or find any interest in life.

5. Behavioral dysfunction: Behaviors that range from involuntary motor movements to complex behaviors involving some degree of volition.

   Involuntary movement disorders: include posturing, mannerisms, rocking, tapping, etc.; they are repetitive.

   Waxy flexibility: where a limb may remain in position in which it is placed.

   Negativism: a more complex behavior involving the client's thought processes. It occurs when a client is asked do one thing and the response is the exact opposite. The client may become increasingly disorganized in appearance and behavior, aggressive, ritualistic, or sexually aggressive. These extremes of behavioral dysfunction may be noted in catatonic stupor or excitement.

   Lack of clue recognition: when a client has problems with abstract tasks such as recognizing cues from another regarding appropriate behavior. When interpersonal cues are missed, the interaction is based solely on concrete facts. For example: There is a cookie; the client sees it. "I want it"; the client takes and eats it. There is no thought or abstraction that it is Mary's and she is planning to eat it later.

   Information processing problems: when a client has difficulty processing information to solve a problem. This also occurs when memory is not effectively avail-

able for problem resolution, such as when events in the morning are not recalled as relevant to what should be done now.
6. Positive and negative symptoms:

Organizing the multiple symptoms of schizophrenia into two groups has aided treatment and research.

Positive symptoms: hallucinations, delusions, bizarre behaviors, e.g., assaultiveness, self-mutualization, suspiciousness, etc.

Negative symptoms: Avoliton (lack of will to do), anhedonia (problems in experiencing pleasure), distractibility or selective inattention, problems in decision making, psychomotor slowness.

▌ Definition/Selected Major Categories*

Schizophrenia

Schizophrenia consists of a group of five subtypes of clinically described symptoms of severely disordered thinking, e.g., hallucinations, delusions, confusion, disorientation, and bizarre behaviors that are accompanied by social or occupational dysfunction. In each instance two or more of the following symptoms are present: psychomotor immobility or stupor; excessive psychomotor activity; extreme negativism or resistance to all instructions or mutism; posturing, grimacing, or repetitive stereotypic behavior; and echolalia or echopraxia. Symptoms are present for 6 months; the active phase lasts for 1 month. Symptoms do not arise from mood disorders, substance intoxication, or a general medical condition.

1. *Catatonic Type*: characterized predominantly by psychomotor disturbances. Positive and negative symptoms are also present. The client's behavior may be described as rigid (does not move even when requested to do so), mute (does not speak), or posturing (assumes various bizarre postures). The client may become overly active or stuporous, posing a danger to self or others. Waxy flexibility may be exhibited. The client may repeat words or phrases (echolalia) or movements (echopraxia) of others

*References 2,10,12,28,30,31,46,59,66

2. *Disorganized Type* (formerly hebephrenic schizophrenia): characterized predominantly by disorganization of speech, behavior; affect is flat or inappropriate. Behavior is described as extremely silly, laughing inappropriately, speaking incoherently, making grimaces, having peculiar mannerisms.

3. *Paranoid Type*: characterized predominantly by delusions or hallucinations; disorganized speech, odd affect, or psychomotor disturbance are less prominent. The client's delusions are frequently paranoid (being persecuted, e.g., the FBI wants him; a neighbor follows him in his car; the food is poisoned). Behavior is generally appropriate. He may or may not act on the delusions.

4. *Undifferentiated Type*: characterized by not meeting criteria for other subtypes. The client exhibits more general symptoms of schizophrenia such as hallucinosis with social or occupational decline. It is the most common subtype.

5. *Residual Type*: characterized predominantly by symptoms of residual phase. The client is withdrawn; affect is flat; communication is limited; behavior is peculiar; thinking is illogical.

Schizophreniform Disorder

Schizophreniform Disorder is characterized by positive and negative symptoms lasting between 1 month and 6 months. The client experiences hallucinations, delusions, disorganized speech, bizarre behavior, and some negative symptoms. The client may or may not be socially or occupationally impaired.

Brief Psychotic Disorder

Brief Psychotic Disorder is characterized by symptoms of an acute or psychotic state lasting between 1 day and 1 month. The client and family have little or no clue that the person is becoming ill. A particular stressor may trigger the episode, such as the birth of a child, losing a loved one, or combat activity. The symptoms are acute and severe; there is a risk of suicide.

Delusional Disorder (also known as Paraphrenia or Paranoid Delusional Disorder):

Delusional Disorder is characterized by having a *non-bizarre* delusion lasting 1 month. The client does not experience hallucinations and is not described as behaving inappropriately. Although the behavior may not be understood, it may be noted as peculiar in some aspect by family and friends. The client's ability to work may not be affected, if the work does not involve the use of many social skills.

Delusional Disorder subtypes are characterized by the content of the delusion as described below:

Erotomania Type is the belief that client is loved by a particular person. This may lead to stalking.

Grandiose Type is the belief that one is exceptionally important, talented, and has a special message to give to the world.

Jealous Type is the belief that a spouse or significant other is unfaithful.

Persecutor Type is the client's belief that someone is after the client, wishes the client harm, or is harassing the client. This belief can lead to violence. It is the most common subtype.

Somatic Type is the belief that a body part is not functioning correctly, e.g., a virus has invaded the body or a sensation is present, e.g., crawling bugs, smelling odor on skin.

Mixed Type is a belief that is not clearly any of the above.

Schizoaffective Disorder

Schizoaffective Disorder is characterized by periods of acute schizophrenic symptoms combined with periods of depression, mania, or a mixture of both. It is reserved for cases in which neither schizophrenia nor Psychotic Mood Disorder can be excluded. Diagnosis is difficult.

Schizoaffective Disorder subtypes are characterized by mood types as described below:

Depressive: symptoms of sadness, hopelessness, loss of interest in all activities of daily life, lack of motivation.

Bipolar: symptoms of elevated mood, speech pressure, distractibility, flight of ideas, decreased sleep pattern.

Shared Psychotic Disorder (Folie a Deux)

Shared Psychotic Disorder is characterized by a shared delusion system of two persons. The client, frequently a woman, experiences the delusional belief of another (spouse) who may have a psychotic disorder. It is uncommon.

▊ Incidence*

- Schizophrenia occurs in approximately 0.85% of the world's population. It is reported at a lower rate in some countries, possibly due to greater tolerance of unusual behavior in some cultures. As diagnostic criteria are refined and methods of case finding are improved, the effect of culture on incidence may diminish and a more accurate incidence will be known.
- Schizophrenia ccurs in 1.1% of the population (1-year prevalence rate) or 0.7% (l-month prevalence rate) in the U.S.
- Schizophreniform Disorder is the most common type, 0.1%.

▊ Course†

A. Early signs
   1. Problems in high risk children are:
      a. poor attention and/or concentration, e.g., problems in arithmetic, listening to teacher
      b. poor motor function and perceptual motor integration, e.g., problems with balance, participating in games
      c. social adaption and self-esteem problems, e.g., withdrawal from activities, getting into fights.
   2. Problems found in adolescence are:
      a. blocking or cutting off conversation, not responding as usual to friends, appearing aloof
      b. expressing various concerns regarding body symptoms, e.g., back pain, digestive symptoms
      c. forgetting and abandoning life goals
      d. disregarding social customs and talking incessantly about abstract ideas such as love, creation, equality.

*References 2,6,15,25,30,31,66
†References 1,17,22,25,30,31,32,48

B. Acute or psychotic state

The first acute episode generally occurs in adolescence. It may be precipitated by a loss, separation, or rejection; by use of street drugs or alcohol; or by other major stressful events such as going away to college, recovery from a virus, or hormonal changes. It may initially be noted in contacts with police or emergency rooms for various reasons; schizophrenia is often confused with drug intoxication. Positive symptoms of hallucinations, delusions, and bizarre behaviors are present in the acute state. These may last a week until moderated by medication and then slowly lessen.

C. Residual or remission phase

Some clients experience the disorder as a continuous psychotic process, whereas others experience an episode or periodic episodes of the disorder throughout their lives. Deterioration does not occur over the life span. Recent studies demonstrate that it is limited to the first 2 years or the first two episodes. Intensity of symptoms also decreases with increasing age. Some symptoms, e.g., anhedonia, avolution, remain throughout one's life. The client may continue to have odd beliefs, speak vaguely or very concretely, act in peculiar ways, and remain severely withdrawn.

D. Exacerbations and relapses

Indications of a recurrence include problems in sleeping, increasing restlessness, lack of appetite, lack of pleasure in anything, depression, and problems in concentration. Relapse is frequently related to failure to take prescribed antipsychotic medications "because of the side effects." Another reason is the extreme sensitivity of the client to stress, which may take the form of ordinary life events (missing an appointment, spilling coffee all over a desk), high expectations of others, subtle expressions of criticism, disagreements, or overinvolvement of others.

E. Prognosis

Schizophrenia is a chronic, disabling disorder. Less than 50% of clients experience improvement after 6 years. Only 20% to 30% of schizophrenics are able to live minimally sheltered lives.

Predictors for good outcome are the presence of insight, which promotes treatment compliance, achievement of some academic and occupational skills that increase the person's ability to meet basic needs, and an acute onset of positive symptoms (how their influence promotes good outcomes is not understood).

▌ Contributing Factors*

- Etiology is unknown.
- Research data point toward Schizophrenia being a neurodevelopmental disorder.
  - Genetic studies of twins, adoptees, and close relatives indicate that there is an alteration in genes. Maternal viral infections, especially in the second trimester, have been suggested as a cause because of their affect on the development of the brain, e.g., the hippocampus, temporal lobe, and interconnections to frontal lobe; this is controversial.
  - Schizophrenia may be related to the influenza virus and to extreme food restrictions because of their impact on the developing brain and nervous system. Other possible factors include lack of oxygen during gestation and birth complications that affect the nervous system.
  - Myelination and continuing maturation of the nerve cells in frontal lobes is not completed until after adolescence. This may be a factor in the onset of Schizophrenia during puberty and adolescence. It also contributes to the vulnerability of the client to stress, the effect of neuroleptic medications on positive versus negative symptoms, and the varied symptoms and course of the illness.
- Theories being researched include:
  - Genetic: Postulates that an alteration in a gene(s) causes Schizophrenia. Strong support exists.
  - Neuroimmunovirology: Postulates the existence of a defect—genetic, environmental, or immunologic—that prevents responding to, detecting, and/or taking action against a virus. There is some evidence to suggest that a viral infection in the second trimester affects the brain of the fetus.

*References 6,7,15,30,31,47,58,59,61,66,71

○ Birth and pregnancy complications: Postulates that a defective gene affects fetal development and the birth process itself, causing immature, abnormal development or injury of the nervous system; that defects can be caused by the influenza virus and/or by extreme restriction of foods; and that defects can be caused by birth complications resulting from a decreased oxygen supply.

○ Structural and functional abnormalities: Postulates that abnormalities in the nervous system that affect function produce symptoms of Schizophrenia. A few examples are (1) lateral ventricular enlargement, wider third ventricle, and sulcus enlargement in cortex; (2) developmental abnormalities as revealed by brain tissue examination; (3) decreased blood flow and glucose supply to frontal lobes; and (4) frontal cortex is not activated when completing some cognitive tests involving problem solving.

○ Pathophysiology: There is some evidence supporting the theory that there is a dysfunction in biochemical processes in the neural network as the electrical impulse passes through the neuron and across synapses; there is excessive dopamine activity as noted in studies of antipsychotic medication.

• Sex: No difference.

• Age: Usually occurs in adolescence but may occur at any age. Males 15 to 25 years old and females 25 to 35 years old. Severity of symptoms decreases with age.

• Culture: Occurs in industrialized countries where poverty is a major factor related to poor maternal nutrition and prenatal care, increased complication in pregnancy and delivery, and decreased rates of perinatal survival. Poor hygiene also increases exposure to infectious agents.

• Socioeconomic class: Occurs more frequently in the lower class. Explanations offered are (1) that the environment increases exposure to infectious agents, job-related accidents, poor maternal–child care, etc., with results on increased stress levels and fetal injuries; (2) that the symptoms of Schizophrenia prevent a client from getting a better job and moving upward; and (3) that the disorder begins in adolescence when education is still being pursued; social and work skills are not fully developed.

Level of tolerance of bizarre behaviors, the point at which an illness is defined, when help is sought, the response to medication as treatment, and the level of support of family and community are all influenced by culture and class.

- Marital status: Only 25% of first admissions to a hospital are married.
- Family: In families with a schizophrenic member, problems in communication have been reported. Interactions with client by the central family figure are described as being overinvolved, hostile, and critical (a negative affective relationship).

▌ Laboratory and Physical Examination Findings*

- Laboratory screening is done to differentiate mental illness from other associated medical conditions (e.g., alcohol intoxication, diabetes), using CBC (complete blood count), electrolytes, blood chemistry, urinalysis, and blood and urine levels of medications and of drugs of abuse.
- Physical examination may reveal soft neurological signs, e.g., poor coordination in movements, mixed response when asked to move to the right or left or move the arms or legs. Persons who are vulnerable to Schizophrenia have problems in smoothly following a moving object with their eyes.
- Diagnostic techniques (e.g., skull series) are used to rule out brain tumors, structural changes, trauma to central nervous system, seizure problems.

▌ Special Assessment Considerations†

- Ruling out the presence of other medical conditions by utilizing various techniques is important because presenting symptoms are similar. It is the first step in the diagnostic process and particularly so in the adult client with no history of previous mental disorder. Psychotic states are associated with many medical conditions

*References 31,33,66
†References 3,13,14,15,29,33,34,40,60,67,69,76

(e.g., cancer, cerebrovascular disease, endocrine disorders, viral illnesses) and with medications (e.g., barbiturates, corticosteroids) or street drugs (e.g., cocaine, amphetamines, PCP). Confirmation of the diagnosis occurs over a period of time—6 months or more. Interpretation of findings is based on careful observation and data collection; this is a difficult process for the client and the family.

- When the client is of a different ethnic group or culture, the assessment of his or her understanding, health beliefs, stigmas frequently associated with psychological problems, presence of guilt and shame, ways in which help/treatment are accepted, and the importance of relationships in family and community need to be carefully considered. Hispanic schizophrenic clients have been reported to require lower neuroleptic dosages; family involvement affected the outcome of disorder.[15] A Hasidic Jewish client may respond to a more medically oriented unit and fewer demands for socialization.[67]

- The perception of Schizophrenia by client, family, and clinician affects the whole assessment and treatment process. The person experiencing Schizophrenia feels pain and a deep sense of loss over a disrupted future, work that might have been done, intimate relationships with loved ones that might have developed, and even the lost ability to express this pain to another. The client is stigmatized even today when the diagnosis is mental illness. The client, family members, and even clinicians have a particular problem in understanding the impact of negative symptoms (e.g., alogia, ambivalence, social isolation) on everyday activities. Only recently have family members had the opportunity to experience the support of mental health systems to cope with severely and persistently ill family members. In the past they were blamed and not always included in the treatment process.

- Thirty to sixty percent of clients on antipsychotic medication report problems in sexual functioning. This may lead to discontinuance of the medication.

- Suicide risk is greatest within 6 years of the first hospitalization. Besides being depressed about the symptoms of Schizophrenia and its consequences, the client may also experience the dampening effects of neuroleptic medications on the dopamine reinforcement and reward systems; therefore he actually feels less pleasure.

- Schizophrenics are prone to substance abuse because they do not have a high motivation to quit; their psychotic symptoms reoccur; they have cognitive impairment; they have decreasing or no social support. The mental health and public health systems may not offer integrated substance abuse programs and psychiatric programs, making treatment coordination difficult.
- PIP (psychosis, intermittent hyponatremia, polydipsia) syndrome is reported mostly in inpatient settings. An increase in intake of water and other fluids is noted first. Symptoms include excessive thirst, constantly seeking fluids, 5% weight gain during the day, increasing psychotic symptoms as the day progresses, decrease in Na serum level, and decrease of urinary specific gravity. Coma and death can occur; other medical complications may develop, e.g., urinary and/or renal dysfunctions, gastric/bowel problems, congestive heart failure. Treatment involves antipsychotic and anxiolytic drug management, supportive measures, restriction of fluid access, behavioral interventions, and teaching client self-monitoring.

▌Treatment*

Only 64.3% of persons with Schizophrenia receive treatment.

Biological/Psychopharmacological Interventions

These focus on controlling the symptoms of the illness through the use of antipsychotic drugs to regulate neurotransmittors and the central nervous system. Thus far no effective drug treatment is available for the negative symptoms (see Chapter 4).

- Involvement of the client and family in the medication regimen is critical.
- Administration of antipsychotics to manage symptoms in acute and maintenance states.

*References 4,5,11,13,16,18,20,21,25,26,27,31,32,36,41,42,50,53,54,55,56,59, 62,63,64,66,67,72,73,74,78

- ○ An acute state may require chlorpromazine 400 to 600 mg (Thorazine) or its equivalent, e.g., medicating violent clients with haloperidol (Haldol) and lorozepan (Ativan). Management of insomnia, psychomotor restlessness, and aggression is achieved in 1 to 2 weeks. Depression, anxiety, and discomfort in social situation are then lessened. Hallucinations, delusions, and other disorders of thinking are the last to abate, usually in 6 to 8 weeks.
  - ○ The lowest dose possible is used for maintenance and to prevent a relapse.
- • Management of side effects of antipsychotic medication is necessary to increase client comfort and enhance treatment compliance. The side effects are described below. (See Chapter 4 for a thorough discussion of treatment.)
  - ○ Common effects—drowsiness and sedation, orthostatic hypotension, anticholinergic effects of dry mouth, blurred vision, bowel and urinary problems
  - ○ Extrapyramidal symptoms—oculogyric crisis, torticollis, opisthotonus, akathiasis, parkinsonism
  - ○ Tardive dyskinesia
  - ○ Metabolic and endocrine (including sexual dysfunction), dermatological, and ophthalmic effects
  - ○ Increased risk for seizures
  - ○ *Life-threatening* side effects (see Chapter 4):
    - Lethal or malignant catatonia
    - Hyperpyrexia
    - Neuromalignant syndrome (NMS)
    - Overdose
    - Agranulocytosis

Behavioral Interventions

Interventions focus on resolving psychotic dysfunctions that are perceived of as behavioral excesses (hallucinations), behavioral deficits (poor grooming skills), and failure of behavior to fit social situation.

There must be a careful analysis of situations to determine what stimuli precede and follow behaviors, to identify behaviors needing alteration, and to teach needed skills.

SOCIAL SKILLS TRAINING

This training focuses on developing social skills by providing specific structured training that uses demonstrations, role modeling, repetition, and positive reinforcement of behavior. With this training improvements in clients has been reported; relapse rates have been reduced. The training provided to schizophrenic clients includes:

• Development of communication skills, e.g., how to carry on conversation, greet others, express thanks, ask for help, and talk about weather or news events.
• Development of assertiveness skills, e.g., how to say no without being confrontive or argumentative, express one's own views without putting down another, continue to seek help, recognize and deal with aggressiveness, and "fight for rights" in appropriate ways.
• Development of relationships with opposite sex, e.g., how to develop friends; what are reasonable expectations of friendships; how to develop boy/girl friend relationships; what are the responsibilities in love, sex and marriage; and how to handle kissing, petting, and sexual feelings/expressions.
• Development of medication management skills, e.g., what are the benefits of taking medication, how to take the medication, what are the side effects, how to manage and report them, and how to talk with a physician about medicines.
• Development of stress management skills, e.g., how to identify stressful situations, how to deal with these situations, how to relax alone or with others, and how to know when one is not managing the stress.
• Development of skills to manage psychotic symptoms, e.g., distraction, self talk, humming, listening to soothing music, participating in some type of physical activity, identifying prodromal cues, and avoiding alcohol and street drugs.

Cognitive Interventions

These interventions focus on improving the deficits in information processing, memory, attention, and problem solving. The process utilizes four steps in teaching clients how to manage the problems of daily living:

1. identify the problem
2. brainstorm for solutions
3. select an action plan
4. act on plan and report results.

The application of cognitive training to everyday functions of the client living in the community has been found to be minimal. More specific techniques focusing on memory or concept formation are being studied.

Interpersonal/Familial Intervention

Family systems–oriented therapy focuses on the function and structure of family organization, as well as the coalitions in the family. It seeks to change the behaviors occurring among the family members. Strategic family therapy focuses on achieving change within the family through the therapist's use of directives and paradoxical interventions. The Bowen family systems theory focuses on the emotional system in the multi-generational family system and seeks to increase the differentiation of the self in the system. Research supports the use of family therapy but provides no clear understanding of why it is effective.

Personal Therapy (PT)

A useful comprehensive approach is described by Hogarty and coworkers.[26] It encompasses social skills, cognitive training, family education, and psychotherapeutic techniques in stages over a 3-year period; medication is inherent also in the program.

Hospitalization

Brief periods of hospitalization assist with evaluation and treatment, with monitoring the effects of drugs or other therapies, with designing strategies for deviant behaviors, and with problems of danger to self or others. Discharge planning to maintain continuity of treatment in the community is important because of the chronic nature of the disorder.

Longer hospitalizations assist in the rehabilitation of clients with complicating medical problems, personality disorders, and/or family and environmental problems. Specific programs designed for the clients who are dually diagnosed (mental disorder and alcohol/drug abuse/dependency; who are elderly; who are children; who need to develop work skills or basic skills for daily living) are available.

Outpatient Treatment Setting

This focuses on comprehensive long-term treatment providing medication monitoring, social/vocational skill development, and crisis intervention to prevent relapses. Treatment planning and interventions need to reflect the stages of life and changing health needs of the client. Currently, the case management model provides the continuity of care so needed by the client. One clinician has the responsibility for coordinating the care provided by several clinicians and/or agencies. Outpatient services in a public or nonprofit center provide the majority of the care given to clients with Schizophrenia.

Community Programs

Halfway houses, group homes, independent living settings, crisis beds, and homeless shelters provide various degrees of supervision of activities of daily living. Programs offering around-the-clock services, intensive case management with a team approach, and assertive outreach ability are designed for clients who are more difficult to maintain in a community setting. One model is the PACT, Program for Assertive Community Treatment.

Failure to follow treatment regimen or attempts to manage symptoms alone can result in a relapse.

The following problems may occur:

- Violence toward others or property: individuals may be hospitalized against their will or jailed. It is to be noted that there is a high prevalence of chronic mental illness in jails and prisons.

- Homelessness and/or problems related to maintaining shelter: between 33% to 50% of the homeless are considered to have a severe and persistent mental illness.
- Development of medical conditions: malnourishment, infections from poor hygiene, exposure to excessive cold/heat, substance abuse, AIDS
- Inappropriate sexual behaviors and exposure to HIV
- Loss of job, unemployment, frequent job change
- Decreased social support system, lack of friends, alienation from family, loneliness
- Frequent visits to emergency rooms

▌ Commonly Occurring Nursing Diagnoses

Coping, ineffective individual
Family processes, altered
Health maintenance, altered
Home maintenance, impaired
Hopelessness
Management of therapeutic regimen, individual:
    Ineffective
Personal identity disturbance
Role performance, altered
Self-care deficit: bathing/hygiene
Self-care deficit: dressing/grooming
Self-esteem, chronic low
Sensory-perceptual alteration (specify)
Social isolation
Thought processes, altered
Violence, risk for: self-directed or directed at others

▌ Selected Nursing Diagnoses, Outcome Criteria, and Nursing Interventions with Rationale*

Example: Client With Schizoaffective Disorder in a General Hospital

NURSING DIAGNOSIS #1: *Risk for violence: directed at others related to overwhelming feelings of anger*

*References 8,9,11,12,18,19,23,24,27,31,32,35,37,38,39,44,45,49,51,52,57,59, 62,63,65,66,75,77

EXPECTED CLIENT OUTCOMES

- Client will demonstrate no hostile acts and will demonstrate several ways to control angry and/or anxious feelings and behavior.
- Client will verbalize or communicate in some understood way with staff that he feels threatened, disrespected, or more anxious.

NURSING INTERVENTIONS WITH RATIONALE

- Provide assistance with controlling anger. *Acknowledging angry feelings and anger-inducing experiences and demonstrating appropriate ways to manage strong feelings and thoughts reduces the likelihood of violence to others.*
  - Assist the client to identify triggers in the environment and to compare them with others that have previously occurred.
  - Identify to the client how shame and injuries to self-esteem are factors in the generation of anger.
  - Discuss feelings of anger and roleplay ways to deal with anger.
  - Encourage the client to schedule physical exercise daily *as a constructive outlet for feelings.*
  - Identify ways that the client can be assisted when anxiety appears to be increasing and a violent act is imminent.
  - Specify the nurse's or staff availability to assist client in anger control.
- Provide environmental management: use violence prevention techniques *to increase the safety factor and contain violence if/and when it does occur.*
  - Identify a staff member to be with the client at times of increased confusion, activity, or noise, e.g., meal time, community meeting
  - Observe the environment for signs of increasing tension between persons or in groups. Use verbal intervention to prevent violence.
  - If the client is anxious, use interventions that *encourage ventilation and that help the client become more hopeful and able to act.* Assume that anxious feelings will exist in crisis situations and demonstrate genuine concern to the client *to assure the client of protection.*

○ If the client is angry, use interventions *that assist the client to obtain attention and power and to feel adequate or respected.* The intervention may be giving advice, suggesting a course of action, or offering choices.

○ If the client is hostile and has lost control, use an intervention such as a direct command, "Stop"; *this gains the immediate attention of the person and most frequently results in compliance.* State the limits of the behavior permitted and the consequences of continued hostile action in a clear, concise, and firm manner; *this is done to obtain client participation in stopping the behavior.*

• Provide interventions of medication, seclusion, or restraint if the client is aggressive *to prevent further injury to the client, to others, or to the environment.* See Protective Interventions: Seclusion, and Protective Interventions: Restraint.

NURSING DIAGNOSIS #2:   *Sensory/perceptual alteration (auditory) related to neurotransmitter deficit, beginning psychotropic medication regimen, lack of symptom management skills*

EXPECTED CLIENT OUTCOMES

• Client will verbalize that auditory hallucinations are a symptom of Schizophrenia and acknowledge that antipsychotic medication is one way to manage the symptom.

• Client will demonstrate at least two ways to manage auditory hallucinations and associated feelings/ thoughts.

NURSING INTERVENTIONS WITH RATIONALE

• Provide hallucination management *to assist the client in coping with the voices and reduce the negative effect hallucinations have on activities of daily living.*

○ Observe client for nonverbal cues that anxiety or discomfort is increasing, particularly when behavior does not appear to be related to anything in the environment.

○ Perform ongoing assessments of hallucinations *to better design interventions that are helpful,* e.g., when do they appear; how does client communicate their existence; what is their duration; how do they intrude on client;

how severe are they; and what are the precipitating factors (e.g., stress, physical tiredness).
- ○ Instruct client in the use of techniques that may be helpful *to reduce or limit the voices/noises, e.g., listening to tapes, relaxation, distraction.*
- Provide information to client and family about prescribed medication *to enhance participation in treatment process that will continue following hospitalization.*
  - ○ Provide the name, dosage, route, and duration of effect of the medication.
  - ○ Identify the effect of antipsychotic medication on positive and negative symptoms; assist client to note the effect of the medication on behavior.
  - ○ Discuss side effects (dry mouth, restlessness, etc.) and ways to manage them, as well as when to report problems to a physician (symptoms of tardive dyskinesia, fever, symptoms of extrapyramidal reaction).
  - ○ Monitor the client's satisfaction with the medication *as noncompliance with medication regimen is a major factor in relapse.*

NURSING DIAGNOSIS #3: *Thought processes, altered related to neurotransmitter deficits, anxiety, problems in information processing*

EXPECTED CLIENT OUTCOMES

- Client will participate in treatment planning meetings with less anxiety and expressions of delusions.
- Client will demonstrate problem solving behavior, particularly in seeking to find out what is happening in reality, e.g., "what are my privileges? my pills?"

NURSING INTERVENTIONS WITH RATIONALE

- Provide delusion management *to decrease distortion, enable client to participate in daily activities, and meet basic needs without undue stress.*
  - ○ Monitor verbal interaction for delusional content; note if the client expresses the material as an actual fact or as a way to communicate what is experienced in order *to increase understanding of delusional material and thereby respond to it more appropriately.*
  - ○ Listen to client's concerns and validate client's statements of reality *to provide comfort and respect.*

- ○ Provide information regarding the effect of the central nervous system dysfunction on client's thoughts; describe the delusions.
- ○ Teach coping mechanisms for managing thoughts:
  - Ways to control thoughts: use distraction to end thinking the same thought repeatedly, and immerse oneself in concrete activities.
  - Recognize when thoughts are becoming disorganized—jumping from subject to subject.
  - Anticipate that there will be increased anxiety in a new situation; think of a way to decrease the anxiety.
  - Check out ideas and thoughts with others.
  - Practice thought-stopping techniques.
  - Engage in thought-switching technique.
  - Dispute irrational thoughts.
  - Learn when, where, and with whom delusional talk can be shared.
- Teach problem-solving skills in order *to manage the confusion experienced when client processes information.*
  - ○ Identify the steps in problem solving and practice using problem-solving steps in situations that arise on the unit.
  - ○ Assist the client in understanding when he or she has missed cues while interacting with others.
  - ○ Emphasize the importance of collecting all facts and finding information.
  - ○ Assist the client in using the problem-solving process to understand and participate in the treatment plan.

NURSING DIAGNOSIS #4:   *Self-care deficit (bathing, hygiene, dressing) related to problems in thought processes*

EXPECTED CLIENT OUTCOMES

- Client will establish a routine for bathing, caring for teeth, and dressing in clean clothes daily.
- Client will consent to help when he or she is unable to do something, e.g., trim nails and hair.

NURSING INTERVENTIONS WITH RATIONALE

- Provide self-care assistance with dressing/grooming *to assist in reestablishing a routine of daily personal hygiene, because routines become habits that require less mental processing and deliberative actions.*

○ As necessary, perform or assist client in bathing, cleaning of teeth, dressing daily; then post reminders *to establish the routine to decrease confusion about what to do and when and how.*

○ Monitor on a daily basis the client's need for assistance to begin and carry through the routine, thus *nurturing the ability to act on behalf of self and maintaining self-respect.*

○ Allow time and set limits for these activities.

○ Encourage the client's verbalization of a lack of motivation or willingness to do something; validate these feelings and beliefs as symptom(s) of the disorder *to demonstrate empathy.*

○ Acknowledge the decrease in negative remarks and the increase in positive statements by others about the client's appearance.

○ Reinforce small steps in establishing a daily routine: "You did it."

○ Assist the client in dividing a task into smaller parts *so that it will not seem so overwhelming and impossible.*

NURSING DIAGNOSIS #5: *Risk for Social Isolation related to lack of contact, delusional system and limited social skills.*

EXPECTED CLIENT OUTCOME

• Client will contact one or two significant family members and begin to discuss the incident preceding hospitalization.

NURSING INTERVENTIONS WITH RATIONALE

• Provide coping enhancement *to help client re-establish relationships with the family, who are needed to provide emotional support as well as contribute to basic needs.*

○ Provide direction by role-playing with the client how to talk to the family about events preceding hospitalization, the client's feelings, and asking for the family's input.

○ Discuss ways to deal with the family's expectations and the client's feelings about them.

○ Give feedback about what is known about events prior to the hospitalization as one way to sort out feelings, delusions, and actual events.

- ○ Discuss the client's basic needs and how the client might request assistance from the family in meeting these needs.
- Provide family process maintenance *because a family dealing with chronic illness may become less functional over time and itself become symptomatic, i.e., increased conflict, projection, distancing, intense closeness, etc.*
  - ○ Listen to and assist the family in dealing with the events leading to hospitalization; help them prepare for the client's return.
  - ○ Provide the family an opportunity for sharing with other families with a schizophrenic member.
  - ○ Provide an opportunity for dialogue between the client, family members, and treatment team.
  - ○ Direct the family to community support groups.

Example: Client With Schizophrenia, Undifferentiated, and Alcohol Abuse Living on Streets

NURSING DIAGNOSIS #1:   *Powerlessness related to the lifestyle of homelessness*

EXPECTED CLIENT OUTCOME

- Client will agree to go to a homeless shelter as an initial way to meet basic needs, i.e., safety, shelter, food, water, love, belonging, and respect.

NURSING INTERVENTIONS WITH RATIONALE

- Assess how client's basic survival needs are being met *to provide clues for actions needed to maintain or improve current state.*
  - ○ Observe client's belongings, immediate environment, and contacts with others *in order to begin to know the person and to assess needs.*
  - ○ Gather data about where and how the client feels safest, can sleep or rest, and can be warm and dry.
  - ○ Gather data about what kinds of foods the client eats and when.
  - ○ Gather data about where and how the client finds places to bathe, use a bathroom, and care for clothing.
  - ○ Listen carefully and learn about the client's basic concerns *because they may be quite different than expected.*

- Provide presence consistently *to demonstrate trustworthiness and concern for the client who is existing marginally.*
  - Contact the client in the park or another place where the client may be found at least twice weekly.
  - Consistently offer the client help in contacting and working with agencies to find satisfactory housing and health care.
- Respond immediately to the client's willingness to visit a shelter and meet with some residents *to support the decision to obtain shelter before the client becomes fearful or less motivated.*
- Provide reality validation as well as belief in individual's ability to change *to assist in re-establishing a reason to be hopeful.*
  - Listen for and verbally acknowledge personal achievement(s) (e.g., "I went to a dinner program at X church last night") or any object(s) in which the client has demonstrated special pride, e.g., a black, intact plastic bag with personal items.
  - Assist in identifying the client's assets.
  - Ascertain with the client what can be done with the assets and what the client would like done.

NURSING DIAGNOSIS #2:   *Thought processes, altered related to neurotransmitter deficit and substance abuse*

EXPECTED CLIENT OUTCOME

- Client will not experience a relapse of Schizophrenia requiring hospitalization.

NURSING INTERVENTIONS WITH RATIONALE

- Initiate surveillance *to obtain clues that indicate the beginning of a relapse so that the relapse can be avoided or the symptoms more quickly managed.*
  - Observe and listen for symptoms of sleeplessness, expressions of fear, increasing argumentativeness, fights with others, and increased use of alcohol.
  - Review triggers of the last relapse experience *to reinforce and review what was learned in hospital and to identify what is happening now.* Include lack of sleep, pressure to drink alcohol from old friends, housing problems, loneliness, "poor me" attitude.

- Provide teaching on the negative symptoms of Schizophrenia *to increase cognitive awareness of what effect the negative symptoms are having on feeling and beliefs and their consequences as noted in behavior.*
  - Help the client learn to identify feeling states in others, their possible reasons, and their implications for the client.
  - Discuss negative symptoms of Schizophrenia and their similarity with feelings generated by homelessness.
  - Discuss the feeling states and behaviors related to alcohol consumption.
- Support problem-solving efforts and coping strategies *to increase feelings of worth and self-respect that assist in preventing relapse.*
  - Listen carefully and acknowledge accomplishments, e.g., obtaining one hot meal daily, taking medicine for 1 week, not taking a drink for 1 day.
  - Offer information and assistance when problems or issues are presented.

CHAPTER 10

Mood Disorders

▌ Definition/Major Symptoms*

Mood disorders include the major categories of Depressive Disorders, Bipolar Disorders, and Mood Disorders Based on Etiology; the predominant feature of all is a disturbance in mood (a sustained emotion that influences the client's view of self, others, and the environment). The disorders are characterized by various mood episodes and involve somatic, cognitive, emotional, and behavioral disturbances.

Mood Episodes

MAJOR DEPRESSIVE EPISODE

Consists of depressed mood, diminished pleasure in activities, weight loss, sleep disturbance, psychomotor retardation or agitation, fatigue, difficulty concentrating or thinking, suicidal ideation, and impaired social and occupational functioning.

MANIC EPISODE

Consists of elevated mood, grandiosity, reduced sleep needs, talkativeness, flight of ideas, decreased attention span, increased goal directed activity/psychomotor agitation, overinvolvement in pleasurable activities, especially those with a potential for negative outcomes, and impaired social and occupational functioning.

*References 2,16,20,22,23,51

MIXED EPISODE

Meets criteria of both depressive and manic episodes, with impaired social and occupational functioning.

HYPOMANIC EPISODE

Similar to a manic episode except that social and occupational functioning are not markedly impaired.

█ Definitions/Symptoms of Selected Major Categories

Depressive Disorders

Major Depressive Disorder, Dysthymic Disorder, Depressive Disorder Not Otherwise Specified—exhibit the presence of depressive episodes but no evidence of manic, mixed, or hypomanic episodes.

Bipolar Disorders

Bipolar I Disorder, Bipolar II Disorder, Cyclothymic Disorder, Bipolar Disorder Not Otherwise Specified—exhibit the presence/history generally of major Depressive Episodes along with Manic, Mixed, or Hypomanic Episodes.

Mood Disorder Based on Etiology

Mood Disorder Due to a General Medical Condition, Substance-Induced Mood Disorder, Mood Disorder Not Otherwise Specified—mood disturbance related to the physiological aspects of a medical condition (e.g., CVA), drug abuse, toxin, or medications. Medications associated with depression include cardiovascular drugs (e.g., reserpine, clonidine, digitalis, propranolol); hormones (e.g., oral contraceptives, corticosteroids); psychotropics (e.g., benzodiazepines, opioids); anticancer agents (e.g., cycloserine); and anti-inflammatory/anti-infective agents (e.g., sulfonamides). Medications associated with mania include, for example, levodopa and corticosteroids.

▌ Incidence[*]

- There is a 10% to 25% lifetime risk of Major Depressive Disorder for women and 5% to 12% for men.
- Major/minor depression occurs in 5% of the elderly in primary care clinics and in 15% to 25% in nursing homes; depression in the elderly is common but often overlooked.
- The mid-20s is the average age of onset for Major Depressive Disorder.
- There is a 15% death rate from suicide in clients with Major Depressive Disorder.
- The incidence of postpartum depression ranges from 3% to 30%.
- There is a 3% lifetime prevalence for Dysthymic Disorder.
- Seasonal affective disorder is most common in young women.
- There is a 1% to 2% lifetime risk of Bipolar Disorder; it is equally common in males and females.
- The peak onset of Bipolar Disorders is between the ages of 20 and 25, with rare onset after 60.
- Cyclothymic Disorder is often diagnosed in adolescence or early adulthood.
- There is a 0.4% to 1.0% lifetime prevalence rate of Cyclothymic Disorder; it is equally common in men and women.
- Between 25% and 40% of clients with selected neurological conditions develop a Mood Disorder Due to a General Medical Condition; about 50% of clients with CVA develop depression; 10% to 25% of clients with Alzheimer's disease have depression in the early stage of the disease; about 30% of clients with Parkinson's disease have depression.

▌ Course[†]

Depressive Disorders

- A variable course is exhibited in Major Depressive Disorder.
- The number of previous episodes predicts the likelihood of subsequent episodes of Major Depressive Disorder.
- The presence of Dysthymic Disorder is a risk factor for Major Depressive Disorder.

[*]References 2,15,16,35,41,52,64,74,79
[†]References 2,8,20,21,44

- A chronic medical condition is a risk factor for Major Depressive Disorder.
- In the elderly with a medical condition, depression may be of longer duration, have additive effects on general functioning, and increase the risk of suicide; untreated depression may lead to increased medical visits and use of ancillary health services, as well as the need for hospitalization or nursing home placement.
- Women with postpartum depression can experience an intense sense of inadequacy, difficulty in coping, loss of interest in normal activities, and anorexia.[77]
- Dysthymic Disorder has an early, insidious onset and chronic course.

Bipolar Disorders

- Bipolar I Disorder is recurrent in nature: over 90% of clients have recurrent Manic Episodes, with decreasing intervals between episodes as client ages.
- Mood lability and functional difficulties are seen in 20% to 30% of clients between episodes in Bipolar I Disorder and in 15% with Bipolar II Disorder.
- Hypomanic episodes are characteristic in 60% to 70% of clients with Bipolar II Disorder shortly before or after a Major Depressive Episode.
- A Bipolar II Disorder that is characterized by a rapid-cycling pattern (four or more episodes per year) has a poorer prognosis.
- An insidious onset with chronic alterations between periods of hypomanic and depressive symptoms is found in Cyclothymic Disorder.
- Clients with Bipolar Disorder may use drugs or alcohol to cover up depression and to manage illness.
- Clients with Bipolar Disorder may stop taking medications because of difficulty in handling "normal mood" and a preference for feeling "high."

▌ Contributing Factors to Mood Disorders*

The causes of Mood Disorders are not known, but several theories have evolved.

*References 3,9,24,25,29,31,32,35,39,48,61,63,65,66,69

Neurobiological/Genetic

- There may be a genetic predisposition for Bipolar and Major Depressive Disorder; Mood Disorders tend to occur in families, and occurrence is greater in identical than in fraternal twins. Current genetic-linkage studies on the genetic predisposition for Bipolar Disorders are searching the entire genome.
- Research is attempting to identify any consistent biochemical abnormalities in clients with Mood Disorders (e.g., acetylcholine system dysregulation or norepinephrine deficit in brain nerve terminals are possible mechanisms for depression).
- Functional and structural imaging techniques are being used in studies to identify mechanisms for Mood Disorders (e.g., studies have found, in white matter in the brain, a greater number of focal signal hyperintensities in persons with Mood Disorders). Functional brain imaging studies are being used to determine the treatment effects of ECT and antidepressant medications.
- Neuroendocrine system research has identified hypothalamic–pituitary–adrenal axis abnormalities in depression and linked thyroid function abnormalities to Mood Disorders.
- Beginning research links neuropeptides to Mood Disorders.
- Sleep studies link Mood Disorders with sleep disturbances, proposing, for example, decreased REM latency as a biological marker.
- Changes in circadian rhythms may contribute to development of Bipolar Disorder.
- A phase delay hypothesis has been offered for seasonal affective disorder, i.e., circadian rhythms are phase-delayed in relation to the onset of sleep.[7]

Psychological Models

- *Psychoanalytic*—theorists (e.g., Freud) propose fixation at oral stage of development; real or perceived loss results in lowered self-esteem and depression.
- *Behavioral*—theorists (e.g., Lewinsohn) propose that a person with a lack of social skills faced with a decrease in positive reinforcement develops dysphoria and depression, the latter being a secondary gain.

- *Cognitive/behavioral*—theorists (e.g., Beck) propose that a person with dysfunctional attitudes, faced with environmental stressors, triggers symptoms of depression.
- *Learned helplessness*—theorists (e.g., Seligman) propose that persons with certain attributional styles are vulnerable to depression, e.g., persons faced with negative events believe they are helpless and their actions useless in dealing with the negative events or in improving their life situation; persons believe their helplessness is due to personal inadequacies (internal factors), to personality deficiencies (global factors), or to their own fixed personality factors (stable factors).
- *Humanistic/existential*—theorists propose that depression may result from not living according to one's own values, from not exercising those choices that lead to self actualization or fulfillment, or from role loss since self-worth tends to be connected to social roles taken in life, e.g., occupational.

Family/Social/Cultural/Environmental/Other Factors

- Severe, persistent, multiple stressors or losses in vulnerable individuals may lead to sadness, demoralization, and depression.
- Recent cohort studies of younger persons have found the onset of major depression occurring at earlier age and at increased frequency. One speculation is that members of the baby boom generation may be experiencing greater economic and social stressors, or perhaps the older cohort is less likely to report symptoms of depression.
- Family experiences such as parental neglect, lack of support, rejection, abuse, family conflict, and the death of a parent have been related to depression in adolescents.
- Poor physical or mental health, disability, and chronic pain are linked to depression in the elderly; low income, life stressors, and difficulties with companionship also increase risk.
- Nonhardiness and a negative attitude towards death may be predictors of depression in institutionalized elderly persons.[13]

▌ Laboratory and Physical Examination Findings[*]

- Laboratory findings specific to a diagnosis of Major Depressive Disorder have not been identified; some abnormal laboratory findings, although not diagnostic, are found in groups of persons, e.g., sleep EEG abnormalities.
- Although structural scans cannot diagnose Mood Disorders, they can exclude other illnesses in which depression is a symptom.
- Research is being conducted to develop reliable biologic markers to identify potential treatment-resistant depression.
- An acute or chronic medical condition (e.g., stroke, myocardial infarction, cancer, dementia, diabetes, fibromyalgia, chronic fatigue syndrome) is a risk factor for a Major Depressive Disorder.
- When a first manic episode occurs after the age of 40, it is frequently linked to a medical condition or substance abuse.
- Suicide risk (10% to 15% death rate) exists for persons with untreated Bipolar I or Bipolar II Disorder.
- Abusive or violent behavior can occur in manic episodes.

▌ Special Assessment Considerations[†]

Assess signs and symptoms to determine the presence of a manic or depressive episode.

- To determine the presence of a *manic episode* assess:
  - emotional state for euphoria, expansiveness
  - behavior for diminished control over own activities, irritability, hyperactivity, description of elaborate, unrealistic activities such as buying sprees or promiscuous sexual activity
  - dressing and grooming for excessive use of make-up, outlandish clothing, poor personal hygiene
  - attitudes for grandiosity or inflated self-importance
  - speech patterns for rapid speech
  - level of concentration for distractibility, frequent changes of topic of conversation, referential thinking
  - general health for sleep disturbances, poor eating habits, and loss of weight.

[*]References 2,16,17,33,40,56
[†]References 2,61

- To determine the presence of a *depressive episode* assess:
  - emotional state for depressed mood, hopelessness, sadness, negativity, feelings of guilt and apathy
  - behavior for inertia, social withdrawal, psychomotor retardation or sometimes agitation, slowed gait, sexual dysfunction, decreased interest in pleasure, inability to feel happiness from experiences that most persons find pleasurable (i.e., anhedonia)
  - dressing and grooming for general lack of good grooming habits
  - attitudes for low self-esteem
  - speech for very slow responses
  - level of concentration for difficulty in thinking, concentrating, indecisiveness
  - general health for sleep disturbance (e.g., early morning awakening, insomnia, hypersomnia) and excessive concerns about health.
- Be extremely attentive to suicide risk, which is ever-present in clients with Mood Disorders.
- Assess for underlying medical conditions that may contribute to Mood Disorder.

■ Treatment*

Psychopharmacologic/Biologic

DEPRESSIVE DISORDERS

- Medications used include tricyclic antidepressants (TCAs) (e.g., amitriptyline, clomipramine, desipramine, doxepin, imipramine, nortriptyline, protriptyline, trimipramine); heterocyclics (e.g, maprotiline, bupropion, amoxapine, trazodone); selective serotonin reuptake inhibitors (SSRI) (e.g., fluoxetine, paroxetine, sertraline); monoamine oxidase inhibitors (MAOIs) (e.g., phenelzine, tranylcypromine); and a non-trycyclic antidepressant, venlafaxine.
- Fluoxetine, an SSRI, is the most widely used antidepressant in the U.S., with increasing use of sertraline and paroxetine; when SSRIs do not work, the dose may be increased, the treatment augmented with another drug, drug combinations may be used, or the antidepressant may be changed to another class of medications.

*References 6,10,11,17–19,26–28,30,34,36–38,46,47,53,61,62,70–73,78

- For acute phase of Major Depressive Disorder, recommended first- and second-line antidepressant medications include amine tricyclics, e.g., nortriptyline and desipramine; bupropion; fluoxetine; paroxetine; sertraline; and trazodone.
- For acute phase of Major Depressive Disorder, alternative antidepressant medications for clients with special needs include tertiary amine tricyclics, e.g., amitriptyline and imipramine if rapid sedation is needed and there is no serious medical illness, and MAOIs if there is nonresponse or intolerance to tricyclics or heterocyclics. The practice is increasing of administering SSRIs first because of their safety profile; serial EKGs are needed with TCAs but not with SSRIs.
- TCAs are most likely to be used if a client is suicidal.
- Antidepressant medications are used for varying lengths of time during the maintenance phase of Major Depressive Disorder.
- For each individual elderly client, the choice of an antidepressant is the one with the least adverse effects at the lowest effective dose; elderly persons experience changes in the pharmacodynamics and pharmacokinetics of psychotropic medications.
- The efficacy of antidepressant medications for children is unknown; some physicians recommend beginning with less risky treatment of psychotherapy. When antidepressant medications are prescribed, the family environment must be such that the medication can be given reliably and predictably, side effects will be monitored, medications will be stored safely, and follow-up appointments will be kept.

NURSING CARE CONSIDERATIONS FOR MAOI
MEDICATION THERAPY

- Teach client about most frequent general side effects of MAOIs: hypotension, dizziness, drowsiness, rapid pulse, sweating.
- Teach client that while taking MAOI there are:
  - *strict* dietary restrictions—avoid cheese except cream, cottage, or American processed cheese; sauerkraut; banana peels; broad bean pods; yeast or meat extracts; nonfresh or fermented protein food products, meat, or fish; pickled herring, anchovies, sardines; processed

meats such as sausages, bologna, Spam, canned ham, pepperoni; liver; tap beer, chianti, and vermouth wine.
- ○ *strict* medication restrictions—avoid local anesthetics containing epinephrine; cocaine; meperidine; clomipramine; fluoxetine; fluvoxamine; paroxetine; sertraline; venlafaxine; amphetamines; stimulants; appetite suppressants; phenylephrine; phenylpropanolamine; pseudoephedrine; oxymetazoline; ephedrine; isoproterenol; other decongestants.
- Instruct client to contact doctor before taking any prescribed or over-the-counter medication while taking MAOI.
- Instruct client to immediately call the doctor or go to an emergency room if the following reactions occur: rapid pulse, increased BP, chest pain, sweating, flushing, dizziness, pounding headache, stiff neck, or convulsions as a result of consuming a food or medication to be avoided.

NURSING CARE CONSIDERATIONS FOR OTHER ANTIDEPRESSANT MEDICATIONS

Teach client side effects of:

- SSRIs—nausea, diarrhea, insomnia, anorexia, headache, nervousness, sexual dysfunction, skin rash
- Tricyclic and heterocyclic antidepressants:
  - ○ cardiovascular—postural hypotension, sinus tachycardia, along with occasional dizziness, hypertension with venlafaxine, pedal edema, premature ventricular beats
  - ○ gastrointestinal—constipation along with occasional nausea, vomiting, heartburn
  - ○ neurologic—drowsiness, seizures, hallucinations, delusions, anticholinergic effects along with occasional muscle tremors, twitches, jitteriness, extrapyramidal symptoms, paresthesias, fatigue, weakness, ataxia
  - ○ anticholinergic—blurred vision, constipation, dry mouth, sinus tachycardia, along with occasional urinary retention, sweating, mental clouding, confusion, delirium, speech blockage

BIPOLAR DISORDERS

- Lithium is used to treat and prevent manic episodes in Bipolar Disorder; effects occur 7 to 10 days after therapeutic blood levels are reached, so antipsychotic drugs may be used initially for symptomatic relief. Lithium can be used as an adjunct in the treatment of depression.

- Between 50% and 60% of clients with Bipolar Disorders relapse when on lithium maintenance.
- Hypomania may be the optimal mood that can be achieved by many bipolar clients.

NURSING CARE CONSIDERATIONS FOR LITHIUM THERAPY

- Collaborate in pre-treatment evaluation—WBC, fasting blood sugar, thyroid function tests, serum electrolytes, ECG, BUN, serum creatinine.
- Teach client and significant others about:
  - the need for frequent measurement of lithium levels, especially initially
  - potential side effects—polydipsia, polyuria, edema, weight gain, fine hand tremors, nausea, mild diarrhea, hypothyroidism, or goiter
  - signs of impending toxicity—nausea, vomiting, diarrhea, coarse hand tremor, dysarthria, vertigo, sluggishness, sleepiness
  - the need to avoid lithium therapy during pregnancy or when conceiving.
- Observe for lithium toxicity—cardiac arrhythmias, oliguria, anuria, convulsions, nystagmus, hyperflexia, muscle fasciculation, impaired consciousness, coma.
- Teach client to discontinue lithium and consult physician immediately if signs of toxicity occur.
- Give with food or milk or after meals.
- Monitor for adequate fluid and salt intake.

ELECTRO-CONVULSIVE THERAPY (ECT)

ECT can be useful in treating selected depressed clients who are not responsive (e.g., to antidepressant medications), whose symptoms are both severe and prolonged, and in whom there is marked functional impairment. It is used to treat selected clients with Bipolar Disorders who are unresponsive to medications or clients who request it.

NURSING CARE CONSIDERATIONS FOR ECT

- Be aware of contraindications, e.g., brain tumors, recent MI or CVA, intolerance to general anesthesia.
- Collaborate in obtaining pre-ECT evaluation data, e.g., physical exam, ECG, X-rays, EEG, CT scan, CBC, blood chemistry, urinalysis.
- Be aware of when it is necessary to discontinue (e.g., lithium) or reduce medications.
- Offer client and significant others an opportunity to express feelings about ECT.
- Explain procedure to client and significant others in terms that are readily understood.
- Teach client to use memory aids prior to ECT.
- Obtain signed consent.
- Place on NPO after midnight.
- Instruct client to wear comfortable clothing, remove contact lenses, dentures, etc.
- Encourage client to void prior to ECT.
- Monitor client for temporary memory loss and confusion after ECT.
- Provide supervision as needed and frequent reorientation.

Psychotherapy

Psychotherapy can be used for clients with Mood Disorders.

- For Major Depressive Disorder, psychotherapy can be used alone if the depressive episode is mild to moderate, or it can be combined with antidepressant medications after a moderate to severe depressive episode has been treated.
- For *acute phase treatment* of Major Depressive Disorder, examples of useful therapies are:
  ○ interpersonal, behavioral, supportive, cognitive— directed at removing symptoms and preventing relapse. Research findings show that short-term, acute-phase psychosocial interventions such as interpersonal psychotherapy, cognitive therapy, and behavior therapy can reduce symptoms of Major Depressive Disorder in adults. Structured cognitive-behavioral group interventions have been found useful in reducing depression in female clients.

- ○ marital, occupational, psycho-educational, cognitive, behavioral—can be used to regain psychosocial and occupational role functioning.
- ○ clinical case management—to increase medication adherence.
- ○ marital—to resolve family dysfunction and marital discord.
- For *maintenance phase treatment* of Major Depressive Disorder, psychotherapy may be added to the medication regimen to improve psychosocial functioning. Psychotherapy used alone for maintenance treatment is not well established.
- Structured cognitive-behavioral group interventions have been found useful in reducing depression in female clients.
- Group cognitive therapy can be effective for the depressed elderly; negative thinking is replaced with more positive and valid perceptions.[83] Group therapy as part of an overall treatment plan that includes antidepressant medications, education, and activities can be very effective.[14] Social support is particularly important for the elderly client.[54]
- Group therapy has been found to be a useful adjunct to psychopharmacotherapy for outpatients with Bipolar Disorders.
- Inpatients respond well to diagnostically homogeneous group therapy.
- A self-management Bipolar Disorder group model for inpatients has shown promise.[57–60]

SUICIDE PREVENTION

- Assess suicide risk by determining the presence of risk factors: presence of plan for committing suicide; prior suicide attempts; substance abuse, family history of substance abuse; general medical illness; hopelessness, living alone, depression; psychotic symptoms; and male gender.
- Hospitalization may be required if client is unable to attend outpatient care because there is insufficient social support, if the medication regimen needs close monitoring, if psychosis is present, or if specific suicide plans are verbalized. (See also Protective Interventions: Observation for Suicide in Chapter 5.)

▌ Commonly Occurring Nursing Diagnoses*

Altered family processes
Altered nutrition: less than body requirements
Altered role performance
Altered sexuality patterns
Aggression
Anxiety
Decisional conflict
Dysfunctional grieving
Fatigue
Hopelessness
Impaired social interaction
Ineffective individual coping
Powerlessness
Risk for violence: directed at others
Risk for violence: directed at self
Self-care deficit (dressing/grooming)
Self-esteem disturbance
Sleep pattern disturbance

▌ Selected Nursing Diagnoses, Outcome Criteria, and Nursing Interventions with Rationale†

NURSING DIAGNOSIS #1:   *Risk for violence: directed at self related to Major Depressive Episode with suicidal ideation*

EXPECTED CLIENT OUTCOME

• Client will remain safe as evidenced by inflicting no harm to self and eliminating suicidal ideation.

NURSING INTERVENTIONS WITH RATIONALE

• Assess the client's current suicide potential by asking such questions as: Have you thought of committing suicide? Are you thinking of committing suicide now? How long have you thought about it? What is the frequency and duration of such thoughts? How would you go about doing it? Do you have the means? Have you ever

*References 42,50,55
†References 1,4,5,12,41,45,49,68,71,75,76,80–82

attempted to commit suicide in the past? What was the deterrent? What is the likelihood that you will commit suicide now? How do you see your future? *A specific, high-lethality suicide plan (e.g., shooting, hanging, poisoning) of recent origin for which the client has the resources available increases the potential of suicide.*

- Identify the presence of the following risk factors: verbalizations of a wish to die with definite plan; highly lethal plan with availability of resources; previous suicide attempts or self-destructive behavior; perception of suicide as a release or escape; recent loss of significant person, possession, or role; physical pain or illness; alcohol or drug abuse; history of or current mental illness, especially Schizophrenia and other Psychotic Disorders; age and sex; domestic difficulties; unemployment; retirement; financial stress; lack of spiritual resources; being an elderly male; being isolated and ill. *The identification of the presence of these risk factors can assist in evaluating suicide potential. Factors especially indicative of high risk for suicide are depressive episodes (especially changing levels of depression), major recent loss, family history of suicide, "putting house in order" by giving away prized possessions, and hopelessness with few plans/goals for the future. It should be noted that (1) suicide ranks among the leading causes of death in 15- to 23-year-olds and is the ninth leading cause of death among the elderly; (2) white males over 65 are at the highest risk; and (3) males outnumber females in actual suicide, while females outnumber males in suicide attempts.*

- Use established scales to assist in assessing suicide potential, e.g., The Los Angeles Suicide Prevention Center Scale for Assessing Suicidal Potential, as well as general mental health status. *Note that (1) more suicides occur during the period of improvement following severe depression than during the period of severe depression itself; (2) a client who experiences hallucinations may respond to, for example, voices that command the client to kill self; and (3) repression has been found to be correlated with the risk of suicide and may be a mechanism by which aggression is focused inward.*

- In a community mental health setting, if suicidal risk is high, arrange for hospitalization immediately unless client can be safely managed in the community setting. In the hospital setting, offer protective intervention and observe for suicide (see also Chapter 5). *About 80% of persons who commit suicide give some type of clue indicative of the suicide: all talk of suicide is of concern, and observation of the client is very important. Suicide can be prevented because clients with the potential for suicide do experience ambivalence sometime prior to actual suicide.*

- In collaboration with the multidisciplinary team, administer antidepressant medications *in order to reduce depressive symptoms. Beware of lethal dose of TCAs; give less than 1 gm.*
- Provide safe environment by discussing with team members what personal items to remove from the client and what specific environmental hazards to eliminate *in order to provide a safe environment for the client, free from sharp objects and other harmful items so that client cannot harm self (see also Protective Interventions in Chapter 5).*
- For those clients not needing constant observation, use "no suicide or self-harm" contracts for intervening periods, and consider having the client take on responsibility by "checking in" at assigned periods with staff (see also Contracting in Chapter 5). *Note that unwillingness to enter into a "no suicide" contract can be indicative of high suicide risk. Written contracts can result in beneficial outcomes such as developing alternative and constructive thoughts and behaviors, gaining problem-solving skills, learning interpersonal skills, and assuming responsibility for one's own behavior.*
- Offer support against self-destructive impulses and suggest alternative behaviors. *It is important to emphasize a protective, non-punitive attitude and milieu for these clients.*
- Set limits to destructive behavior toward self or others, but permit the client to express anger and hostility within these limits. *Limit setting is very important in establishing to the client that behavior harmful to self or to others will not be tolerated and that constructive channels of expressing anger and other emotions will be encouraged. At times it may be necessary to directly intervene with the client in order to redirect the focus of a perceived threat.*
- Prevent isolation and seek out client *because client may withdraw from others and isolate self.*

- Encourage client to increase physical activities previously enjoyed, emphasizing actual involvement instead of enjoyment initially; collaborate with client to set a daily schedule, allowing for flexibility but making the most out of each part of the day *in order to deal with problem of inactivity and anergia.*
- Help client to recognize the possible recurrence of suicidal thoughts and emphasize the importance of client's talking with health care professionals and/or significant others.

NURSING DIAGNOSIS #2:   *Hopelessness related to major depressive episode*

EXPECTED CLIENT OUTCOME

- Client will develop adaptive methods to cope with stress and emotions and achieve hope as evidenced by demonstrating adequate role functioning and positive self-concept, verbalizing a plan for accessing emergency services if symptoms recur after discharge, and verbalizing hope for own future.

NURSING INTERVENTIONS WITH RATIONALE

- Assist the client in identifying anxiety, depressed mood, anger, and other emotions. *Exploration of the basis for emotions increases the client's awareness of appropriately channeling these emotions.*
- Help client to identify ways to decrease intensity of emotions, e.g., talking with supportive person.
- Listen with sensitivity to expressions of unworthiness, without insisting that words are false: convey message that having bad thoughts and making mistakes does not mean one is a "bad person."
- Avoid imposing one's own feelings, values, and moral judgments. *What is perceived by the nurse as a mild stressor can be perceived by the client as an extreme stressor.*
- Offer hope; point out that other ways are available to cope with what is happening; offer opportunity to reevaluate the situation when client is not overwhelmed by desire to die; do not use a jubilant, cheerful approach in interacting with client. (See also Supportive Therapy: Offering Hope in Chapter 5.)

- Teach client strategies for maintaining emotional control (e.g., walking, listening to music, etc.) when emotional tension increases and to seek assistance from professionals or significant others when needed.
- Encourage client to participate in group therapy such as group psycho-education. *A group approach can increase feelings of independence, especially in women, as well as offer peer support for developing skills and improving self-esteem.*[46,47]
- Enhance client's learned resourcefulness by encouraging positive self statements, believing in personal ability to cope, delaying immediate gratification, and enhancing problem-solving skills. *Resourcefulness appears to be learned; learned resourcefulness may enhance client's ability to interact with others, fulfill expected occupational and social roles, and perform self-care activities.*
- Teach client decision-making and coping skills (see also Decision Making in Chapter 5).
- Teach client to:
  ○ explore present situation *since helping the client think and talk about problems can correct myths, misperceptions, and distorted ideas.*
  ○ establish realistic goals.
  ○ minimize distraction of immediate desires and self-indulgence by recognizing that each day is an opportunity to increase self-confidence and movement toward realistic goals.
  ○ use personal goals as an overall frame of focus in order to put complex situations into perspective.
  ○ master daily activities and rely on self as much as possible.
  ○ identify potential solutions to problems.
  ○ evaluate consequences of different alternatives and change alternatives when necessary.
  ○ role play options when possible.
  ○ evaluate impact of actions.
  ○ demonstrate courage, persistence, and self-possession *in order to minimize negative feedback from others.*
  ○ be assertive *so that other people's opinions do not prevent the accomplishment of activities or personal goals* (see also Assertiveness Training in Chapter 5).

- ○ develop relationships through shared activities; resist compromising self-identity or trying to remold others in case of differences.
- ○ focus on positive, not negative, thoughts.
- ○ avoid feeling obligated to reveal self to others continually.
- ○ find solitude *in order to gain strength and focus on personal direction and goals.*
- ○ recognize that in future stressful situations, feelings of suicide may recur; talk to a professional staff member or to a significant other *since this is an important strategy for prevention.*
- ○ list crisis line and other phone numbers *since these may be very useful in an emergency.*
- Enhance interpersonal relationships, social network, and social resources; involve the family and significant others; and improve social skills *in order to enhance social support. Strengthening of social support can reduce feelings of isolation and hopelessness and suicidal ideation.* (See also Social Skills Training in Chapter 5.)
- Recognize influence of cultural factors on development and expression of depression and suicidal behavior.
- Integrate cultural factors in providing care and be sensitive to the needs of clients of minority status. *Cultural differences may result in challenges in the therapeutic situation. For example, Chinese Americans tend to express symptoms of depression somatically.*[75] *Since relationships and community support are very important for African-American women, these aspects must be central in developing interventions for this group.*[80] *Immigrant women may be at particular risk for developing depression; members of ethnic groups may associate a stigma with reporting psychological symptoms.*[43]
- Instruct client about illness and its treatment; explore beliefs about medication treatment as well as role of significant others in medication regimen *to maximize compliance.*
- Encourage client to avoid substance abuse, taking sedatives or other medications that are not prescribed, or becoming overly exhausted.

• Stress the importance of taking antidepressant medications as ordered and keeping scheduled follow-up appointments after discharge (see also Discharge Planning in Chapter 5).

NURSING DIAGNOSIS #3:   *Self-care deficit (dressing/grooming; bathing/hygiene; feeding)*

EXPECTED CLIENT OUTCOME

• Client will perform activities of daily living as evidenced by adequate hygiene, appropriate dressing and grooming, and adequately meeting nutritional needs.

NURSING INTERVENTIONS WITH RATIONALE

• Reflect a caring, concerned attitude.
• Assist client with bathing, hygiene, grooming and dressing, and meeting nutritional needs as much as needed while in the acute phase of a depressive episode.
• Convey expectation/hope that client will once again be independent in these activities of daily living as condition improves.
• Encourage as much independence as possible while respecting the boundaries of the client's capabilities, which should increase as depression and suicidal ideation decrease.
• Encourage simple decision making based on client's strengths and abilities.
• *During the acute phase of a depressive episode the client may lack interest in performing activities of daily living as well as lack an appetite and interest in eating so assistance may need to be provided.*

CHAPTER **11**

Anxiety Disorders

∎ Definition/Major Symptoms*

Anxiety Disorders are characterized by pathologic emotional responses that "range from excessive worrying about everyday problems regarding work, relationships, or finances to acute, intense episodes of fear (Panic Attacks) usually accompanied by a multitude of cognitive, behavioral, and physiologic symptoms".[35] Panic Attacks and Agoraphobia are two common major symptoms of an Anxiety Disorder. Panic Attacks are characterized by the sudden onset of relatively short-lived periods of intense anxiety or fear with a sense of imminent danger, impending doom, and a urge to escape that is frequently accompanied by somatic symptoms. The diagnosis of Panic Attack requires the presence of 4 of 13 somatic or cognitive symptoms that develop abruptly and peak within 10 minutes:

1. Palpitations, pounding heart or accelerated heart rate
2. Sweating
3. Trembling or shaking
4. Sensations of shortness of breath or smothering
5. Feeling of choking
6. Chest pain or discomfort
7. Nausea or abdominal distress
8. Feeling dizzy, unsteady, lightheaded, or faint
9. Derealization (feelings of unreality) or depersonalization (detachment from oneself)
10. Fear of losing control or going crazy
11. Fear of dying

*References 2,16,18,35

12. Paresthesias (numbing or tingling sensations)
13. Chills or hot flushes

Symptoms of Agoraphobia include anxiety about being in public places or situations from which rapid exit would be difficult or in which no person would be available to help during an experience of Panic Attack or panic-like symptoms; avoidance of being alone in or away from own house, being in a crowd or an elevator, traveling away from home; and the need for a companion to help manage a feared situation. Avoidance of these situations is a major source of disability in persons with Panic Disorder.

▮ Definition/Symptoms of Selected Major Categories

Panic Disorder (PD) Without Agoraphobia[*]

This category includes recurrent, unexpected Panic Attacks that do not include phobic avoidance but may include ongoing worry about further attacks, worry that attack means person is going crazy or may be having heart attack; and avoidance of social situations because of fear or embarrassment of attack occurring in front of others.

Panic Disorder (PD) With Agoraphobia[†]

This category includes recurrent, unexpected Panic Attacks that include rigid phobic avoidance of anxiety-producing situations.

Agoraphobia Without History of Panic Disorder[‡]

This category includes Agoraphobia related to fear of experiencing sudden onset of incapacitating or embarrassing panic-like symptoms, such as losing control of bodily functions, fainting, and lying helpless.

Specific Phobia[§]

A phobia is an obvious and persistent fear of identified and specific objects or situations with an immediate anxiety

[*]References 2,16,18,46   [‡]References 2,16,18
[†]References 2,18   [§]References 2,16

response when exposed to feared stimulus, e.g., fear or avoidance of animals, insects, storms, heights, water, blood or injury; fear cued by invasive medical procedures; fear of public transportation, enclosed places; crying, tantrums, freezing, or clinging in children who are exposed to phobic stimulus; recognition by adults and adolescents that fear is excessive or unreasonable (children may not be able to discern); avoidance of situations that could result in contracting an illness; avoidance by children of loud sounds or costumed characters; intensification of fear, anxiety when forced to face phobic stimulus or perception that escape is limited.

Social Phobia (Social Anxiety Disorder)[*]

Social Phobia is an intense fear and/or avoidance of social or performance situations perceived as potentially humiliating or embarrassing in the presence of others, e.g., public speaking; immediate increase in anxiety or distress when forced to endure feared situation; expressed in children by crying, having tantrums, avoiding situations with unfamiliar people; recognition by adults and adolescents that fear is excessive or unreasonable; noticeable distress from phobia.

Obsessive-Compulsive Disorder (OCD)[†]

Obsessions are conscious, intrusive, inappropriate, recurrent, unwanted ideas, thoughts, or impulses that often cause anxiety or discomfort to the person experiencing them; sometimes referred to as "ego-dystonic," they are perceived to be outside one's own control but coming from within one's own mind. Examples include fears of contamination or committing a horrifying act; repetitious thoughts of reprehensible sexual or aggressive acts; and fear that harm may come to self or others because of own actions. Attempts to ignore or neutralize obsessions may lead to compulsive behaviors. Compulsions are conscious, recurrent, repetitive actions or behavior, e.g., time-consuming rituals such as checking locks, gas stove, mailbox; cleaning of hands, dishes, floors; trichotillomania (compulsive hair pulling); nail biting; or constant requests for reassurance.

[*]References 2,16,38,39
[†]References 2,16,18

Thoughts and actions are recognized as illogical but attempts to suppress them result in extreme psychological discomfort (children may lack cognitive awareness to recognize). Obsessions or compulsions are often complicated by Major Depression.

Posttraumatic Stress Disorder (PTSD)[*]

PTSD refers to the development of distinctive symptoms that follow an individual's exposure to and personal experience with a traumatic stressor of actual or threatened death, serious injury, or other threat to the person's physical integrity. Additional examples of traumatic stressors are "witnessing an event that involves death, injury, or threat to the physical integrity of another person; or learning about unexpected or violent death, serious harm, or threat of death or injury experienced by a family member or other close associate".[2, p. 424] PTSD is identified as *Acute* if symptom duration is less than 3 months, *Chronic* if symptom duration is more than 3 months, and *With Delayed Onset* if symptoms do not begin until at least 6 months after the stressor. Common symptoms in adults include:

1. Reenactment and avoidance, e.g., recurrent, distressing daydreams or nightmares of event; vivid images, flashbacks, illusions, hallucinations associated with stressor; intrusive recollections of event(s); numbing of general responsiveness; avoidance of thoughts, feelings, conversations, activities, places, or people associated with traumatic event(s); amnesia of varying periods of time associated with trauma; dissociative states ranging from minutes to days with perception of reliving event
2. Physiological symptoms, e.g., increased arousal that may include problems falling or remaining asleep
3. Psychological symptoms, e.g., intense fear, helplessness, horror; intense distress, anxiety, anger when exposed to cues that symbolize or resemble traumatic event; markedly diminished interest or participation in significant activities; feeling detached, estranged from others; difficulty experiencing intimacy with significant others; constriction of feelings of affection; sense of foreshortened future, e.g., no expectations of having career, family, nor-

[*]References 2,4,13,16,44

mal life span; irritability or angry outbursts; problems with concentration; hypervigilance, e.g., fear of going out alone, precaution of sitting with back to wall in public place; exaggerated startle response; survivor guilt, guilt about inability to prevent traumatic event. Common symptoms in children include disorganized, agitated behavior as a result of their intense fear, helplessness and horror, and flashbacks, e.g., repetitive play that may include themes or aspects of trauma-specific reenactment.

Acute Stress Disorder*

Acute Stress Disorder is the development of characteristic anxiety, dissociative and other symptoms that occur within a 1-month period after an individual has been exposed to a traumatic event with the person experiencing or witnessing situation(s) of an actual or threatened death or serious injury, or a threat to the physical integrity of the person or others. Specific (dissociative) symptoms may include numbing, detachment, absence of emotional responsiveness, sensation of being "in a daze," decreased awareness of surroundings, derealization, depersonalization, inability to recall important aspect of trauma, as well as other symptoms that are characteristic of PTSD.

Generalized Anxiety Disorder (GAD)†

Generalized Anxiety Disorder is persistent anxiety and worry over minor matters, everyday routines, and responsibilities with an intensity, duration, or frequency that is far out of proportion to the actual probability or effect from the feared happening. Excessive worry interferes with attention to and concentration on current tasks and is often accompanied by additional symptoms such as muscle tension, irritability, feeling keyed up or on edge, being easily fatigued, problems falling or remaining asleep, restless and unsatisfactory sleep, and experiencing clinically significant distress or impairment in important areas of functioning. Children worry about their performance or competence, even when not being evaluated by others; they may also worry about catastrophic events (e.g., natural disasters, nuclear war), be overly conforming, perfectionist, unsure of

*References 2,4,44
†References 2,8,16

self, and overly eager to seek approval and reassurance about performance.

Anxiety Disorder Due to a General Medical Condition*

This category refers to anxiety that is the direct result of the physiological effects of a general medical condition (e.g., endocrine, cardiovascular, respiratory [COPD], metabolic, neurological). Client history, physical examination, or laboratory findings indicate that anxiety is a direct physiological consequence of the general medical condition. The most common manifestation is a syndrome similar to PD; the least common manifestation is a syndrome similar to phobia.

Substance-Induced Anxiety Disorder†

This category includes anxiety symptoms, e.g., those associated with Generalized Anxiety, Panic Attacks, obsessions, or compulsions that occur within approximately 4 weeks of intoxication or withdrawal syndrome and do not occur within the course of delirium (Acute Confusion) determined to be due to direct physiological effects of ingested substance (e.g., alcohol, drugs, caffeine) and are in excess of those usually associated with intoxication or withdrawal syndrome.

▌ Incidence‡

Anxiety Disorders are the most frequently occurring psychiatric disorders in the general population; symptoms are common in general hospital populations. Phobias are the most frequently occurring Anxiety Disorder, affecting women two to three times more often than men; Agoraphobia and other Anxiety Disorders are common in elderly women. The prevalence of PD (1% 6-month, 1% to 2% 1 year, and 1.5% to 3% lifetime) is likely underestimated because of the difficulty differentiating among many medical illnesses during evaluations in medical settings. OCD has a 10% occurrence in outpatient settings with a lifetime prevalence of 2% to 3% and an earlier onset in males (6 to 15 years old) than females (20 to 29 years old). The incidence in PTSD varies from 1% to 14% in the general popu-

*References 2,18
†References 2,18
‡References 2,14,16,18,31–33

lation to 3% to 75% lifetime prevalence for at-risk individuals, e.g., combat veterans, victims of violence. GAD is a frequent comorbid disorder with Social Phobia and Simple Phobia as well as other mental disorders.

Course[*]

The course varies from acute, severe onset with a brief wave of intense anxiety accompanied by marked cognitive, physiologic, and behavioral components to lower-grade persistent distress. It may occur in conjunction with medical illness or other psychiatric disorders; there is considerable functional impairment and distress if untreated, e.g., interference in ability to accomplish expected routines and maintain occupational or academic responsibilities; social relationships are impaired. Complications of PTSD include Panic Attacks, depression, Substance Abuse, somatic complaints, self-injury, suicide attempts; marital discord; and impairment in social, occupational, or other important areas of functioning. The course of an Anxiety Disorder is often complicated by Major Depression and may overlap, as in agitated depression.

Contributing Factors to Anxiety Disorders

Neurobiological/Genetic[†]

- Cardiovascular, gastrointestinal, and respiratory symptoms are associated with stimulation of autonomic nervous system, e.g., hypoxia.
- Neurotransmitters such as norepinephrine in poorly regulated noradrenergic system with occasional bursts of activity have been associated with Anxiety Disorders; there is a possible association between increased serotonin and anxiety; it is hypothesized that some Anxiety Disorders may result from abnormal functioning of gamma aminobutyric acid (GABA) receptors; PD often worsens in the first week of treatment with antidepressants and then improves.
- Functional cerebral pathology may be causally relevant to symptoms of Anxiety Disorder in some clients.

[*]References 16,31,34,35
[†]References 16,31,34,35

- There is increased risk of PD among first-degree relatives of clients with PD, e.g., over one-half of clients with PD have an affected relative(s).
- There is a possible involvement of the cerebral cortex in the production of Anxiety Disorders; increased activity in septohippocampal pathway in limbic system could cause anxiety and possible implication of cingulate gyrus in limbic system with pathophysiology of OCD; possible role of locus ceruleus as primary source of noradrenergic innervation of limbic system cerebral cortex, cerebellum, and hypothalamus in memory retrieval facilitation as manifested by flashbacks, traumatic nightmares associated with PTSD; possible association between trauma-induced dysregulation of multiple neurobiologic systems and PTSD-related symptoms, e.g., chronic hyperarousal, recurrent intrusive memories, impulsivity, and numbing, as well as substance abuse.
- Fight-flight response is closely involved with serotoninergic and dopaminergic systems.
- There is a possible cerebral basis for OCD, e.g., onset after head trauma, EEG abnormalities, occasional findings of frontal lobe dysfunction.
- An unknown mechanism in sodium lactate causes Panic Attacks in clients with PD with no effect on normal controls.
- An association between Panic Attacks and abnormalities in respiratory function has been hypothesized.
- There is a possible autonomic dysfunction in PTSD.
- Adenosinergic dysfunction is hypothesized because of hypersensitivity to caffeine in clients with PD.

Psychological Model[*]

- Intrapsychic conflict with anxiety arouses ego to mobilize repression and other defenses to offset threat against pressures from within.
- Stressful events may have unconscious meaning, leading to Panic Attacks that may be related to neurophysiological factors precipitated by psychological reactions.
- Developmental factors such as overprotective parents, stressful life events may be involved.

[*]References 16,18

Conditioned Reflex Theories[*]

- Phobic anxiety is seen as a conditioned response in the emergence of some phobic symptoms.
- Obsessions and compulsive rituals serve as escape/avoidance responses to decrease anxiety associated with a specific environmental event.
- Learned helplessness model is used to explain negative symptoms of avoidance and social withdrawal in PTSD.

Cultural Factors[†]

- Cultural variations in presentation, expression of and impairment from anxiety.
- Anxiety-related behaviors may be an expression of distress when client feels overwhelmed.
- Culture-bound syndromes may be related to PD.

▌ Laboratory Findings[‡]

Laboratory tests, e.g., CBC, vitamin B_{12} and folate levels, EKG, drug levels of currently prescribed medications, thyroid function tests, blood sugar, pulse oximetry (less invasive than blood gases), as well as drug and alcohol screening, are used to diagnose underlying conditions that can cause signs and symptoms of anxiety.

Toxicology screen may be ordered if client is suspected of surreptitious drug use.

▌ Physical Examination Findings

Increased pulse rate, rapid breathing, sweating, and trembling, and dermatologic problems from excessive washing/cleansing.

▌ Special Assessment Considerations[§]

- Look for possible underlying medical problem as source for anxiety, especially in a client with late onset and no previous history of anxiety.

[*]References 18,28   [‡]References 2,15,34,35
[†]References 2,21,24,29   [§]References 2,7,11,14,15,21,22,24,29,32,34,35

- Review prescribed and illicit medication, caffeine, nicotine, and alcohol history to determine possible contributing factors to signs and symptoms of anxiety; marijuana commonly triggers Panic Attacks.
- Focus on history of current and past illness as well as family history for indications of remissions and relapses indicative of PD.
- Assess for Major Depression and suicide risk, particularly in client with PD.
- Conduct a brief cultural assessment to determine if anxiety responses to a situation are excessive, exceed cultural norms, or interfere with social role functioning.
- Obtain history of recent major stressful events to detect possible unrecognized post-traumatic stress symptomatology.
- Assess for consequences of civilian stressors in rape and motor vehicle accident victims, police, firefighters, body handlers, health care providers.
- Be attentive to the presence of medical stressors that increase the risk for Acute and Chronic PTSD in clients with catastrophic medical illness.
- Observe for presence of dermatologic problems that could be due to excessive washing with water or caustic cleaning preparations in clients with OCD.

▌ Treatment

Psychopharmacologic*

SPECIFIC DISORDERS AND DRUG TREATMENT

See Chapter 4 for drug class, action, and dosage.

1. PD with Agoraphobia: antidepressants are the first line of choice; tricyclics, e.g., imipramine and monoamine oxidase inhibitor (MAOI), phenelzine; selective serotonin reuptake inhibitors (SSRIs), fluvoxamine plus gradual exposure to anxiety-producing situations have been effective in decreasing agoraphobic avoidance. A benzodiazepine, alprazolam, may be prescribed.
2. Social Phobia: minimal pharmacological research. Medications used include high-potency benzodiazepines, e.g.,

*References 3, 10,12,18–20,26,28,30,34,37,40,41, 45,46,48

alprazolam, clonazepam, and an MAOI, e.g., phenelzine. Propanolol, a beta blocker, reduces fear associated with performance anxiety (medication is taken prior to anxiety-producing activity).

3. OCD: TCAs and SSRIs are drugs of choice; another SSRI may be selected if client is refractory to initial SSRI; SSRI, fluoxetine, is widely prescribed; MAOIs are beneficial for some OCD clients with concurrent Panic Attacks; benzodiazepines are rarely useful.

4. PTSD: Medication focus is on treating adjunctive symptoms (depression and impulsivity) rather than core symptoms (hypervigilance and intrusive memories).

TCA, imipramine or MAOI, phenelzine: helpful for management of nightmares and intrusive memories; there is evidence that SSRIs such as fluoxetine and fluvoxamine alleviate chronic symptoms of nightmares, insomnia, anxiety, and intrusive recollections; sertraline is helpful in reducing dysphoria, irritability, and social volatility.

Benzodiazepines: adjuncts to antidepressant treatment of free-floating anxiety and sometimes for alleviation of sleep difficulty.

Anti-convulsant: carbamazepine for impulsivity, hyperarousal, intrusive recollections, sleep impairment, and hostility.

Beta blockers: propanolol for clients with persistent symptoms of autonomic arousal when there are no medical contraindications.

Antipsychotics: for severe impulsivity and psychotic-like symptoms.

5. GAD: Anxiolytic options include benzodiazepines and buspirone for short-term management of symptoms; there is controversy about their use for long-term treatment. Specific drug selection is based on drug potency, half-life, and side effects. Buspirone has a slow onset (full effect at 3 to 6 weeks), which is a major drawback. Imipramine, a TCA, is used for anxiety associated with depression; SSRIs with treatment effectiveness after 1 month or longer on medication.

CONTRAINDICATIONS/CAUTIONS

See Chapter 4.

GENERAL NURSING IMPLICATIONS[*]

- Obtain history of possible allergic and adverse reactions to all medications client has taken in the past as well as history of preexisting conditions, e.g., cardiac, kidney, visual, neurologic, endocrine.
- Ensure ongoing monitoring of client's overall physical status, e.g., appetite, weight, vital signs, vision, bowel sounds, elimination; obtain liver and kidney function tests, as well as specific and routine laboratory findings.
- Obtain a baseline mental status and be alert for subtle as well as obvious changes, e.g., mood and affect, suicidal ideation/intent, changes in attention, concentration, alertness.
- Observe for indications of paradoxical effect, e.g., increased excitability, anxiety.

SPECIFIC NURSING IMPLICATIONS[†]

- Benzodiazepines: Potential for problems with abuse, dependence, withdrawal, and tolerance; physical withdrawal from abrupt discontinuation of medication; rebound of original symptoms with discontinuation in some cases; minimal risk for overdose unless taken in conjunction with alcohol; increased risk for mental status changes in elderly, especially benzodiazepines with active metabolites, e.g., diazepam, chlordiazepoxide.
- TCAs: Minimal potential for dependence; serious potential for overdose (most commonly prescribed drug used in suicide attempts) and for sudden occurrence of cardiovascular reactions that can cause acute heart failure; major cardiovascular risk is orthostatic hypotension; serious drug interactions with CNS depressants, e.g., antipsychotics, benzodiazepines, sedatives, anticonvulsants, alcohol, and certain antihypertensive drugs; need for lag time of minimum of 14 days when changing from TCA to MAOI to avoid potential hypertensive crisis; need for attentiveness to overall anticholinergic effects from all medications prescribed for client to minimize "atropine-poisoning" effect; elderly are particularly vulnerable to interaction from central and peripheral effects of anticholinergic medication.
- SSRIs: Use with caution with any medication that causes CNS depression.

[*]References 19,20
[†]References 3,19,20,22,30

- MAOIs: Require close monitoring for compliance, particularly in area of dietary management, as well as avoidance of non-prescribed medication. (See Chapter 4 for a listing of specific precautions, including dietary management and drug interactions.)
- Anticonvulsant, carbamazepine: Reduce the likelihood of gastrointestinal upset by giving with food; arrange for monitoring of serum levels.
- Azaspirone, buspirone: Improvement of target symptoms, e.g., decreased agitation, improved concentration within first several days of administration, delayed onset of 3 to 6 weeks to achieve maximal therapeutic effect as anxiolytic; minimal likelihood of overdose fatality; cannot be readily substituted for benzodiazepines, which must be tapered gradually during initiation of buspirone; no impairment of cognitive and motor functioning during treatment; minimal additive effects with alcohol.

GENERAL CLIENT/FAMILY EDUCATION[*]

- Take medication exactly as prescribed and do not stop taking medication without discussing plan with health care provider; do not take over-the-counter medication without provider's knowledge.
- Avoid alcohol while taking medication.
- Encourage use of hard candies, sugarless gum, frequent sips of water or ice chips when taking medication that causes a dry mouth.
- Implement precautions to reduce likelihood of injury if medication affects vision, e.g., use caution driving and avoid use of heavy equipment until side effects subside; remove objects in home environment that are conducive to falls.
- Monitor food and fluid intake and elimination to minimize problems with urinary retention, constipation; encourage high fiber diet and large amounts of water to be taken in conjunction with medication that has anticholinergic effect.
- If orthostatic hypotension is a problem, teach the client to avoid abrupt changes from lying to standing, beginning by sitting on side of bed, dangling feet, and rising slowly.

[*]References 19,20

SPECIFIC CLIENT/FAMILY EDUCATION[*]

- TCAs: Report eye pain immediately (possible acute glaucoma attack); wear appropriate clothing and exercise sensibly if anhidrosis is a problem; blurred vision is common owing to anticholinergic side effects.
- MAOIs: Full therapeutic effect of medication may require 10 days to 4 weeks; inform all health care providers when taking this medication (consider use of MedicAlert bracelet as well); discuss with health care provider extent of dietary adherence in avoiding tyramine-rich foods to prevent food–drug interactions. (See Chapter 4 for specific listing.)
- Benzodiazepines: Emphasize the potential for abuse and that the medication is not intended for management of everyday life stresses; emphasize potentiation of alcohol and other CNS depressants when taking benzodiazepines; hypersensitivity to one benzodiazepine may mean hypersensitivity to another; do not abruptly discontinue.
- Anticonvulsant, carbamazepine: Avoid alcohol or over-the-counter drugs; always use contraceptive techniques; notify health care provider of unusual bleeding, bruising, jaundice, abdominal pain, pale stools, darkened urine, impotence, CNS disturbances, edema, fever, chills, sore throat, or mouth ulcer.
- Azaspirone, buspirone: Emphasize delayed achievement of full therapeutic effects with expectation of improvement of target symptoms within a few days prior to increasing initial dosage.

Psychotherapy/Self Regulation Methods[†]

- Traditional psychotherapy is of limited usefulness with the possible exception of GAD; insight-oriented psychotherapy is beneficial for clients with PD and Agoraphobia.
- Hypnosis and supportive therapy are useful to clients with phobias.
- Family therapy is helpful for clients with phobias and OCD.
- Cognitive/behavioral therapy, individual or group, is useful for treatment of OCD, PTSD and phobias; relaxation training (see Stress Management in Chapter 5), cognitive restructuring techniques and real life (in vivo) exposure

[*]References 19,20,22
[†]References 1,5,6,9,12,15,16,18,28,32,34–36,43, 47

or fantasy (in vitro) exposure using imagery scenarios to recreate phobic situation; meditation.

- Symptom hierarchy for OCD to facilitate client's breaking down fears and anxieties into manageable goals for working with behavioral interventions.
- Substance Abuse treatment is often recommended for clients with PD and PTSD because of the high rate of abuse for these populations.
- Psychoeducational/supportive treatment may include referral to local support groups, e.g., Recovery Inc., and organizations.
- Cognitive/behavioral therapy for Panic Attacks includes focus on breathing retraining to control acute and chronic hyperventilation; voluntary hyperventilation followed by breathing retraining.
- Group therapy (group-centered analytic, psychoanalytically oriented psychotherapy, psychoanalysis in group, psychodrama, time-limited, behavior therapy, transactional analysis, Gestalt, and combined individual and group therapy) may be useful for selected clients, e.g., those with a history of some level of gratification in significant early relationships, with severe anxiety in one-to-one relationships and with significant dependency needs. Clients with PTSD benefit from group interventions.
- Crisis intervention is used for PTSD.
- Electromyographic feedback (EMG) can be beneficial.

▌Commonly Occurring Nursing Diagnoses

Altered thought processes
Anxiety
Altered social interaction: compulsive behaviors
   (Accepted by NANDA for development, NANDA 1994)
Compulsive behaviors
Fear
Impaired skin integrity
Impaired social interaction
Ineffective individual coping
Post-trauma response
Powerlessness
Rape-trauma syndrome

Rape-trauma syndrome: compound reaction
Rape-trauma syndrome: silent reaction
Risk for infection
Risk for impaired skin integrity
Risk for loneliness
Sleep pattern disturbance
Social isolation

▍ Selected Nursing Diagnoses, Outcome Criteria, and Nursing Interventions With Rationale

NURSING DIAGNOSIS #1:[*]   *Anxiety related to perceived failure of adaptive coping skills*

EXPECTED CLIENT OUTCOME

- Client will experience reduced level of anxiety as evidenced by increased recognition of factors that predispose to or precipitate anxiety and development of adaptive coping strategies for prevention and management of anxiety.

NURSING INTERVENTIONS WITH RATIONALE

- Encourage description of perceptions of distress or uneasiness, *to determine level of anxiety as it may impact client's ability to engage in specific treatment strategies.*
- Assess for presence of undetected physical or mental disorder; *anxiety symptoms often accompany undetected physical illness as well as mental disorders, e.g., depression.*
- Obtain specific information about prescribed, over-the-counter, and illicit drugs, as well as tobacco habits, alcohol, and caffeine intake *to determine possible influence on anxiety.*
- Have client describe daily routines, including rest, activity, and sleep pattern *to determine the impact of anxiety in general and in specific areas of functioning.*
- Determine client's current ability to recognize the presence of anxiety, *a prerequisite for increased awareness of anxiety-provoking situations.*
- Engage client in health teaching that includes content such as recognition that a degree of anxiety is part of living and that mild levels of anxiety can enhance learning

[*]References 16,18,25,28,50,51

and problem-solving; development of a realistic physical activity program that can be followed through on a regular basis; establishment of sleep hygiene practices; minimization or avoidance of caffeine intake; and assertive communication skills (see Assertiveness Training in Chapter 5), *to promote client's perception of constructive management of anxiety.*

- Encourage incorporation of selected stress management techniques, e.g., progressive relaxation (client must be taught specific techniques), music, or reading (see also Stress Management in Chapter 5) *to prevent or minimize anxiety.*
- Encourage client to explore possible solutions for preventing or alleviating anxiety, e.g., change in rest and activity, engaging in pleasurable social interactions, making dietary changes.
- Develop a specific discharge plan based on client's achievement of mutually determined treatment goals (see also Stress Management in Chapter 5).

NURSING DIAGNOSIS #2:[*] *Fear related to anticipatory anxiety about Panic Attacks*

EXPECTED CLIENT OUTCOME

- Client will experience increased sense of control in management of Panic Attacks, using health-promoting strategies for the prevention and alleviation of attacks.

NURSING INTERVENTIONS WITH RATIONALE

- Obtain specific information about prescribed, over-the-counter, and illicit drug use, as well as tobacco habits, alcohol and caffeine intake *to determine possible influence on exacerbation of attacks and management; marijuana is an often unreported cause of Panic Attacks.*
- Collaborate with treatment team in looking for possible underlying medical problems *that may be contributing factors to Panic Attacks.*
- Assess for presence of stressful life events, particularly loss; *clients with history of Panic Attacks may experience greater distress about life events.*
- Assess suicidal ideation/intent; *clients with history of Panic Attacks are at increased risk for suicide attempts;*

[*]References 16,18,23,49,50,51

they have a 15% lifetime risk of suicide, especially if they have co-existing Alcohol Abuse.

- Encourage client's specific description of the frequency and severity of attacks and occurrence of hyperventilation (*a central feature in pathophysiology of Panic Attacks*) and what actually occurs, *to obtain information for appropriate treatment planning and interventions.*
- Determine extent to which client has been able to discuss the problem with the family; *people with PD often maintain secrecy about symptoms, resulting in worry by family and friends about the meaning of behavioral changes.*
- Encourage client to talk about concerns with family and friends *to minimize possible feelings of stigma and helplessness.*
- Collaborate with the treatment team regarding a plan that includes client and family; *pharmacologic and cognitive-behavioral management are considered the most effective treatments; group therapy may be helpful for both client and family in management of related psychosocial difficulties.*
- Encourage client description of areas of perceived control, as well as helplessness, in current anxiety management.
- Offer realistic hope for improvement in client's ability to manage symptoms.
- Based on interdisciplinary treatment plan:
  - incorporate stress management techniques that include behavioral retraining *to decrease frequency of Panic Attacks by not hyperventilating* (see also Stress Management in Chapter 5);
  - ensure client knowledge of medication management, purpose, dosage, side effects, dietary considerations;
  - encourage development of individual plan for physical activities that is realistic for follow-through on a regular basis *to ensure client's success in achieving increased control over symptom management*;
  - refer client to resources, such as Anxiety Disorders Association of America (ADAA).
- Provide opportunity for client to review progress in development of constructive coping strategies.
- Collaborate with interdisciplinary treatment team for coordination of discharge plans, as appropriate (see also Discharge Planning in Chapter 5).

NURSING DIAGNOSIS #3:[*] *Altered Social Interaction: Compulsive Behaviors Related to OCD*

EXPECTED CLIENT OUTCOME

- Client will experience reduced anxiety and need for ritualistic behavior as evidenced by decrease in use of ritualistic behavior and use of effective anxiety-reducing techniques.

NURSING INTERVENTIONS WITH RATIONALE

- Use calm, quiet, caring approach when interacting with client *to help client become more comfortable in talking about thoughts and feelings.*
- Encourage client to talk about compulsive behaviors, including the extent to which rituals interfere with the performance of activities of daily living and role expectations.
- Observe for expression of feelings of distress associated with ritualistic behaviors, including client perception that compulsions are not within his or her control.
- Assess for behaviors indicative of co-morbid Major Depression *because the client's prognosis is directly related to the recognition and appropriate management of depression.*
- Avoid judgmental attitude or disapproval of client's behavior; *client may already feel embarrassed about irrational aspects of compulsive behaviors.*
- Avoid confrontation of compulsive, ritualistic behaviors *to minimize client attempts to maintain secrecy about self.*
- Provide opportunity for discussion of anxiety-provoking situations and client's responses to them *to increase client awareness in management of his or her anxiety.*
- Assist client to increase range of strategies to decrease anxiety, e.g., identifying feelings, controlling unwanted accompanying thoughts, developing schedule of daily activities that includes exercise, and planning for leisure time and hobbies *to increase client's sense of control in minimizing or extinguishing unwanted behaviors and to increase level of comfort in social interactions and relationships.*
- Encourage client to avoid introducing too much change in daily routine *to minimize the feeling of being overwhelmed with new activities.*

[*]References 16,18,27,49,59

- Teach client to engage in normal activities that allow time for rituals that client is not ready to relinquish; *total abstinence from compulsive behaviors is usually an unrealistic expectation.*
- Convey recognition of client accomplishments.
- Teach client to learn to reward self for engaging in non-ritualistic behaviors.

NURSING DIAGNOSIS #4:[*]   *Post-trauma Response (PTR), related to traumatic combat experiences*

EXPECTED CLIENT OUTCOME

- Client will experience increased self-control over post-trauma responses and will develop constructive strategies for "living well" with residual symptoms as evidenced by expressing feelings appropriately, refraining from Alcohol Abuse, experiencing improved sleep patterns, and identifying constructive resources for working with PTR.

NURSING INTERVENTIONS WITH RATIONALE

- Elicit information about client's current psychological functioning and trauma exposure *to obtain necessary factual information for appropriate treatment planning. Limit exploration of details that should be deferred to formal individual or group treatment sessions. There is a risk of worsened outcome if client is pushed too quickly to delve into trauma history.*
- Determine impact of symptoms on family, vocational, and social functioning.
- Obtain specific information about sleep pattern disturbances, including likelihood of startle reflex; *combat PTR can include client's automatically striking out when suddenly awakened, particularly if client is awakened by being touched*; post sign at bedside (for inpatients) informing staff that client startles easily, should be called by name only, and not be touched to awaken.
- Encourage description of client's initial treatment expectations.
- Evaluate need for brief supportive discussion following initial assessment *to provide opportunity for client to focus on thoughts and feelings generated by interview.*

[*]References 1,9,13,16,36,41,42

- Collaborate with interdisciplinary team *to avoid possible interdisciplinary conflict that would compromise treatment;* determine:
  - appropriate treatment setting, e.g., inpatient or outpatient, for client to focus on PTR management, including Alcohol Abuse;
  - pharmacologic management of client's intrusive recollections and recurrent nightmares;
  - specific treatment modalities, e.g., individual, group, alcohol treatment, family therapy; cognitive restructuring, skills training; relaxation techniques for management of underlying anxiety and insomnia (see also Stress Management in Chapter 5, Referral to a Veterans Center).
- Encourage appropriate expression of feelings; set realistic limits as necessary if feelings of anger or rage are indicative of impulsive acting-out behaviors.
- Teach client to learn constructive coping with excess negative feelings and energy by engaging in physical activities, such as working out in a gym or walking.
- Collaborate with team in development of treatment plan that incorporates family system issues, e.g., psychoeducation *to provide framework for working with family problems as a family challenge*; family therapy *to focus on supportive energy instead of traumatogenic* and to promote focus on identified actual client needs instead of playing non-helpful auxiliary roles in client's traumatic reenactment.

NURSING DIAGNOSIS #5:[*]   *Post-trauma response (PTR) related to physical assault on elderly male adult by trusted adult granddaughter*

EXPECTED CLIENT OUTCOME

- Client will experience reduced anxiety as evidenced by verbalization of strengths for managing aftermath of assault and identification of appropriate discharge plans that ensure personal safety and availability of supportive resources for continuing trauma follow-up.

NURSING INTERVENTIONS WITH RATIONALE

- Permit client to proceed at his own pace in verbalizing perceptions, thoughts, and feelings associated with assault (see also Crisis Intervention in Chapter 5). *Allow-*

[*]References 25,41,42

ing client to proceed at his own pace increases the sense of control, which often serves to enable client to provide additional information with minimal increase of anxiety.

- Listen for client's explanation of what occurred before, during, and following assault *to clarify client's current perceptions, to detect possible pattern of previous abuse by family or others, and to determine appropriateness of client's returning to previous living situation.*
- Assess extent of physical injury *to determine need for medical intervention.*
- Provide opportunity for concerned family members to discuss their perceptions and concerns about the assault *to facilitate their understanding of the client's adjustment as well as their own adjustment.*
- Collaborate with treatment team in obtaining sufficient history from client and other family members *to substantiate factual information about event, ensuring a coordinated treatment plan that addresses legal and safety issues during hospitalization as well as continuity of care after discharge.*
- Determine client's level of PTR as it impacts on his sleep patterns, overall perception of safety in hospital environment, and perception of safety after discharge.
- Encourage client identification of currently perceived coping resources, e.g., beliefs about self and others, energy level, morale, family and social support; *there is an increased likelihood of favorable outcome when client sees traumatic situation as manageable.*
- Collaborate with treatment team in coordination of client's return to previously established family and community social support (see also Abuse Protection in Chapter 5).
- Provide client and family with written information about additional available community resources (see also Discharge Planning in Chapter 5).

CHAPTER 12

Somatoform Disorders

▊ Definition/Major Symptoms

The Somatoform Disorders are a group of disorders characterized by multiple somatic complaints with no actual physical illness, although complaints may closely resemble a physical disease. It involves use of physical symptoms to communicate feeling states to others.

The major symptoms are:

- Physical symptoms associated with the gastrointestinal, sexual, and neurological systems
- Pain
- Symptoms that are inexplicable by physical or laboratory findings
- Emotional distress; the client may have a history of another psychiatric disorder.

▊ Definition/Major Symptoms of Selected Categories*

Somatization Disorder

This is characterized by a history (before the age of 30) of multiple physical complaints with no medical basis. The individual experiences emotional distress and has impaired functioning in various family, social, and work roles.

*References 1,2,4,5,8,10,13,16,22,24,27,31,32,36

Symptoms occur in different body systems:

- Gastrointestinal symptoms: Minimum of *two*. Example: Nausea, diarrhea
- Sexual symptom: Minimum of *one*. Example: Menstrual irregularity, erectile problems
- Pseudo-neurological symptom: Minimum of *one*. Example: Amnesia, problems in swallowing
- Pain symptoms. Minimum of *four* sites or functions. Examples: Sites—head, abdomen, back, joints; functions—urination, sexual intercourse.

Conversion Disorder

This is characterized by complaints of a change or loss of function not explicable by a known pathophysiological mechanism.

- Types include:
  - *Motor symptoms or deficit*: Paralysis, mutism
  - *Sensory symptoms or deficit*: Paraesthesia, blindness, stocking and glove anesthesia of hands or feet, seizure or convulsions
  - *Mixed motor and sensory symptoms or deficit*
- Symptom occurs after stress or conflict.
- Symptoms may be associated with secondary gain, i.e., with a way to have another person do something or to avoid participation in an unpleasant situation.
- Symptoms may not be acknowledged openly by client; client may convey a lack of concern or a stoic attitude.

Pain Disorders

These are characterized by four pain factors:

1. Pain that is so significant, it requires clinical investigation
2. Pain that causes distress and interferes with social and occupational functioning
3. Pain that is affected by psychological factors, e.g., when it begins, how severe it becomes, how long it lasts, what causes it to occur.
4. Pain unassociated with other psychiatric disorders.

The disorders are classified as:

- Pain Disorder Associated with Psychological Factors; Acute (6 months or less) or Chronic
- Pain Disorder Associated With Both a Psychological Disorder and a General Medical Condition
- Pain Disorder Associated With a General Medical Condition. Note: This condition is noted on Axis III and is not a separate disorder.

Hypochondriasis

This is characterized by the presence of fear(s) of having a disease based on misinterpretations of symptoms lasting at least 6 months. This causes distress for the individual and impairment of social and work roles. Despite a medical evaluation and assurance that no disease exists, the client's distress continues. Anxiety and depression are also frequently present.

Body Dysmorphic Disorder

This is characterized by the presence of an imagined defect of one's body, primarily facial defects, e.g., wrinkles, too much hair, something wrong with eyebrows, lips, or nose. Other areas of imagined body deficits are the genitals, breasts, buttocks, abdomen, etc. The client experiences distress sufficient to interfere with social life and work. The disorder may be associated with Obsessive-Compulsive Disorder.

Body-checking behaviors may be noted, e.g., looking in mirror, frequently asking "Do I look alright?"; they are almost a compulsion.

The client is intent on hiding the defect, may compare the "ugly" feature with another person, and/or may repeatedly seek confirmation that he or she looks great.

■ Incidence*

Somatization Disorder

- The disorder occurs among 0.1% of the general population.

*References 1,12,13,22,25,32

It is the fourth most common diagnostic group seen in medical outpatient clinics.

Conversion Disorder

- This is found among 20% to 25% of patients in medical settings.

Pain Disorder

- It is believed to be common, but there are no reliable statistics. For example, it is found in 10% to 15% of cases in which back pain causes a disability.

Hypochondriasis

- This is found in perhaps 4% to 6% of clients in medical outpatient clinics.

Body Dysmorphic Disorder

- Incidence is unknown but probably not rare, because more clients are treated in medical settings, e.g., plastic surgeon's office, than by psychiatrists.

▌ Course*

Somatization Disorder

Onset may be noted in adolescence, with symptoms of the disorder clearly present by the age of 30. Multiple visits to the doctor(s) for vague and striking symptoms in various body parts are noted. New symptoms may arise at times of increased stress. The client has a poor health record and may have had multiple tests, treatments, or surgeries. Medications are minimally effective. Physicians may have prescribed a benzodiazepine or barbiturate that has led to addiction.

Conversion Disorder

Onset generally occurs between the ages 10 to 35 years, with an acute episode leading to evaluation in an emergency room

*References 1,3,5,8,13,19,22,31,35

or outpatient clinic. Generally the symptoms last a few days, perhaps months, before spontaneous recovery. It is important to note that 25% of clients have underlying medical condition(s) that may not be recognized on initial evaluation. Some clients have more than one Conversion Disorder episode, or the condition may become chronic.

Pain Disorders

Chronic Pain Disorder is variable in onset, and a psychiatrist may not be involved for years. Prognosis is affected by the client's ability to maintain daily activities without allowing his or her lifestyle to be controlled by the presence or absence of pain. Note: Chronic pain may lead to a depressive disorder. The presence of depression may also be an important predictor of chronic pain. Malingering is to be considered in the differential diagnosis.

Hypochondriasis

Onset may occur in adolescence or adulthood when the client becomes obsessed with the idea that he or she is ill. Shopping for a doctor occurs even though tests are normal. Psychiatrists are not sought. Prognosis is not good.

Body Dysmorphic Disorder

Little is known regarding the disorder; some personality traits may predispose a person to the disorder, e.g., obsessive-compulsive, schizoid, narcissistic, insecure, sensitive. Clients are frequently seen by dermatologists, plastic surgeons, and primary care physicians because improvement in their perceived ugliness or deficit is sought. Most clients avoid social situations; a few may refuse to leave home. The disorder may last several years or become increasingly worse over time. The client may experience depression and may become suicidal.

▌ Contributing Factors*

Etiology is unknown for all disorders in this group.

*References 2,7,10,13,16,22,25,26,30,35,36

Somatization Disorder

GENERAL

- Sex: Five times as many women are affected as men.
- Genetic Deficit: It has been found that 10% to 20% of first-degree relatives of the client have Somatization Disorder.
- Biological deficit: Studies suggest a deficit in cytokinese, a essential messenger in the immune system.
- Severe stress: Natural disasters, sexual trauma.

PSYCHOLOGICAL

Theories postulate the following about the disorder:

- It functions as a defense that allows a limited expression of discomfort in the form of physical symptoms; the symptoms are a way to communicate feelings and wishes, e.g., not wanting to go to a party or not wanting to talk to a mother-in-law because of angry feelings, and/or to make an indirect general statement about a situation as being disgusting or impossible.
- It functions as an amplification of the client's style in information processing. Some body sensations are greatly exaggerated, e.g., noise, presence of blood, temperature, body fluids, intestinal peristalsis.
- It functions as a means of seeking care for common symptoms or bodily sensations.
- It occurs as a result of the health care system, cultural forces, and medical procedures that serve to positively reinforce certain illness behaviors and the reporting of symptoms.
- It functions as an expression of depression or equivalent distress that the client is experiencing rather than a defense against the awareness of the distress.

CULTURE

In certain countries the disorder is associated with symptoms of particular diseases as follows:

- United States: Viruses, environmental disease, chemical sensitivity
- England: Constipation, red blotches on skin
- Germany: Low blood pressure, fatigue, poor circulation
- France: Headache, general fatigue, liver crisis

- Eastern Jews: Hypochondriasis, neurasthenia
- Latin America: "Nervios" with headache, trembling, heart palpitations, stomach problems, numbness, fainting, disturbed sleep
- Iran: "Narhati" or being depressed, anxious, not at ease

Conversion Disorder

- Biological studies suggest impaired communication between the cortex and brain stem.
- Psychoanalytic theory postulates that anxiety is caused by conflict between the expression of sexual and aggressive impulses and their repression. The resulting symptoms are an expression of the "bad" impulse and the client's need to obtain help (a solution). There is an element of secondary gain in that the conversion symptom may protect the client from others' blame or may help the client to obtain help and comfort from others.
- Interpersonal theory postulates that the behavior/symptom is a demand for attention, nurturing, and protection from pressure or obligation that occurs in the context of a perceived absence of a significant person(s) or relationship(s).
- Stress or trauma theory postulates that the conversion symptoms follow traumatic events, e.g., death, disaster, intense combat during war.
- Learned behavior theory postulates that the behavior is reinforced in family, community, and culture, thus becoming part of the client's behavior pattern as a way to deal with life.

Pain Disorder

- Sex: Twice as many females are affected as men.
- Socioeconomic: Lower class.
- Severe trauma and stress: Pelvic pain is associated with sexual or physical abuse. Orofacial pain is related to Major Depressive Disorder and Post-Traumatic Stress Disorder.
- Psychodynamic theory postulates that the symptoms are ways to express intrapsychic conflicts, express feeling states, meet dependency needs, deal with feelings of guilt, and be punished.

- Behavioral theory postulates that symptoms are reinforced or inhibited by others in the environment.

Hypochondriasis

- Psychodynamic theory, which is controversial, postulates that aggressive impulses that have been generated in the past are expressed when the person requests help for a physical problem but then refuses to accept the help. Another way to view this is that the person has low self-esteem. Feelings of unworthiness, badness, and then guilt are unconsciously dealt with through symptoms of hypochondriasis. It is postulated that the mother had problems helping the child individuate or separate self; therefore, the client remains in an infantile, regressive, physical realm.
- Cognitive theory postulates that misinterpretation of symptoms creates concern about the state of health for which the client seeks help. There is an exaggeration of bodily sensations. Health is believed to be a symptom-free state; many common and ambiguous symptoms are understood as indicators that a disease is present.
- Learning theory postulates that obtaining acceptance as a sick person relieves the client of problems and others' expectations.

Body Dysmorphic Disorder

BIOLOGICAL FACTORS

Biological theory postulates an involvement of serotonin neurotransmitter since the disorder is associated with Mood and Obsessive-Compulsive Disorders.

CULTURAL FACTORS

Physical attractiveness may be highly prized in some highly dependent relationships with a mother, within certain families, and in some cultures. A person may feel rejected or unloved if this criterion cannot be met.

PSYCHOLOGICAL FACTORS

- Several psychodynamic theories have been suggested, because the condition is not well understood. These include a displacement of sexual or emotional conflict into the body part; a defense against weak ego or overwhelming anxiety; a masking of disturbances in interpersonal communication and/or social relationships, e.g., offers explanations of failure to find boyfriend/girlfriend, explains the distress being experienced.

- Stress or trauma theory postulates that a casual remark made about a body feature or a more traumatic event, e.g., a fight with boyfriend, acts as a trigger for the development of the disorder.
- Growth and development theory suggests that the secondary sexual characteristics developing at adolescence could act as triggers, causing a weakening of ego and symptoms. Teasing, joking, or rejection experienced in early years also may increase the perception of a body part as ugly.

▌ Laboratory and Physical Examination Findings[*]

- *The client needs to be carefully screened for physical causes of the presenting symptoms.* A detailed description of symptoms, e.g., seizures, parasethesias, or pain, will assist in the diagnosis because the symptoms appear suddenly and are difficult to decipher or to understand. For example, a client may almost fall and hurt self but avert injury by avoiding falling on the chair or wall; a client who has lost consciousness may respond to painful stimuli; a client who is unable to obtain wanted medicine will cease to have pain in the leg and walk away freely; a client facing a stressful court case complains of chest pain, resulting in postponement of the case.
- The Minnesota Multiphasic Personality Inventory (MMPI) adds to data but should not dictate a primarily psychological focus. Clients with Pain Disorder may have high scores in MMPI on three scales: hypochondriasis, depressive, and hysteria.
- Amobarbital given IV may assist the physician in diagnosis of Conversion Disorder; the symptom will disappear under the influence of the medication.

[*]References 13,22,33,35

▌ Special Assessment Considerations*

- Physical symptoms must be carefully examined to determine their cause. There is always a possibility of a misdiagnosis. Over time a disease may develop as part of life events. Treatments for "a condition" may produce little or no improvement and no explanation can be found. Treatment can cause an iatrogenic injury, which compounds the problem of diagnosis and treatment, e.g., drug addiction.
- Presentation of symptoms of degenerative diseases, central nervous system and endocrine disorders, ulcers, or tuberculosis should lead clinicians to careful examinations.
- Several mental disorders also present with somatic symptoms, e.g., Major Depressive Disorder, Generalized Anxiety Disorder, and Schizophrenia. However, over time a cluster of symptoms will be apparent. When criteria are met for Hypochondriasis and other mental disorders, both diagnoses are given.
- Somatization has several meanings. The term is used to describe an immature defense mechanism in which psychological conflicts are converted into bodily symptoms. It is also a process that describes a more conscious use of physical symptoms to deal with problems in interpersonal relationships, such as a person hoping to obtain monetary gain by assuming a sick role. It can be viewed as a self-handicapping strategy. Society does give a sick person some relief from everyday demands; a sick person needs help from family and friends and more easily receives it in the sick role.

▌ Treatment†

Treatment occurs more frequently in outpatient settings than in psychiatric hospitals or clinics.

General Guidelines

- Treatment focuses on symptom management in three areas:
  1. Predisposing factors, e.g., past tendencies to somatize, problems in communicating, psychological conflict

*References 13,22,33,35
†References 2–4,6,9–11,13,14,17,18,20,21,30,34–36

2. Precipitating factor, e.g., sexual abuse, death
3. Factors perpetuating the conversion symptom, e.g., sick role

- Investigate and treat the underlying physical illness that the client presents most frequently, e.g., recurring pain, gastrointestinal problems, dizziness, and fatigue.
- In children, the presence of physical symptoms may indicate a medical condition, psychiatric disorder, e.g., Anxiety or Depressive Disorders, or maltreatment.
- Recognize the risk of misdiagnosis.
- Investigate and treat any new symptom(s) as they present.
- Management of treatment should be confined to *one physician/case manager* to foster development of a therapeutic alliance and to reduce focus on physical complaints.
- Reassurance is a process that conveys an attitude of acceptance of the validity of the client's symptom experience. It is communicated through an ongoing, trusting relationship with the client. It is not confrontational. It also implies continued review of data so that inappropriate reassurance is not given.
- Regularly scheduled appointments generally begin as a review of physical symptoms, after which psychological issues are approached.
- Review how symptom(s) are affecting important relationships and social and occupational functioning.
- Recognize the possibility of psychiatric disturbances, e.g., Malingering, Major Depressive Disorder (frequently present), Dissociative Disorder.
- Refer to psychiatric consultation when there is increasing severity of symptoms, especially depression; more disturbed behavior or relationships; or discovery of severe trauma/stress related to symptom presentation, e.g., sexual assault.
- Recognize the client's risk for addictive and self-destructive behaviors.
- Recognize the client's risk for iatrogenic complications.
- Involve the family and significant others in recognizing and changing expectations and behavior toward the client to avoid reinforcing sick role behaviors and secondary gain from bodily symptoms.

Somatization Disorder

- As rapport develops, more attention is directed toward life problems, coping styles, and the possibility that psychological stress may be a factor to consider. Eventually the client may be willing to see a mental health clinician.
- Psychotherapy focuses on assisting the client to manage the physical symptoms and to express and cope with underlying feelings. Positive reinforcement is given for behavior that is not "complaining" and not focused on bodily symptoms.
- If the client believes that symptoms are environmentally caused, e.g., a spray for insects, electromagnetic fields, working at a computer, the following suggestions are offered:
  - Review carefully the client's psychosocial history to identify stressors.
  - Note the presence of increased anxiety or alexithymia as indicators for psychiatric treatment.
  - Differentiate the disorder from a hygienic problem in the environment.
  - Avoid any suggestion that the spray, the work, etc., may be a cause until a differential diagnosis is completed.

Conversion Disorder

- Develop an authoritative-directive relationship with the client.
- Provide assurance that the problem/condition is not dangerous, will not cause an impairment, and can be easily corrected.
- Hospitalization may shorten the duration of treatment because it removes client from the stressful situation.
- Behavior modification: Assist the client in focusing on issues of secondary gain from assuming a sick role if he or she continues to experience episodes of Conversion Disorder.
- Family therapy focuses on resolving enmeshment, protection of the "sick" member, inflexibility within the family, and continued conflict; this is especially indicated if symptoms are reinforced by other family members and a number of episodes occur.

- If Conversion Disorder becomes chronic, it is treated in a similar manner to Somatization Disorder.

Pain Disorder

- Pain management, not pain reduction, is the focus of treatment.
- Psychological management focuses on learning to live with the pain and not to continue to search for a cure. The client may fear that an underlying condition exists and/or that when activity is increased, pain will also increase.
- The clinician–client relationship is very important because the client probably has experienced abandonment in the past or is currently experiencing abandonment and/or rejection. The client and clinician need to work together to manage the suffering.
- Coordinate care of the client's complaints with one physician/case manager because of the client's tendency to manipulate and to overuse medical facilities, tests, etc.
- Maintain an ongoing assessment of stress and trauma experienced, e.g., poor interaction with workers' compensation program, parts of the health care system, work, or family.
- Risk for suicide: Suicide ideation may increase when pain management is inadequate. Collaboration with other professionals to improve the management of pain is recommended.
- Pharmacological treatment: Guidelines for pain treatment:
  - Cancer, recovery from surgery and acute pain: Try nonsteroidal anti-inflammatory agents (NSAIDs) first; use mild opiates, e.g., acetaminophen with codeine, Vicodin, Percodan, before using stronger ones, e.g., morphine, hydromorphine; give medication on a fixed schedule.
  - Acute and chronic pain, especially bone cancer or metastasis, arthritis: Use NSAIDs.
  - Neuropathic pain, diabetic neuropathies, rheumatoid arthritis, osteoarthritis, migraine and cluster headaches, facial pain, fibromyalgia: Use antidepressants; tricyclics may be helpful if sleeplessness is experienced.
- Behavior psychotherapy focuses on reinforcing health behaviors and reducing self-defeating behaviors, which

include demanding that family member give medication or care, complaining about pain, using a wheelchair when it is not necessary, or refusing to go out. By receiving rewards for other alternatives, healthier behaviors are increased. Praise what the client can do; do not emphasize what he or she cannot do or does slowly. For example, give medication on a fixed schedule so that the client does not have to complain and display other behaviors to get medicine. The family and significant others are vital to the success of therapy. All need to promote healthy behaviors.

- Cognitive psychotherapy focuses on helping the client to understand the relationships among physiological, affective, and cognitive factors and the pain experience, to alter the techniques used to manage pain, and to learn new strategies; thus the client gains the knowledge and experience for controlling the pain. Relaxation techniques may be useful.
- Pain-control programs using a variety of treatment methods are effective in improving the management of chronic pain.
- Nerve blocks and surgery are used only after other modalities have proved ineffective, e.g., acupuncture, physical therapy, transcutaneous electrical nerve stimulation (TENS).

Hypochondriasis

- The physician–client relationship is the most important factor; only *one* physician/case manager should be involved to provide consistency. It is difficult to manage a long-term relationship with a client who is/has been doctor shopping or who is perceived to be a nuisance, dependent, and/or manipulative. The client is seeking care, not a cure. The physician is not going to "get rid" of the symptoms. It is essential to allow the client some dependency on the doctor/case manager but to be alert for regressive behaviors.
- Place the psychosocial history in a prominent place in client's chart to alert others to his or her behavior.
- Continue inquiry and data gathering regarding the context of the symptom experience to identify themes of

dealing with a loss, being disappointed or rejected, or feelings of helplessness.

- Refrain from additional laboratory tests and other procedures to check out new symptoms until more data are available.
- Other disorders must be treated first, e.g., major depression, Schizophrenia, cognitive impairment disorders, disorders secondary to general medical conditions or Substance Abuse, Malingering.
- Use palliative techniques for benign symptoms, e.g., a brief physical examination for current symptom, a vitamin or antihistamine, a special exercise, a bandage.
- Recognize that the presentation of physical symptoms is an attempt to communicate the client's emotional state. Involve the client in discussion of how work and other relationships add to his or her burden, e.g., "Is something else happening? Something is missing . . . It is difficult to understand." Improvement may be noted when communication is not focused only on the symptoms. The client needs to gradually accept stress as one reason for condition.
- Group cognitive psychotherapy focuses on managing stress and coping with the chronic illness/disability. Emphasis is placed on how attention paid to bodily symptoms increases their intensity. Explore new explanations for aches, pains, etc., experienced; explore how the client can tolerate a risk without worry; how circumstances increase the discomfort and what cues are being used to decide what may increase discomfort; the effect of anxiety and depression on bodily symptoms, e.g., increased awareness, anticipation of danger, misinterpretation.
- Pharmacological treatment: The use of fluoxetine and other antidepressants has been effective. If antianxiety drugs are used for temporary relief of anxiety or to avoid panic attacks or increasing fear, it is recommended that they be used in conjunction with psychotherapy.
- If hospitalization is indicated to assess a possible medical condition, the focus of treatment must remain on precipitating stressors.
- Limit referrals to specific symptoms and only after careful analysis. The client may experience additional rejection if the motivation for referral is frustration with the treating physician/case manager.

Body Dysmorphic Disorder

- Treat any co-morbid disorders, e.g., Anxiety or Personality Disorders.
- Behavior/cognitive psychotherapy focuses on developmental and current sources of focus on body image; realistic description of the defect; use of relaxation, exposure, thought-stopping techniques to manage distress; recognition and interruption of negative thoughts about self; specific ways to manage body checking, e.g., limit dressing time; relapse prevention.
- Plastic surgery is recommended only after collaboration with a psychiatrist and other appropriate medical specialist(s). Dermatological, surgical, and other techniques tried by clients are often perceived as ineffective.
- Pharmacological treatment: Use of antidepressants, particularly serotonin-specific drugs, e.g., fluoxetine and clomipramine, has been reported to be helpful.

▌Commonly Occurring Nursing Diagnoses

Anxiety
Body image disturbance
Caregiver role strain
Coping, defensive
Coping, ineffective individual
Denial, ineffective
Family processes, altered
Fear
Grieving, dysfunctional
Health maintenance, altered
Injury, risk for
Knowledge deficit (specify)
Management of therapeutic regimen, individual: ineffective
Noncompliance
Pain
Pain, chronic
Post-trauma response
Powerlessness
Rape trauma syndrome
Relocation stress syndrome
Self-esteem disturbance or chronic low

Self-mutilation, risk for
Sexual dysfunction
Sexual pattern, altered
Social isolation
Violence, risk for, self-directed

▮ Selected Nursing Diagnoses, Outcome Criteria, and Nursing Interventions With Rationale*

Example: Client With Somatization Disorder in a Medical Outpatient Setting and Participating in Group Cognitive Therapy Program

NURSING DIAGNOSIS #1: *Ineffective individual coping related to situational stressors at work and lack of resources to manage resulting anxiety*

EXPECTED CLIENT OUTCOMES

- The client will present to clinic with just one physical complaint.
- The client will make several remarks indicating an awareness of the variety of stressors being experienced.

NURSING INTERVENTIONS WITH RATIONALE

- Provide coping enhancement *to assist in the management of the emotional components of stress at work.*
  - Ensure coordination of treatment *to provide increased support.*
  - Encourage continued involvement in group therapy program.
  - Provide positive reinforcement when client describes event of day or work without referring to somatic symptoms, e.g., high blood pressure, pain in back, or pain on urination.
  - Provide positive feedback when client attends social events or has a pain-free work day.
- Provide emotional support to convey acceptance and empathy with the frequent presentation of client with complaints that may change from appointment to appointment, *recognizing that the client is seeking care and not just expressing complaints.*

*References 2,9,13–15,23,24,26,28,34,35

- ○ Listen actively to demonstrate respect and concern.
- ○ Gather data on new symptoms as they develop, *remembering that misdiagnosis is a risk*.
- ○ If the symptoms are evaluated and the client does not have a medical condition, the symptoms should be considered a way for the client to express the emotional need for caring.
- ○ Allow dependency in the relationship; *this contributes to feelings of self-worth and a sense of control, leading to more independence; the goal is for client to manage own behavior and care.*

NURSING DIAGNOSIS #2: *Altered family processes related to intensity of sick role assumed by family member*

EXPECTED FAMILY OUTCOME

- The client will identify ways to give support to member in sick role without reinforcing sick role behaviors.

NURSING INTERVENTIONS WITH RATIONALE

- Provide family process maintenance *to decrease the effect of the inability of client to fulfill role in family*.
  - ○ Identify what behaviors are troublesome to the members.
  - ○ Develop strategies with family, including the client, to manage the behaviors.
  - ○ Discuss realistic needs for help and expectations of care.
- Provide family support *to promote maintenance of family as a unit*.
  - ○ Engage entire family in treatment planning *to avoid misunderstanding of interventions and interference with treatment process*.
  - ○ Respond to questions and concerns, especially when client begins independent actions, *because any change is disruptive to a family system*.
  - ○ Refer to support groups *so family can receive support from others, not only from the health care agencies*.

Example: Client With Hypochondriasis in Medical Outpatient Setting

NURSING DIAGNOSIS #1: *Fear related to misinterpretation of symptoms and perceived rejection in environment*

EXPECTED CLIENT OUTCOMES

- The client will limit time spent discussing symptoms at school and with family and will not be preoccupied with fears over the nature of bodily symptoms.
- The client will keep regularly scheduled monthly appointments and report no visits to other clinics or emergency rooms.

NURSING INTERVENTIONS WITH RATIONALE

- Provide emotional support that *offers a non-threatening, continuing presence in which to explore psychological and social factors contributing to the fear.*
  - Maintain consistency in appointments *because client may seek change or demand more frequent contact.*
  - Listen carefully to current physical complaints; take vital signs and assess other symptoms. Avoid devoting the entire appointment time to a bodily complaint; focus on overall functioning.
  - Inquire about aspects of client's life and how it is made more complicated or burdensome by the symptom.
  - Assist client to begin to acknowledge that health problems might be indicative of something other than a disease with dire consequences.
  - Encourage continued appointments with primary provider for check-ups, and discuss how this in itself is useful, *because it further validates that a medical condition is not present and the client is being cared for and attended to.*
  - Emphasize wellness, i.e., nutrition, exercise, rest, hobbies, pleasurable activities.
- Provide problem-solving assistance when client reports visits to other health care agencies *to assist in determining the need for the help being sought.*
  - Gather information about the need to seek help, i.e., who, what, why, when, where.
  - Review the days preceding the client's seeking help *to identify experiences of loss, rejection, disappointment, and helplessness.*
  - Raise question of stress and its possible effect on client.

EXPECTED CLIENT OUTCOME

- The client will accept referral to and participate in group psychotherapy program.

NURSING INTERVENTIONS WITH RATIONALE

- Arrange for referral to group psychotherapy program *because the client needs support to take a risk and become involved.*
  - Encourage client to accept the referral as a way of dealing with stress *because stress is a more acceptable reason for attending.*
  - Provide orientation of what topics and issues may be explored in the group *to allay fears and prevent failure to attend.*

EXPECTED CLIENT OUTCOMES

- The client will verbalize a basic knowledge of the anatomy and physiology connected with the major body symptom and how it relates to self.
- The client will identify symptoms that are perceived as "dangerous."

NURSING INTERVENTIONS WITH RATIONALE

- Provide teaching about the disease process. Include anatomy and physiology associated with bodily symptom *to assist in allaying fear from misinterpretation, false beliefs, lack of knowledge.*
  - Carefully explain the anatomy, physiology, and function of body part involved in symptoms.
  - Provide appropriate reading materials as necessary.
  - Seek feedback *to determine understanding and need for further information or understanding.*
- Support self-awareness enhancement *to explore application of knowledge about the disease/symptom to self.*
  - Encourage questioning of experience, events, stress.
  - Question the difficulty client has in getting mind off "dangerous" symptoms.

CHAPTER 13

Factitious Disorders

▌ Definition/Major Symptoms*

Factitious Disorders are characterized by the intentional production or feigning of physical or psychological signs and symptoms that are under voluntary control and serve to help the client assume or take on the sick role. Characteristic features include:

- Dramatic historical presentation of complaints
- Pathological lying (often referred to as pseudologia fantastica)
- Fabrication of nonexistent physical or psychological symptoms
- Vague and inconsistent answers when pressed for details about complaints
- Above-average knowledge of medical information and hospital routines
- Willingness to undergo multiple examinations, treatments, and invasive procedures
- Drug-seeking behavior with complaints of pain and requests for pain medication (opioids)
- Few or no visitors when hospitalized
- Rapid discharge from treatment center after confrontation
- A pattern of travel and ongoing admissions to multiple health care systems in numerous cities, states, and other countries
- No ulterior motives, material advantages, or secondary gain other than to achieve status as a patient and to assume the sick role.

*References 1,3,6,8,9,15

These symptoms are part of a spectrum of illnesses, encompassing Somatoform Disorder, Factitious Disorder, and Malingering.

▌ Definition/Symptoms of Major Categories

Factitious Disorder With Predominantly Psychological Signs and Symptoms*

Clinical presentation is characterized by predominance of intentionally produced, wide-ranging psychological signs and symptoms that do not follow a typical pattern and may have an unusual course, as well as an unusual response to treatment. Simulated symptoms suggestive of a mental disorder usually represent the client's concept of mental disorder and do not necessarily conform to actual recognized diagnostic categories. Symptoms are typically worse when the client is aware of being observed. Other characteristics include:

- Endorsement of symptoms brought up during initial evaluation
- Feigned bereavement—reporting depression after death of loved one when, in actuality, there was no death
- Reporting dramatic past losses (all family burned in fire on Christmas Day) resulting in no living family members
- Complaints of Post-Traumatic Stress Disorder associated with combat experiences when client has never served in combat or may not be a veteran.

Clients are often negativistic and uncooperative when questioned for details.

Factitious Disorder With Predominantly Physical Signs and Symptoms†

This subtype entails a convincing clinical presentation with signs and symptoms predominantly indicative of a general medical condition. Clients may fabricate their past medical history. Actual client history often includes multiple attempts to be admitted or to remain within a hospital ("Munchausen Syndrome") and a wide range of physical symptomatology, e.g., fever of unknown origin, skin lesions, acute abdominal pain (when in actuality the client

---

*References 1,6,9,11,13,15,22,23
†References 1,5,6–9,14–16

has no pain) with nausea and vomiting; and reporting history of HIV positive (with no HIV) or "lupus-like" syndromes. Self-inflicted injuries are sometimes seen, including infection from self-injection of a contaminated substance such as own saliva; urinary tract infection from introduction of contaminated material into urethra; surreptitious use of medication, e.g., diuretic to cause electrolyte imbalance, anticoagulant to cause hematuria; or exacerbation of preexisting medical condition, e.g., stasis ulcers or wound infections that respond well to treatment within hospital and rapidly return after discharge. Clients will often complain of new physical or psychological problems when initial complaints prove negative.

Factitious Disorder With Combined Psychological and Physical Signs and Symptoms[*]

This encompasses clinical presentation with both psychological and physical signs and symptoms with neither category predominating.

Factitious Disorder Not Otherwise Specified[†]

This category is reserved for factitious symptoms "that do not meet criteria for Factitious Disorder," Factitious Disorder by proxy, "the intentional production or feigning of physical or psychological signs or symptoms in another person who is under the individual's care for the purpose of indirectly assuming the sick role."[1, p. 474] For example, an outwardly caring and attentive parent or caregiver of an elder person provides a false medical history for or creates illness in the child or elder. These feigned disorders may include seizures, allergies, deliberately adding blood to urine sample, and poisoning with emetics or other drugs to induce a variety of medical problems. Suspicion of Factitious Disorder by proxy is raised by a history of hospital and doctor "shopping," persistent or recurrent illness in child (sometimes adult) that cannot be explained, and discrepancies between actual clinical findings and history provided by parent/caregiver. There is often an absence or abatement of signs and symptoms when the perpetrator is not present. The caregiver may deny knowledge of the eti-

[*]References 1,6
[†]References 1,3,6,10,15–18,20,21,25

ology of the client's illness. Clinical presentations may be viewed as a rare disorder, or symptoms may not respond to what has been determined to be appropriate treatment.

Incidence*

Information on actual prevalence is limited because clients travel ("wander") from physician to physician, appear at different hospitals, often use different names, and are unreliable historians; their average age is 30 to 40 years. This disorder is more commonly seen in males and persons in medical and related professions; Munchausen's syndrome by proxy usually affects infants and children in the age range of 7 weeks to 14 years, although there may be a possible future increase of factitious disorder by proxy in the elderly.

Course†

The course is usually chronic with poor prognosis. Onset often follows hospitalization for a general medical condition or for another mental disorder; a lifelong pattern of successive hospitalizations is seen in clients with a chronic form of the disorder.

Contributing Factors to Factitious Disorders

Neurobiological/Genetic

- There is no evidence of a direct neurobiological or genetic basis for the disorder, although some evidence exists of central nervous system dysfunction in cases with pseudologia fantastica.[3,15]
- Frontal lobe and nondominant hemisphere dysfunction has been reported (deficits in client's ability to conceptually organize and manage complex information, impaired judgment) in clients with Munchausen's, even though they may appear intellectually intact on the basis of verbal skills.[12] The role of frontal or parietal dysfunction has not been proved, however.

*References 1,3,6,9,14,15,17
†References 1,6,16,24

Psychological Model (proposed but not systematically studied)*

Mental disorders or childhood or adolescent illness with extensive medical treatment and hospitalization

Important past physician relationship

Grudge against the medical profession

Abuse, neglect, abandonment, lack of nurturance during childhood

Unmet needs for nurturing, dependency, attention as adult

Past history of physical and sexual abuse

Fear of abandonment as adult

Anxiety related to fear of disintegration or fragmentation of the self

Inability to experience subjective sense of reality of emotions or perceptions

Severe sexual or marital stress

Inward direction of aggressive impulses (sadomasochistic personality)

▌Laboratory and Physical Examination Findings†

- Laboratory findings are consistent with specific self-inflicted conditions, e.g., sepsis, fever, electrolyte disorders, urinary tact infections, anemia, and hypoglycemia.
- Scar tissue, sometimes referred to as a "gridiron abdomen," is evident from unnecessary multiple surgeries,
- Chronic, non-healing wounds and purpura are evident.
- Self-induced bruises are evident.
- Findings of diagnostic tests, procedures, and surgeries are negative, e.g., no infection, no basis for complaints of seizures or loss of consciousness.

▌Special Assessment Considerations

- Do not overlook the possibility of an actual medical or psychiatric condition. Diagnosis of Factitious Disorder is based on the exclusion of actual general medical conditions and mental disorders.
- Observe the client for an atypical or dramatic presentation that does not meet the usual criteria for identifiable general medical conditions or mental disorders.

*References 1,5,6,14,15,25
†References 1,5,15,16

- Observe the client for symptoms that occur only when client is knowingly being observed; pseudologia fantastica; pattern of arguing with health care providers; or an above-average knowledge of medical terminology and hospital routines.
- Be suspicious of a client whose medical history includes multiple treatment interventions, e.g., surgeries, ECT, or multiple diagnostic workups; with extensive history of traveling from state to state and hospital to hospital; or who has few or no visitors while hospitalized.
- Observe for fluctuations in the clinical course with a pattern of rapidly developing "complications" or new "pathology" when clinical workup proves to be negative.
- Observe for indications of the client's need to assume the sick role and the lack of ulterior motives or material advantages for the client's behavior, e.g., economic gain, avoidance of legal responsibility.
- Verify data provided by the client to the extent possible, e.g., review of previous medical history, interview with family or friend, contact with known health providers, reported military history.
- Obtain a neurological workup to evaluate for possible pathology.

▌ Treatment

General

Restrict care as much as possible to one primary provider.

Psychopharmacological

- Provide no specific pharmacological intervention unless the client has a concomitant disorder such as depression, psychosis, infection, or electrolyte imbalance.[3]
- Avoid the unnecessary use of prescribed medication, such as opioids, for complaints of pain.

Psychotherapy

- Clients may be reluctant to engage in psychotherapy.
- Interpersonal, cognitive, and behavioral therapy is beneficial for some clients.

- It is difficult to establish a therapeutic alliance (important factor).
- Neutrality regarding etiology of medical difficulties rather than direct confrontation is preferable in some situations.

▎ Commonly Occurring Nursing Diagnoses

Altered parenting (Munchausen's by proxy)
Anxiety
Impaired tissue integrity
Ineffective individual coping
Personal identity disturbance
Risk for infection
Risk for injury
Risk for self-mutilation
Violence, directed at others (Munchausen's by proxy)

▎ Selected Nursing Diagnoses, Outcome Criteria, and Nursing Interventions With Rationale

NURSING DIAGNOSIS #1:* *Personal identity disturbance, related to impaired sense of reality about emotions or perceptions, disturbance in the sense of self, fear of disintegration or fragmentation of self*

EXPECTED CLIENT OUTCOME

- Client will develop and maintain a consolidated, integrated sense of self and recognize the reality of emotions or perceptions as evidenced by responding to personal, situational, and environmental stressors without resorting to medical imposturing or use of other factitious symptoms.

NURSING INTERVENTIONS WITH RATIONALE†

- Strive to establish a therapeutic alliance by conveying a calm, accepting, and non-demanding approach *to minimize client's need for continuation of deception, to encourage client to verbalize concerns and anxieties related to personal identity, and to reduce likelihood of abrupt termination of treatment.*

*References 19,24
†References 2–5,13–16,23,24

- Encourage client to give examples of problems related to management of emotional and/or physical health and well-being *to convey interest in client's concerns and perceived needs.*
- Maintain therapeutic stance of sustained empathic inquiry and persistent therapeutic curiosity about client's emotional life, *to facilitate client's identifying, communicating, and validating emotional experiences and to decrease likelihood of behavioral enactments of emotional states.*
- Collaborate with health care team in decisions related to confrontation about factitious behaviors *to minimize staff suspicion, alienation, and disputes; to ensure certainty regarding specific factitious behaviors; and to promote staff unity and consistency in implementation of client's plan of care.*
- Do not attempt to force client to admit recognition of factitious behaviors *to minimize client's prematurely discharging self from treatment and to avoid client's experiencing humiliation and perceived rejection.*
- Assess client's motivation for learning about improved management of emotional and/or physical health.
- Create individual assessment and interdisciplinary treatment plan for client that could include the following:
  - Engage client in discussion of principles of normal growth and development *to facilitate client's recognition of stressors that are associated with specific developmental phases.*
  - Suggest that client keep a daily written record of thoughts and feelings *to provide the client with the opportunity for autonomous ongoing view of self that is not solely dependent on external feedback from others; to increase the client's awareness of personal, situational, and environmental stressors that may be threatening to client's self-identity; and to facilitate the client's recognition of the tendency to indirectly express emotions through behavior and somatic complaints.*
- Collaborate with client in the development of a mutually agreed-upon treatment contract *to encourage the client's recognition of and responsibility in the development of problem-solving skills and strategies that promote and maintain integration of personal identity* (see also Contracting in Chapter 5).

- Collaborate with client and members of the mental health team in the development of a discharge plan that includes specific information regarding mental health after-care appointments (for inpatients) (see also Discharge Planning in Chapter 5).

NURSING DIAGNOSIS #2: *Risk for injury related to fabrication of nonexistent physical symptoms and/or nonexistent psychological symptoms; simulation of physical symptoms of disease, e.g., seizures, acute abdominal pain, acute leukemia; exaggeration of previous medical problems*

EXPECTED CLIENT OUTCOME

- The client will not experience unnecessary or dangerous diagnostic evaluations and treatments. The client will demonstrate problem-solving skills and strategies without resorting to use of self-injurious behaviors, e.g., surreptitious use of medication, deliberate reinfection of self with contaminated substances.

NURSING INTERVENTIONS WITH RATIONALE[*]

- Conduct a comprehensive nursing assessment and collaborate with the health care team to determine presence of behaviors such as atypical presentation that does not conform to identifiable general medical condition or mental disorder or needing to assume the sick role (see also Special Assessment Considerations). *Use this information to verify and confirm likelihood of client deception and probability of Factitious Disorder with risk for injury.*
- Collaborate with the health team to ensure adherence to ethical practices, e.g., maintenance of client confidentiality while trying to verify diagnosis of Factitious Disorder, respect of client privacy, and not searching client's room without permission. *Avoid invasion of privacy and violation of the client's right to self-determination.*
- Collaborate with the health care team to ensure that an adequate work-up has been conducted to rule out actual additional mental disorders or medical or surgical conditions. *Clients with Factitious Disorders may have a verifiable medical or surgical illness that requires prompt attention and treatment.* For example, a client with a his-

tory of multiple previous abdominal surgeries is at increased risk for actual intestinal obstruction.

- Collaborate with health care team to minimize implementation of unnecessary, dangerous procedures or diagnostic tests.
- Encourage ventilation of feelings.
- Assess for suicidal ideation/intent.
- Observe for behaviors indicative of increased anxiety. *Client willingness and eagerness to undergo invasive procedures and surgical interventions may be associated with attempts to avoid fragmentation or with disintegration anxiety.*
- Collaborate with mental health team in the development of a treatment plan that provides structure and support, as well as focuses on helping the client to identify and begin to discuss emotional experiences. *This should minimize the client's perceived need to simulate illness that might result in unnecessary and potentially harmful diagnostic tests and procedures.*
- Refer to previous interventions and rationale under Personal Identity Disturbance.

CHAPTER **14**

Dissociative Disorders

▋ Definition/Major Symptoms*

The Dissociative Disorders are a group of mental disorders presenting as a temporary alteration in conscious awareness, identity, or behavior.

Major symptoms include:

- Amnesia is the most common symptom in adults.
- Inattention and lack of sensitivity to their environment are the most common symptoms in children.
- Symptoms of dissociation, i.e., amnesia, depersonalization, are found in other psychiatric disorders, i.e., Schizophrenia, drug intoxication or withdrawal, Borderline Personality Disorder, and Factitious Disorder.
- When stress is experienced in areas of the client's life, the client copes through dissociative symptoms and function is impaired.
- Classification is based on the presenting symptom and psychological mechanism employed.

▋ Incidence†

- Rare.
- Dissociative Amnesia is the most common disorder of the group.
- Disasters and wars contribute to the increased incidence of Dissociative Amnesia and Dissociative Fugue Disorders.
- Dissociative experiences are common in the general population. They may take the form of daydreaming, an

*References 1,5,14
†References 1,5,10,12,14

awareness that one does not know what has occurred, finding oneself dressed to go somewhere that one does not know, being unable to recall certain events, feeling that one's leg is not one's own, acting differently in similar situations ("like two people"), feeling others are far away and unavailable, abusing drugs, and abusing others.

- A dissociative experience, an alteration in consciousness, is more common in Latin America, the Far East, and Africa. The person may be observed "falling out," immobilized, screaming, crying, behaving in bizarre ways, or having changed sensory control, i.e., sword swallowing. The person may behave as if possessed by a spirit or an ancestor. In countries where the behavior is accepted by relatives, friends, and the community, the person does not appear distressed; in these instances the behavior is not considered a disorder.

▋ Course*

The course is varied, with sudden or slow onset. It may be acute or chronic or episodic and tends to be self-limiting.

▋ Definition/Major Symptoms of Major Categories†

Dissociative Amnesia

- This disorder was previously called psychogenic amnesia.
- It is characterized by the client's inability to recall pertinent information in the absence of an organic cause.
- The client cannot remember an experience that was physically and/or emotionally traumatic. He or she is unable to describe what followed an event for a few hours, cannot remember certain events, or cannot recall a period of time prior to the event. This is commonly noted in patients who come to emergency rooms.
- The course of the disorder is short and self-limited.

Dissociative Fugue

- This disorder was previously called psychogenic fugue.
- It is characterized by a sudden memory loss and confusion about the client's own identity.

*References 1,5,14
†References 1,3,5,9,10,14,15

- Professional help may not be sought until the episode is over and the client is wondering about what happened and wants to find out. Assistance may be sought in behalf of the client because he or she may appear confused, worried, disoriented. The client may suddenly leave home or work or travel. A new identity and life may be assumed. The fugue may last from a few hours to days or months.

Dissociative Identity Disorder

- This was previously called multiple personality disorder.
- It is characterized by the presence of two or more personalities controlling the behavior of the person.
- The client displays several personalities, each having distinct behaviors, thoughts, and perceptions. They may even differ in age, sex, race, friends, and associates. They may or may not know of the existence of the alter (other personality) or may seek to hide the fact. Scars from self-inflicted injuries or abuse may be noted. Symptoms may first appear in adolescence and last into adulthood.

Depersonalization Disorder

- This disorder is characterized by the experience of perceiving oneself as unreal, with thoughts and feelings unattached to anything; the environment may be experienced in the same way.
- The client reports a sense of estrangement from the self, a loss of meaning, a perception of things being different, a perception that the body is foreign or deformed, or of watching oneself. The symptoms tend to be chronic.
- Young adults, especially women, experience transient episodes, or the condition may become chronic.

▌ Contributing Factors to Dissociative Disorders[*]

- Etiology is unknown; there may be a dysfunction in the temporal lobe.
- Psychodynamic theory: When an emotionally traumatic event or intense conflictual situation occurs, mental mechanisms are activated to manage the environment.

[*]References 1–3,5,9,12,14

- Learning theory: When a painful emotional state is experienced, memory is also affected so that the event is not accessible to the person.
- Neurobiological processes: There may be a dysfunction in the temporal lobe that affects the temporal-limbic systems.
- Psychological trauma may be associated with natural disasters, war, or intrapersonal conflicts.
- Childhood trauma involving sexual, physical, and/or emotional abuse may have been experienced. Dissociative Identity Disorder is also associated with Borderline Personality Disorders.
- A learned conditioning occurs altering how one receives, remembers, and processes the traumatic events.
- Dissociative Identity Disorder occurs when the environment does not offer protection. Parents and others do not provide an experience of caring and love; there is an absence of role modeling; there is a lack of opportunities to deal with stress in a variety of ways; there is an absence of a support system.

▌ Laboratory and Physical Examination Findings[*]

Diagnosis is to be made only after ruling out medical conditions by blood work and electrolyte, serum glucose, and blood alcohol levels.

▌ Special Assessment Considerations[†]

- Observe and record signs and symptoms carefully because they are frequently associated with other psychiatric disorders (Malingering, Borderline Personality Disorder, Antisocial Personality Disorder, PTSD, Major Depression, Substance Abuse) or medical conditions (diabetes, drug abuse, alcohol abuse, epilepsy, head injury).
- Note that children experiencing severe trauma frequently present with multiple symptoms of psychosis, Post-Traumatic, Conduct, and Dissociative Disorders. After careful evaluation the diagnosis may be Dissociative Disorder, a disorder of lesser severity than Schizophrenia.

[*]References 1,5,14
[†]References 5,9,12,13,14

- Be prepared to participate in the diagnostic process over a long period of time; this may involve data collection and several evaluations and diagnoses before consensus is reached.
- Note that some cultures may accept a range of behavior patterns.
- Events such as medical and surgical procedures or diagnostic testing also produce increased stress and psychological reactions such as depersonalization. Provide emotional support and teaching during technical procedures to prevent the dissociation.

▌ Treatment*

Psychodynamic Treatment

Provide brief, immediate assistance in recalling an event and managing the anxiety. Hypnosis and/or an amytal interview is usually effective in helping to remember the event.

DISSOCIATIVE IDENTITY DISORDER

Treatment focuses first on establishing a sound working relationship with the client in order to begin the necessary and difficult treatment process. There is controversy regarding whether the goal of therapy should be resolution or reintegration. Resolution focuses on developing some degree of communication amongst the alters, increasing the client's control over dysfunctional behaviors, and establishing a collaboration among the alters. Reintegration attempts to blend the alters into a single personality for the client. The original experience that overwhelmed the self and the current sources of conflict and stress are explored. Hypnosis or an amytal interview may be helpful in gathering data or recalling the traumatic event. Antidepressive and antianxiety medications may be used to treat symptoms. Hospitalization may be indicated when treating a violent or self-destructive personality, but this may worsen symptoms and encourage regressive dependency.

DEPERSONALIZATION DISORDER

Therapy offers support, reviews the stressors related to the event(s), and assists client to modify defenses/conflicts.

*References 5,7,9,12,14,15

█ Commonly Occurring Nursing Diagnoses

Anxiety
Coping, ineffective individual
Coping, ineffective family
Fear
Injury, high risk for
Personal identity disturbance
Post-trauma response
Rape-trauma syndrome
Rape-trauma response
Relocation-stress syndrome
Self-mutilation, risk for
Sleep pattern disturbances
Violence, risk for, self-directed

█ Selected Nursing Diagnoses, Outcome Criteria, and Nursing Interventions With Rationale*

Example: Dissociation Identity Disorder in a Hospital

NURSING DIAGNOSIS #1: *Risk for self-directed violence related to anxiety aroused by alter personality*

EXPECTED CLIENT OUTCOME

• Client will be free of self-inflicted injury during hospitalization.

NURSING INTERVENTIONS WITH RATIONALE

• Provide surveillance. *Careful observation of the behaviors occurring in the hospital setting contributes to the understanding of the dynamics of behavior, development of effective interventions, and prevention of suicidal actions.*
  ○ Monitor patient's behavior and environment during the appearance of the alter personality.
  ○ Facilitate data collection regarding present stressors or abusive events in the past.
• Prevent suicidal acts. *Clear communication about the risk for self-harm for certain clients and about actions that can be taken to reduce risk of self-harm contribute to a decrease in the risk.*

*References 4–8,11,13–15

○ Establish rapport.
○ Monitor behavior constantly, particularly the verbalization of feelings of hopelessness.
○ Contract with client to do no harm to self.
- Provide limit setting. Establishing the parameters of acceptable behavior increases the possibility that the client will choose a more effective response.
  ○ Explain hospital routines to the client in a firm and consistent manner.
  ○ Recognize that testing and manipulative behaviors are not deliberate but reflect the client's need to experience safety and security.
- Assist in self-awareness enhancement. *Aid client to verbalize and clarify feelings, then thoughts and behaviors, and finally possible motivations of behaviors.*
  ○ Assist patient to verbalize feelings of trust or distrust of others.
  ○ Assist patient to verbalize increasing anxiety and to take action to decrease it.

NURSING DIAGNOSIS #2: *Sleep disturbance related to psychological stress*

EXPECTED CLIENT OUTCOME
- Client will sleep 5 to 6 hours without waking.

NURSING INTERVENTIONS WITH RATIONALE
- Provide sleep enhancement. *A regular sleeping pattern will enhance overall health.*
  ○ Promote the client's use of new or established bedtime routines to prepare for sleep.
  ○ Establish a routine bedtime hour with the client.
  ○ Determine what awakens client and respond to the feeling state presented.

NURSING DIAGNOSIS #3: *Coping, ineffective individual, related to lack of skills in allaying anxiety*

EXPECTED CLIENT OUTCOME
- Client will identify two successful ways to reduce anxiety experienced in hospital.

NURSING INTERVENTIONS WITH RATIONALE

- Provide presence. *An empathetic, accepting, respectful nurse or other staff member contributes to an environment in which a client can experience security.*
  - Provide a calm, safe environment.
  - Respect the client's personal space while remaining quickly accessible.
- Provide anxiety-reduction strategies. *Strategies that lessen emotional reactivity to threats of harm or loss assist the client in lowering the tension or distress being experienced.*
  - Assist the client in describing the expected appearance of the alter personality.
  - Assist the client in making a list of things to do when anxious, angry, or experiencing an alter personality.
  - Use listening techniques.
- Provide autogenic training. Strategies that promote relaxation by self-suggestion can be taught to the client as an appropriate coping response to reduce tension.
  - Use a specific technique or tape to assist client to become relaxed.
  - Practice autogenic training once daily.
- Provide exercise therapy. Providing the client with instruction, role modeling, practice, and an opportunity to exercise promotes health and reduces tension.
  - Instruct the client on the beneficial effects of exercise on stress reduction, as well as on overall health improvement.
  - Identify and engage in two methods of exercise, e.g., brisk walking and step dancing.

Example: Dissociative Amnesia in Outpatient Service

NURSING DIAGNOSIS #1:   *Fear related to lack of knowledge regarding treatment methods and benefits*

EXPECTED CLIENT OUTCOME

- The client will demonstrate and verbalize changed feelings about seeing a psychiatrist and gain insight into efforts to avoid therapy.

NURSING INTERVENTIONS WITH RATIONALE

- Provide emotional support. *Responding to the client's feelings is experienced by the client as care and concern, which enhances further problem solving.*

- Listen to client's expressions of fear of being mentally ill.
- Be available to answer questions.
- Point out that fear can mobilize client to take appropriate action.

EXPECTED CLIENT OUTCOME

- The client will verbalize knowledge of the major treatment methods and benefits for dissociative amnesia.

NURSING INTERVENTIONS WITH RATIONALE

- Provide teaching about disease process. *Providing information to the client about a disease process decreases the unknown factor and enables the client to problem solve more efficiently.*
  - Describe the severe stressors generally involved in a dissociative reaction.
  - Assist client in understanding the major reactions to stress and the current method of treatment.
  - Assess for alcohol or drug abuse *because this may be a factor affecting the treatment process and indicate an area for further teaching.*
- Provide teaching focused on the individual. *Planning and implementing strategies to meet a client's needs or desires increases the client's motivation to achieve a healthier state.*
  - Determine the client's previous experiences with therapists and beliefs about mental diseases.
  - Identify the motivator for treatment, e.g., recalling lost memory, gaining more knowledge of self, improving relationships with significant others.

EXPECTED CLIENT OUTCOME

- The client will keep scheduled weekly appointments with therapist.

NURSING INTERVENTIONS WITH RATIONALE

- Provide counseling. *Establishing a regular period to discuss a problem enables the client to address emotional and cognitive issues.*
  - Assist client in making a list of reasons for and against keeping appointments with the therapist, and then explore each one.
  - Ask client to report the making and keeping of appointments with the therapist and any related concerns.

NURSING DIAGNOSIS #2:   *Coping, ineffective family, related to over-concern for family member with dissociative amnesia*

EXPECTED FAMILY OUTCOME

• The family will verbalize a reason for the apparent disregard of the client's recall problem.

NURSING INTERVENTIONS WITH RATIONALE

• Provide teaching about the disease process. *Providing explanations of behavior may assist family members to change their response to the client's behavior.*
  ○ Discuss the nature of stress reactions and common defenses, e.g., dissociation, denial.
  ○ Facilitate the family's understanding of the dissociative process and how it relieves the traumatic stress, but also why it is necessary to support the client's attempt to integrate the experience into client's reality.

EXPECTED FAMILY OUTCOME

• Family will describe ways to be supportive to client.

NURSING INTERVENTIONS WITH RATIONALE

• Provide support system enhancement. *Strategies to help the family to support client in effective ways facilitate the functioning of the family system.*
  ○ Determine availability of client's spouse, his or her usual method of giving support, and his or her comfort level in doing so.
  ○ Assist client in communicating to spouse what is comforting and supportive.
• Promote family involvement. *Assisting in the way emotional and physical needs are met in the family promotes support provided by each member to all the others.*
  ○ Identify the family's expectations before and after the severe stress as a way for family members to experience the expression of needs and boundaries of others.
  ○ Encourage the discussion and modification of expectations as appropriate.
  ○ Role play two methods of giving mutual support.

CHAPTER 15

Sexual and Gender Identity Disorder

Three major groups are included in the Sexual and Gender Identity Disorders: Sexual Dysfunction, Paraphilia, and Gender Identity Disorders.

▌ Definition/Major Symptoms

Sexual Dysfunction Disorders[*]

These are a group of disorders of the sexual response cycle ranging from desire, to excitement and plateau, to orgasm, and to relaxation. Categorization of specific disorders is based on the major symptoms experienced by the client, such as:

- Hypoactive desire or aversion to sexual activity
- Inability to become aroused or excited associated with mental and/or physiological changes
- Lack of or delay in achieving orgasm
- Pain at some point in the sexual response process
- Distress affecting client's self-esteem
- Disturbances in relationships with others

Paraphilias[†]

These are a group of Sexual Disorders that exhibit recurring strong urges, fantasies, and behaviors directed toward an object, a child, or a nonconsenting adult; these disorders continue over time, frequently causing pain and distress to others. These urges continue to occur for a minimum period

[*]References 3,7,21,22
[†]References 2,3,14,21,22

of 6 months. Impairment in personal daily functioning and personal distress are present. The disorders interfere with the ability to pursue relationships with consenting sexual partners.

Gender Identity Disorders (Transsexualism)*

These are a group of disorders in which the person experiences an ongoing discomfort with self as male/female and/or with the role attached by society to being male or female.

▌ Definition/Major Symptoms of Selected Major Categories

Sexual Dysfunction Disorders

SEXUAL DESIRE DISORDERS†

- Hypoactive Sexual Desire Disorder. This disorder is characterized by a lack of interest in sex, manifested by loss of desire and absence of sexual fantasies or daydreaming. The client may report personal distress or a variety of responses such as indifference or denial. The sexual partner may be very distressed, and interpersonal problems may be apparent.
- Sexual Aversion Disorder. This disorder is characterized by disliking, avoiding, or being unwilling to have sexual activity with the partner. The client experiences distress, e.g., anxiety, fear, distaste; no pleasure is felt. Personal problems result due to phobic avoidance, e.g, ..."the kids, too tired, lack of time..." This disorder may also be associated with Anxiety Disorder.

SEXUAL AROUSAL DISORDERS‡

- Female Sexual Arousal Disorder. This disorder is characterized by the lack of ability to maintain psychological arousal, vaginal lubrication, and vasocongestion of the external genitalia with swelling for the completion of sexual act; the client is distressed and interpersonal problems are intensified.
- Male Erectile Disorder. This disorder is characterized by impotence or inability to achieve or maintain an erection

*References 3,7,21,22
†References 3,7,8,12,21,22
‡References 3,7,17,18,19,21,22

to complete the sexual act. The client experiences personal distress, frustration, anger, anxiety and a lack of satisfaction along with interpersonal difficulties. This disorder is commonly caused by general medical conditions and use of substances, e.g., alcohol, drugs. Impotence is the most common complaint of men seeking treatment; its incidence increases with age. Many men fear impotence.

ORGASMIC DISORDERS*

- Female Orgasmic Disorder. This disorder is characterized by the inability to achieve an orgasm during sexual intercourse concurrent with the experience of distress and/or interpersonal problems. Confirmation of the diagnosis is based on client's age, sexual history, and presence of sufficient stimulation to achieve an orgasm.
- Male Orgasmic Disorder. This disorder is characterized by inability to achieve an orgasm after the excitement phase of sexual activity concurrent with the experience of distress and/or interpersonal problems. Both the client's age and sufficiency of stimulation are considered in making the diagnosis. It is associated with the use of some antidepressants, particularly SSRIs.
  - Premature Ejaculation. This disorder is characterized by inability to control the ejaculation at penetration or as the client desires. The client is distressed, may become fearful or isolated, or may seek another sexual partner; relationships are stressed.

SEXUAL PAIN DISORDERS†

- Dyspareunia. This disorder is characterized by genital pain at some point in the sexual act; the client experiences personal distress and interpersonal problems.
- Vaginismus. This disorder is characterized by spasms of the muscles of the outer third of the vagina during intercourse, preventing achievement of the sexual act. The client experiences distress and the sexual partner is upset; interpersonal problems coexist.

Paraphilias‡

The type of stimulus causing the sexual urge, fantasy, or behavior determines the diagnostic label as described below:

*References 3,7,12,17,19–22   ‡References 2,3,14,21,22
†References 3,7,16,21,22

Exhibitionism—involves the exposure of genitals.

Fetishism—involves inanimate objects.

Frotteurism—involves rubbing or touching a noncon-senting person.

Pedophilia—involves a prepubescent child; client is at least 16 years old and at least 5 years older than child.

Sexual masochism—involves self-inflicted suffering or humiliation.

Sexual sadism—involves inflicting suffering, distress, or humiliation on another.

Transvestic fetishism—involves cross-dressing of male/female.

Voyeurism—involves watching another undress or per-form a sexual act.

Gender Identity Disorders[*]

GENDER IDENTITY DISORDER IN CHILDREN

This disorder is characterized by a child's consistent, con-tinuing identification with the opposite sex in thought and behavior. Behavior includes statements of "I am a man...a lady"; cross-dressing; assuming the role of the opposite sex in make-believe stories and plays and in fantasies; a strong wish to play games typically associated with the opposite sex; and having best friends of the opposite sex. There is a consistent, continuing distress about the child's sex or the role assigned to that sex, which he or she believes to be peculiar, unconnected, and unsuitable. For example, a boy says, "Penis is ugly" or avoids playing soccer with other boys; a girl believes that she will not menstruate or insists on urinating in a standing position.

GENDER IDENTITY DISORDER IN ADOLESCENTS OR ADULTS

This disorder is characterized by the consistent, continu-ing desire to be or become the opposite gender. Behaviors include statements of "I wish I were.."; assuming attitudes and behaviors of and passing for the other sex; and state-ments of "I enjoy, like, hate...just like men/women." The client exhibits consistent, continuing distress about his or her sex, believing the role to be peculiar, unconnected, and unsuitable. Behaviors include cross-dressing, seeking or

[*]References 7,21,22

taking hormones, and/or requesting surgery to change sexual characteristics or as part of a total sex change. There is impairment in work and social functioning.

Incidence

Sexual Dysfunction Disorders[*]

- 20% of the general population experience hypoactive sexual desire.
- 36% to 38% of males experience premature ejaculation.
- These disorders are prevalent in the medically ill but may not be a treatment focus.

Paraphilias[†]

- These disorders are rare; little information exists.
- Pedophilia is the most common of these disorders.
- Pedophilia, Exhibitionism, and Voyeurism account for 80% of those seeking treatment.
- These disorders occur mostly in males.

Gender Identity Disorders[‡]

- Incidence is unknown.
- Adults seeking surgical sex change are predominantly male.
- Children in treatment are predominantly male.

Course

Sexual Dysfunction Disorders[§]

- Sexual Desire Disorders usually begin in adulthood; they may follow a period of stress related to a major life change, loss, or personal or relationship problems.
- The course may be specified in the diagnostic statement as "Lifelong Type" in which the dysfunction occurs after the onset of sexual functioning (prognosis is less favorable) *or* "Acquired Type" in which the dysfunction develops after a period of sexual functioning (prognosis is more favorable).

[*]References 3,7,21,22
[†]References 1–5,7,13,14,21,22
[‡]References 7,21,22
[§]References 3,7,21,22

- The prognosis is better when the Hypoactive Sexual Desire Disorder is a situational type (see Contributing Factors), e.g., a particular person (wife) must be present for the dysfunction to occur.
- The disorder may occur once, recur during periods of acute stress, or continue during the sexual life of the client.
- As the adult woman matures, some problems may be resolved because of her increased interest in sex.
- Variations in interest and function are related to age.
  - The aging process produces some loss of interest and function; however, this is variable.
  - The young male may experience premature ejaculation, but with increasing knowledge, experience, and time, he may or may not need help.
- The overall course of the disorder is influenced by the relationship with the sexual partner.

Paraphilias*

A more positive treatment outcome is related to later age of onset, a history of normal sex prior to Paraphilia, completion of a few sexual acts, the absence of substance abuse, self-referral for treatment, and experience of some guilt and shame.

With Pedophilia there are frequent relapses over long periods; the outcome is poor.

Gender Identity Disorders†

These disorders begin early in life with symptoms appearing by the age of 4 years. During school years, conflicts with peers and problems in fitting in with the group are noted. Children are often referred for treatment because of concern of parents and/or teachers. Some children, however, may be mistreated or rejected by parents, peers, physician, or minister. Homosexuality is usually present in adolescence. For some persons the disorder is transient. By adulthood it is considered chronic with noticeable impairments in work, play, and love relationships. Few seek treatment. Prognosis is related to the age of onset and the severity of symptoms.

*References 1–5,7,13,14,21,22
†References 3,7,12,13,14,21,22

▌ Contributing Factors

Sexual Dysfunction Disorders*

Contributing factors may be specified as part of the diagnostic statement in two ways as subtypes:

- *Generalized Type* describes a dysfunction that may occur with different partners, in various situations, or with a variety of sexual stimuli. *Situational Type* describes a dysfunction that occurs with a certain partner, in a particular circumstance, or only when there is a particular sexual stimulus.
- *Due to Psychological Factors* is used to indicate that no other reason can be found for the dysfunction. *Due to Combined Factors* is used to indicate that psychological factors, medical conditions, and/or substance abuse are all contributing to the sexual dysfunction, as outlined below:
  - Anatomical or physiological abnormality, e.g., estrogen deficiency
  - General medical conditions:
    - Endocrine disorder—e.g., diabetes, Addison's disease
    - Neurological disease—e.g., multiple sclerosis, head trauma, spinal cord injury
    - Renal, hepatic, pulmonary disorders, vascular disease
    - Infectious diseases—e.g., mumps
  - Surgical procedures—e.g., prostatectomy
  - Medications—e.g., antihypertensives, anticholinergic, antipsychotics, benzodiazepines, antidepressants
  - Drug abuse—e.g, alcohol, cocaine, marijuana, tobacco
  - Stress related to illness, relationships, sexual affairs, changes in job, life cycle events (marriage), crises
  - Sexual trauma or abuse, particularly during childhood
  - Restrictive environment—moral prohibitions, lack of opportunity to learn sexual facts, misinformation and myths, experiencing effect of parental conflict
  - Fears—loss of control, vulnerability, closeness, hostility
  - Inexperience
  - Feelings of sexual inadequacy, criticizing of self
  - Lack of sexual skills or knowledge
  - Inability to maintain continuous stimulation of sexual desire leading to sexual act

*References 7,8,16–22,24

○ Interruption of sexual stimulation—e.g., telephone, child's cry
○ Abstinence from sex for a long period of time
○ Relationships with partner:
  – Problems in communicating sexual desires and wishes
  – Use of poor technique
  – Problems of commitment, intimacy, power, and lack of trust

- The psychodynamic theory centers on a conflict regarding separation from the love object and fears of rejection by the mother or father. This conflict generates anxiety and the symptoms of sexual dysfunction, which serve as a defense.
- The social learning theory emphasizes sexual attitudes, ways to express love to others, and sexual behaviors as learned early in everyday family life. Attitudes are reinforced and/or changed throughout the growing years. Dysfunctional behaviors are learned, e.g., the stereotyping of sexual role/behavior, the use of sex as power in relationships, and the inability to express affection develops.
- Cognitive theory, rather than seeking a cause from the person's past, emphasizes the beliefs that cause him or her to feel and act in sexually inadequate ways in the current situation or with sexual partners.

Paraphilias*

- No factor has proved to be significant, although a history of sexual abuse may be a risk factor.
- The role of the male in society, requiring him to be aggressive, dominant, and to meet his emotional needs in sexually aggressive ways, has been suggested as a causative factor.
- There is a question of a temporal lobe disorder because of its function in sexual behavior.
- Psychoanalytic theory, which is controversial, posits a failure to resolve the oedipal crisis. The anxiety created may be experienced as castration or mutilation anxiety and further displayed in sexual urges, fantasies, and behaviors. There is also a defending against dissolution of ego boundaries because of the weak ego and lack of identity.
- Social learning theory holds that early childhood sexual experiences condition or mold the child's behavior.

*References 1–5,7,13 14,21,22

There is little communication of thoughts or urges with others and less chance to transform these thoughts into more acceptable expressions.

Gender Identity Disorders[*]

- Etiology is unknown.
- Levels of the hormones testosterone and estrogen are believed to affect aggressiveness and libido. The effect of these hormones on the development of these disorders is controversial.
- Disorders may result from childhood experiences of learning about gender roles from parents, school, TV, community, and culture.
- Disorders may result from the devaluing of self in the process of separating from the mother. This may be caused by hostile mothering, abuse, rejection, and death or absence of the father. This theory is controversial.
- Psychoanalytic theory, which is controversial, posits that conflicts during the oedipal phase of development are not resolved. Further conflict and anxiety are triggered in the present that threaten the love of child/adult towards a parent/love object and the identification with the same-sex parent's role. The disorder itself is used unconsciously to alter the emotions felt and the effect on self-esteem.

▌ Laboratory and Physical Examination Findings[†]

- Physical examination of genitals is particularly important to determine any abnormality.
- Routine blood work, e.g., levels of estrogen and androgen, should be done to begin the process of ruling out any medical conditions that might cause the dysfunction.
- Nocturnal penile plethysmography measures changes in the size of the penis.

▌ Special Assessment Considerations[‡]

- Sexual Dysfunction Disorders are common results of general medical conditions; therefore, the clinician

[*]References 7,14,21,22
[†]References 7,21,22
[‡]References 1,7,21,22

needs to acknowledge the importance of the sexual experience of a client when collecting assessment data.

- The most common medical conditions causing sexual dysfunction are diabetes and other endocrine disorders, vascular disease, multiple sclerosis, trauma and fractures, and radical surgeries. Examples are Male Erectile Disorder Due to General Medical Condition, diabetes; Dyspareunia Due to General Medical Condition, surgical procedure; and Hypoactive Sexual Desire Due to a General Medical Condition, mastectomy/prostatectomy.
- Substance-Induced Sexual Dysfunction is also common and occurs about 4 weeks after intoxication or withdrawal.
- Sexually dysfunctional clients may have another psychiatric disorder, e.g., Obsessive-Compulsive Disorder.
- Pedophilia is a sex crime. The legal system requires the reporting of the occurrence of sexual abuse or other types of abuse to the proper authorities. Guidelines for reporting to legal and treating agencies must be sought and followed.
- It is important to consult with experienced clinicians to determine the legal, community, and health systems' effects on the treatment program designed for the client.
- The designation "tomboy" or "sissy" is not sufficient for a diagnosis of gender identity disorder. It must include more than a few behaviors or identification with the opposite sex at one point in a client's life; it is more than being a nonconformist.
- Clients with Gender Identity Disorders may become depressed or anxious; they may attempt suicide or even genital self-mutilation.
- Hermaphroditism (one person having both ovaries and testes) is rare. In cases of pseudohermaphroditism the infant is examined and the sex determined at birth; surgery is then performed within 5 years.
- Homosexuality, or being sexually attracted to a person of the same sex, is not a DSM-IV mental disorder. Its incidence rate is 5% to 10% in the U.S. Owing to the social stigma, an individual may become very distressed about being homosexual and may experience anxiety, shame, hopelessness, and despair. He or she may be classified as Sexual Disorder NOS.

▌Treatment

Treatment generally includes the treatment of any underlying physical problem and the provision of basic sex education as needed.

Sexual Dysfunction Disorders[*]

SEXUAL DESIRE DISORDERS

Treatment focuses on questioning, identifying, and exposing negative attitudes and/or beliefs (e.g., that men are not trustworthy or that women are demanding), and reducing interfering thoughts that prevent sexual pleasure. It works on increasing the client's control over thoughts and correcting misbeliefs about sex. The client is taught to recognize that low desire can be self-generated (e.g., recalling unpleasant scenes from the past) or generated by the partner (behaviors, lack of attractiveness, lack of courtesy, or sloppiness). Negative sexual behaviors are identified and new behaviors are practiced and encouraged. Ways to enhance positive feelings and satisfaction and to feel sexy are explored. If the person is tense, techniques to relax before the sexual act are taught.

Specifically, treatment focuses on increasing libido by (1) use of masturbation and fantasy using erotic material, and (2) preparation for lovemaking, e.g., bathing, setting a special time, courting, flirting with the partner. *Sensate focus exercises* are used to increase physical stimulation; these special techniques and exercises allow a couple to learn to be comfortable with their sexuality in the presence of each other by progressively looking at and touching each other, then using touch to increase the pleasure to the self and other. In using this technique the anxiety level of both persons is reduced because they are concentrating on the sensation, not the goal. The couple is finding pleasure at the moment in a touch or a kiss, with minimal focus on the goal, or orgasm, at a later time. If the client focuses on the orgasm, he or she may focus on potential failure or on being unable to perform or experience pleasure. Genital

[*]References 7,8,14,16,18–22,24

self-stimulation techniques are taught to practice and share, as well as to prolong pleasure.

SEXUAL AVERSION DISORDERS

Treatment focuses on decreasing the fear of or aversion to sex. Desensitization techniques are used that gradually present the sexual triggers that cause the fear, phobia, avoidance, or strong distaste; this is done until the client experiences no symptoms and can participate in sexual activities. When an Anxiety Disorder is also being treated, the desensitization period takes much longer. Antianxiety drugs may also be used. Techniques to increase one's desire are taught.

If there is resistance to this treatment, the focus then shifts to trauma experienced earlier in life, using dream work and transference experienced in therapy.

SEXUAL AROUSAL DISORDERS

These disorders are the most common causes for seeking treatment in a sex clinic. Therapy focuses on the following:

1. Improving the total environment for healthy sexual experiences
2. Identifying thoughts linked to unpleasant emotions, changing distortions, reframing negative qualities of other, or issues of power or closeness
3. Techniques to achieve and maintain stimulation by maintaining thoughts, feelings, fantasies, and positive sexual images, and not allowing interruption of the thought or stimulation process
4. Teaching the squeeze technique to males to assist in preventing premature ejaculation.

Also included are techniques of dating and courting, sensate focusing, and genital stimulation. Men with erectile dysfunction are often advised to initiate sex in the morning, when they are more likely to awaken with an erection.

Special Techniques for Male Erectile Disorder

- Intracavernosal injection therapy uses injection of medication into the penis to relax the muscle and increase arterial blood flow, thus causing an erection. The method is effective, but the client may fear injections, pain, or the interruption. The cost also may be prohibitive.

- External vacuum devices use a cylinder placed around the penis to draw blood into it, creating an erection; a tight band at the base of the penis is used to maintain the erection.
- A surgical implant into the penis to assist erection may give some satisfaction to the client.

SEXUAL PAIN DISORDERS

Therapy for Vaginismus focuses most frequently on the resolution of psychological causes, e.g., pain from the experience of rape or sexual abuse. The client is taught relaxation techniques.

Therapy for Dyspareunia first treats the physical cause (50% of cases may be related to a medical condition). Psychotherapy that uses desensitization and relaxation techniques to allow touch and penetration is emphasized.

Paraphilias[*]

- Treatment is difficult because the client is receiving pleasure and reinforcement in the act itself, and the paraphilia fulfills deeper emotional needs. Denial of the problem is a barrier to treatment.
- It is necessary to treat the personality disorder that is commonly associated with this diagnosis.
- An antiandrogen may be administered.
- Cognitive therapy (sex offender programs) deals with cognitive distortion or denial (e.g., "she wasn't hurt," "it's not my fault") of the offending act through group confrontation, by quoting the victim, and by use of medications. It teaches the client (1) how to deal with triggers to the sexual abuse; (2) self-control techniques, e.g., thought shifting and stopping, covert sensitization, masturbation satiation; (3) assertiveness and social skills; (4) not to interfere with the rights of others; and (5) new ways to meet needs for affection and intimacy.

Gender Identity Disorders[†]

- Careful evaluation of information from parents, significant others, psychometric testing, physical examination, behavior studies, and a history of abuse are necessary

[*]References 1,5,7,10,11,13,14,21–23
[†]References 3,7,12–14,21,22

to rule out personality disorders (e.g., borderline, narcissistic) or neurological or endocrine disorders.

- Supportive psychotherapy focuses on dealing with identity, being a self; it may explore sex surgery using a problem-solving approach, e.g., listing pros and cons, alternatives to hormone use and sex change surgery, etc. This client may be difficult to treat because the disorder is meeting other emotional and identity needs.
- Play therapy for a child combined with parental counseling focuses on learning acceptable behavior patterns and ways to manage cross-gender behaviors, not foster it.
- Feminizing/masculinizing hormones: Both sexes have reported feeling better on hormones. Changes that have occurred in the male-to-female transsexual after taking estrogen include fewer erections, decrease in sex drive, and a small increase in breast size. The nurse must observe the client for possible complications: hypertension, increased coagulation tendency, hyperglycemia, liver dysfunction, and thrombophlebitis and associated problems. Changes that have occurred in the female-to-male transsexual after taking androgen include increasing sex drive, amenorrhea, tingling in clitoris, hoarseness, and increase in body hair. The nurse must observe the client for thrombophlebitis with associated problems and liver problems.
- Sex-reassignment surgery is a controversial treatment. Before surgery is performed certain criteria must be met, including living and dressing as the desired gender and taking hormones for a period of time, e.g., 3 to 12 months.

▌Commonly Occurring Nursing Diagnoses

Anxiety
Body image disturbance
Coping, ineffective individual
Family processes, altered
Pain
Personal identity disturbance
Powerlessness
Self-esteem, situational, low

Sexual dysfunction
Sexuality patterns, altered
Social interaction, impaired
Violence, risk for, self-directed or directed at others

▋ Selected Nursing Diagnoses, Outcome Criteria, and Nursing Interventions with Rationale*

Example: Client With Dyspareunia in Outpatient Setting

NURSING DIAGNOSIS #1: *Altered sexuality pattern, related to fear of pregnancy and role change, lack of physical cause, lack of family support system*

EXPECTED CLIENT OUTCOME

- Client will describe process of contraception and at least two methods she can use.

NURSING INTERVENTIONS WITH RATIONALE

- Provide family planning and contraceptive teaching *to ensure accurate information about the process of conceiving and methods used to control conception, thereby increasing the client's sense of control and lessening her fear of pregnancy.*
  - Refer client to agency offering classes on family planning.
  - Review client's knowledge of physiological processes and together identify misinformation.

EXPECTED CLIENT OUTCOMES

- Client will report lessening of painful intercourse after efforts at relaxation and positive imagery exercise.
- Client will state effect of his medication regimen on sexual desire and behavior.

NURSING INTERVENTIONS WITH RATIONALE

- Provide emotional support *to enable client to risk using relaxation techniques and/or imagery to lessen tension and increase sexual desire.*
  - Teach client simple relaxation technique.
  - Encourage recall of previous pleasurable sexual experiences.

*References 7–9,12,14,15,18–22,24

EXPECTED CLIENT OUTCOME

- Client will report contacting family weekly and will attend a women's group at her church.

NURSING INTERVENTIONS WITH RATIONALE

- Provide support system enhancement *to facilitate feelings of connectedness and security and lessening fears of change and being alone.*
    - Encourage and seek report on phone calls to family members.
    - Discuss reasons for expanding and maintaining a circle of friends.
- Identify support groups in community.
- Question client about her reluctance to associate more with others as one technique *to help her explore the beliefs and thoughts related to that behavior.*

Example: Client With Male Erectile Disorder in Outpatient Setting

NURSING DIAGNOSIS #1:   *Sexual dysfunction related to beliefs about psychotropic medication, impairment of sexual desire, unknown fears or misbeliefs, and poor self-esteem*

EXPECTED CLIENT OUTCOME

- Client will participate in sexual counseling within 3 months.

NURSING INTERVENTIONS WITH RATIONALE

- Provide teaching about prescribed medication in order *to give accurate information about effect and side effects of psychotropic medications and specifically the medication(s) he is taking.*
    - Review positive effects of medication on his ability to think.
    - Explore his beliefs about the affect of antipsychotic medication on his sexual ability.
- Provide support in decision making for seeking help with a sexual problem.
    - Act as liaison to the agency offering sexual counseling.

- ○ Emphasize the positive outcomes of being involved in learning and in therapy: the value of knowing newer, safer sexual techniques, being more in control, and feeling less anxious.
- ○ Restate availability.
- Facilitate self-esteem enhancement *to assist him in seeking help and to be more open to new ideas and information.*
  - ○ Identify strengths in coping with daily situations brought up for discussion.
  - ○ Question client's reason for self-negating remarks as they occur.
  - ○ Discuss difference between dependency that promotes personal growth and dependency that stifles exploration and change.

CHAPTER **16**

Eating Disorders

▌ Definition/Major Symptoms[*]

Eating Disorders are severe disturbances in eating behaviors characterized by preoccupation with weight, refusal to maintain minimally normal body weight, inappropriate attempts to lose weight or to prevent weight gain, and pathological extremes of eating too much or too little.

▌ Definition/Symptoms of Selected Major Categories[†]

Anorexia Nervosa (AN)

This category includes clients who binge and purge as well as clients who only restrict food intake; preoccupation with body weight and food; refusal to maintain body weight that is considered to be minimally normal for individual's age and weight; weight loss through omitting foods that are perceived to increase weight; extreme concern of gaining weight that continues even when person is actually losing weight; lack of insight and denial of serious, life-threatening aspects of emaciation, cachexia, with resistance to treatment; fasting, hoarding food and surreptitiously attempting to get rid of it; rigorous exercise routines; pattern of binge eating and/or purging behaviors, e.g., vomiting, taking laxatives, using diuretics or enemas; problems with delayed psychosocial development in adolescents and decreased interest in sex in adults; dissatis-

[*]References 1,2,34,35
[†]References 1,8,11,35

faction with entire body or selected parts of body, with self-worth based on erroneous perception of body shape and weight; frequent checking in mirrors to see if body is "thin enough"; amenorrhea prior to noticeable weight loss; behaviors indicative of mood disturbance or obsessive-compulsive patterns; impulsivity associated with bulimic anorectic client, e.g., suicide attempts, self-mutilation, Substance Abuse, sexual promiscuity.

Bulimia Nervosa (BN)

Bulimia Nervosa consists of binge eating, recurrent episodes of uncontrolled, rapid ingestion of large quantities of food within a short period of time that is usually followed by inappropriate attempts to prevent weight gain, e.g., self-induced vomiting, use of laxatives or diuretics; attempts to conceal eating behaviors from others, to be as inconspicuous as possible; termination of binge eating is prompted by abdominal pain or discomfort, self-induced vomiting, or social interruption, e.g., unexpected presence of another person; feelings of guilt, shame, disgust are associated with eating episodes; fasting; rigorous exercise that is inappropriate because of medical condition or injury or interference with important activities; self-esteem that is based on self-evaluation of body shape and weight.

▋ Incidence[*]

Eating Disorders are more common in female adolescents and young female adults, particularly in those who are athletes, ballet dancers, and long-distance runners.

- Overall there has been an increase in Eating Disorders in women of all age groups, males, and minorities, e.g., African Americans in the U.S., working-class women in Hong Kong.
- An increase has been noted in upper-middle-class families whose ethnic backgrounds view food as a preferred means for conveying feelings.
- There is a wide variation (2% to 60%) of comorbidity rates for Borderline Personality and Eating Disorders.

[*]References 1,2,12,21,22,24,25,28,30,33,34

Anorexia Nervosa

- There has been an increased incidence in the U.S. and Western Europe over the past 30 years.
- Comorbid disorders: 50% to 75% with Major Depression and/or Dysthymia; 10% to 13% Obsessive-Compulsive Disorder with lifetime prevalence about 25%.

Bulimia Nervosa

- Incidence is highest in large cities, with lowest incidence in rural areas; majority of clients are female high school and college students, with increasing number of males; it is controversial whether male homosexuals are at greater risk than heterosexual males.
- Comorbid disorders: 43% anxiety; 49% chemical dependency; 12% bipolar; personality or substantial personality trait disturbances, 50% to 75%.

▌ Course[*]

Prognosis is poor for both of these disorders, particularly when the client has a concomitant problem with Substance Abuse.

Anorexia Nervosa

Onset: 17 years is the mean age of onset, rarely occurs in women over 40; onset is often associated with a stressful life event; course varies from a single episode to an unremitting course that results in death from medical complications (starvation, electrolyte imbalance) or from suicide. Eating Disorders are "reputed to have the highest death rate of any psychiatric disorder"[22,p.677]; some clients experience improvement in medical condition with ongoing difficulties in psychological aspects of illness; poor outcome is associated with older age at onset, longer length of illness, previous history of psychiatric admissions, and problematic relationships with family.

[*]References 1,11,16,22,24,28,33,34,35

Bulimia Nervosa

Onset: late adolescence or early adulthood, often after episode of dieting; strong social support network found to be predictor of positive treatment outcome; long-term outcome is unknown.

▌ Contributing Factors*

Neurobiological/Genetic

- Rigid diet, a common precipitant of binge-eating behavior, "may influence peptide and neurotransmitter secretion, which may in turn affect appetite and satiety mechanisms."[11,p.868]
- There is an association between an increase in food intake and mood changes to transient alterations in serotonin activity in women with BN who experienced acute tryptophan depletion.
- There is an association between adult obesity and genetic and developmental determinants.
- It has been hypothesized that Eating Disorders may be variants of Affective Disorders.
- Studies of families with Eating Disorders have found higher rates of AN and BN in families of AN and BN subjects than in control populations; there is an increased rate of AN in first-degree female relatives of clients with AN; preliminary findings show that AN is more likely to be inherited than BN, especially with early onset of AN; there are increased rates of BN in twins of clients with BN; there are increased rates of Substance Abuse (particularly alcoholism), Mood Disorders, and obesity in families of clients with BN.

Psychodynamic

- Interrelationships are found with the following developmental factors: adolescent need for autonomy and control that may include eating, dieting, and weight loss; identity searching that may result in strategies to look like a model or actress; binge eating as a way to deal with

*References 2,7,11,25,28,33–38

separation and individuation; associations between physical appearance and popularity.

- Volitional abstinence from eating occurs to postpone sexual maturity, repress sexual drives, e.g., attraction from males leads to unwanted end of childhood.
- There are findings of negative early mealtime and food-related experiences in women with BN, e.g., use of food as reward or punishment; emphasis on importance of weight, physical appearance, and attractiveness; encouragement from family to diet.
- There are some indications of role of body image distortions in women with AN and BN, who overestimate their body size.

Cultural Factors

There is an association between self-worth and attractiveness and diet and weight control for women in Western culture; value is placed on being thin, having a "toned" body as an ideal of feminine beauty, careers that require a thin body type, e.g., ballet, gymnastics; media focus on being thin.

▌ Laboratory and Physical Examination Findings[*]

Laboratory

- Use CBC, urinalysis, BUN/creatinine levels, electrolyte balance to determine electrolyte abnormalities, e.g., elevated serum bicarbonate, hypochloremia, hypokalemia, hyponatremia, magnesium, pre-albumin.
- Studies of malnourished and severely symptomatic clients include measuring calcium, magnesium, phosphorus, and serum amylase levels to detect persistent or recurrent vomiting in client who may deny these behaviors, liver function, and ECG.
- Bone mineral densitometry assesses risk for pathological fractures from osteoporosis in client with chronic AN as well as estradiol levels in amenorrheic clients; low values are indicative of possible bone loss.
- Assess levels of luteinizing hormone (LH) and follicle-stimulating hormone (FSH) when amenorrhea continues at normal weight.

[*]References 1,2,6,11,14,17,19,24,28,31

- Obtain MRI and CT scans of head and EEG for evaluation of abnormalities of brain function.

Physical Findings

- Even if findings from ECG, laboratory studies, and physical examination appear to be normal, the client may be significantly compromised if more than 15% below healthy body weight or if client has had rapid weight loss, has dental caries or swollen parotid glands.
- Other abnormal findings include below-normal weight for age and height, amenorrhea, and menstrual irregularity.

ANOREXIA NERVOSA

Complaints may include constipation, abdominal pain, weakness, lethargy; emaciation; dry skin with yellowish discoloration at times; skin may appear to be "dirty"; brittle hair and nails; scalp and pubic hair loss; low body temperature (below 96.6°F); reduced pulse rate (below 60); intolerance to cold (failure to respond with characteristic shivering); lower-extremity edema; pathological fractures (rare). Associated significant medical conditions, e.g., impaired renal function, osteoporosis, and cardiovascular problems.

BULIMIA NERVOSA

Nonspecific complaints may include fatigue, lethargy, weakness, dizziness, abdominal fullness, feeling bloated, constipation and frequent sore throat; may outwardly appear to be healthy; "Russell's sign", i.e., trauma-induced abrasions and scars on back of hands from persistent efforts to induce vomiting by sticking fingers down throat; hypertrophy of salivary glands; damaged, discolored teeth with enamel erosion from acid from vomitus that causes decalcification, dental caries, and periodontal disease; pharyngitis and hoarseness from gastric acid reflux in mouth; conjunctival hemorrhages and small broken blood vessels on cheeks; swelling of hands and feet; esophagitis.

Medical emergencies include esophageal tears from self-induced vomiting, cardiac failure caused by cardiomyopathy from ipecac intoxication, cardiac arrhythmias associated with electrolyte disturbances and ipecac intoxication.

▌ Special Assessment Considerations*

- A comprehensive multidimensional assessment make take several hours over a period of time. The client and family may be reticent to reveal pertinent information initially; increased sharing of information occurs after establishment of trusting relationship with health care provider.
- Assess for depression, present or past suicidal tendencies, and signs of self-mutilation.
- Obtain information about the client's food intake, preferences, dislikes, and cognitive distortions about food.
- Obtain information about client's laxative use; monitor for common complications from chronic laxative use in client with BN, e.g., cathartic colon, ileus, rectal prolapse, hemorrhoids.
- Inquire about legal history; binge eating is often followed by impulsive shoplifting of food, clothing, and jewelry.
- Obtain descriptions of family history, e.g., knowledge of and attitude toward Eating Disorder, obesity, family interactions in relation to client's Eating Disorder, as well as client descriptions of current living situation.
- Observe for concurrent comorbid psychiatric disorders and inquire about previous treatment for Eating Disorders as well as other psychiatric disorders, including a history of Substance Abuse and Dependency; Alcohol Abuse is common, as is Amphetamine Abuse for weight loss.
- Obtain a developmental history that includes sexual history as well as a history of physical and sexual abuse.
- Semi-structured interview instruments, e.g., the Eating Disorders Examination, or self-report questionnaires, e.g., Diagnostic Survey for Eating Disorders, are sometimes used during initial data gathering.
- Psychological testing may be ordered to clarify personality and/or neuropsychological disturbances.

▌ Treatment†

The initial priorities of treatment focus on nutritional rehabilitation and restoration of normal eating patterns. Longer-term, concurrent interventions focus on assessment and resolution of associated psychological, family,

*References 2,4,10,11,17,22,28,30,36
†References 2,4,5,11,13,17,19–24,26,28,31–33,36

social, and behavioral problems to reduce risk of relapse after biological and psychological sequelae have been corrected.

Psychopharmacologic

ANOREXIA NERVOSA

Phenothiazine, chlorpromazine (CPZ) in liquid form, low dose (10 mg tid with gradual increase) is used with severely delusional and overactive client; antihistamine, cyproheptadine, in liquid form (4 mg bid with increase to 8 mg tid if necessary) is used to stimulate appetite in severely overactive anorexic who does not binge and purge. Selective serotonin reuptake inhibitor (SSRI) (fluoxetine) is preferred after weight restoration due to its tendency to induce arousal in severely obsessive-compulsive behaviors related or unrelated to Eating Disorders and for AN clients with severe depression. Tricyclic antidepressant (TCA) (clomipramine) is used in very low doses due to hypotension side effects, preferably given after weight restoration for AN client with severely obsessive-compulsive behaviors; other TCAs are used with the same considerations as clomipramine for client with severe depression. Estrogen replacement is used for some clients with chronic amenorrhea to reduce calcium loss and risks of osteoporosis; an exception is made for adolescents with recommendation of waiting at least 1 year, during which time the focus is on increasing weight and achieving resumption of menses.

BULIMIA NERVOSA

Antidepressant medications, e.g., TCAs (desipramine, imipramine, amitriptyline, nortriptyline), monoamine oxidase inhibitor (phenelzine), and SSRI (fluoxetine), are used to improve mood and decrease psychopathological preoccupation with body shape and weight. Antidepressant medication without psychotherapy is inadequate treatment.

SPECIFIC NURSING IMPLICATIONS

- Malnourished clients with concurrent depression are more prone to the side effects of antidepressant medication, e.g., hypotension, arrhythmia.

- Assess for the following: CBC in conjunction with all preceding medications; CBC with platelets for client taking cyproheptadine; lying and standing blood pressure for clients taking CPZ, clomipramine, and TCAs; observation of total sleep and activity for client taking fluoxetine; serum electrolytes and amylase and ECG for BN clients taking antidepressants. (See also Chapter 4 for additional specific and general nursing implications for client taking antidepressant medications.)

Hospitalization

- Partial hospitalization in day hospital programs is sometimes used for milder cases or to decrease inpatient hospitalizations. Partial hospitalization requires client motivation to participate in intensive treatment program with mutually agreed-upon criteria for symptom change; client must be able to participate in a group setting.
- Hospitalization in an Eating Disorders unit may be needed for monitoring and interrupting life-threatening behaviors of purging and food restricting. Inpatient admission to a psychiatric, medical, or critical care unit is recommended for clients who are suicidal or have severe concurrent Substance Abuse or life-threatening medical problems that cannot be managed in an outpatient setting; the stabilization of a client with binge–purge cycle may require several weeks of inpatient treatment.

Psychotherapy/Self Regulation Models

- For clients with AN, therapy begins with obtaining client's cooperation in a treatment program with goal to restore client's nutritional state to normal; outpatient treatment is recommended for client with less than 6 months' history of AN, client who is not bingeing and purging, and client with family who are likely to cooperate with treatment plan and participate in family therapy; hospitalization is indicated for clients whose medical management is difficult, e.g., need for weight restoration, rehydration, and correction of serum electrolytes.
- Family therapy is more beneficial for AN clients under age of 18.

- Cognitive therapy is used with AN to help client evaluate automatic thoughts and examine erroneous assumptions that affect client's perception of body weight or shape, result in denial of seriousness of low body weight, and lead to relentless pursuit of thinness as an attempt to control environment.
- Psychodynamic therapy is used with cognitive and behavioral techniques in individual and group therapy modalities.
- Cognitive-behavioral therapy is used for client with BN in group or individual settings, with focus on self-monitoring (daily record of times and durations of meals, binge eating and purging, moods and situations in which binge–purge occurs), cognitive restructuring, and psychoeducation on bulimic disorder.
- Behavior therapy is used to stop binge eating and purging, with focus on restricting exposure to cues, developing strategies of alternative behaviors, and learning to prevent vomiting.
- Operant conditioning is a form of behavior therapy that begins with a behavioral analysis and is followed with positive reinforcements that may include increased physical activity, visiting privileges, and social activities based on client's weight gain.
- Interpersonal therapy focuses on interpersonal relationships.
- Overeaters Anonymous and groups with a 12-step program focus are controversial for clients with BN, e.g., benefits from networking and sense of group connectedness versus lack of focus on nutritional considerations and psychological/behavioral deficits. None of these groups should be used for sole initial treatment.

▌ Commonly Occurring Nursing Diagnoses*

Activity intolerance
Activity intolerance, risk for
Altered nutrition, less than body requirements
Altered oral mucous membrane
Altered social interaction: compulsive behaviors
    (accepted by NANDA for development[29])
Anxiety

*References 10,15,22,23,28–33

Body image disturbance
Constipation
Constipation, perceived
Decreased cardiac output
Diarrhea
Fatigue
Fear
Fluid volume deficit
Fluid volume deficit, risk for
Impaired skin integrity
Impaired social interaction
Ineffective denial
Ineffective individual coping
Personal identity disturbance
Powerlessness
Risk for impaired skin integrity
Risk for altered body temperature
Risk for infection
Risk for injury
Risk for self-mutilation
Risk for violence directed toward self
Self-esteem disturbance

▌ Selected Nursing Diagnoses, Outcome Criteria, and Nursing Interventions With Rationale*

Client With Anorexia Nervosa on Inpatient Unit

NURSING DIAGNOSIS #1:   *Alteration in nutrition, less than body requirements, related to restricted food intake, bingeing and purging*

EXPECTED CLIENT OUTCOMES

• The client will increase food intake to achieve specified appropriate weight gain, interrupt binge–purge cycle, and be able to discuss long-term effects and consequences of starvation and purging behaviors.

NURSING INTERVENTIONS WITH RATIONALE

• Determine client's motivation for agreeing to inpatient treatment. *Motivation may be inversely proportional to*

*References 3–5,9–11,15,16,20,22,23,26–28

the client's level of ambivalence about changing behaviors. It may be helpful to have client rate level of motivation on scale of 1 to 10, with 10 as high motivation for wanting to change and the lowest numbers representing seeking treatment because others want client to change.

- Assess for presence of depression and present or past suicidal tendencies, as well as obsessive thought processes or ritualistic behaviors that interfere with client's choices of dietary intake.
- Inquire about Substance Abuse.
- Obtain specific information about client's weight history, restricting behaviors, and eating and purging behaviors, e.g., laxative, diuretic, emetic abuse; use matter-of-fact, nonjudgmental approach, *recognizing that client may be unaccustomed to discussing these practices.*
- Collaborate with treatment team, client, and involved family to obtain specific information about family involvement, family history of Eating Disorders, Substance Abuse, depression, and family decision-making process *to determine the influence of family on client's motivation and participation in treatment.*
- Assess for client's knowledge about long-term health-damaging consequences of diet restriction, purging; *use information obtained in development of individualized psychoeducational approaches, e.g., acquiring new skills for managing dietary intake, correcting misinformation about normal physiology, weight loss, and regulation. This educational plan might also include referral for assertiveness training as well as group therapy to practice social skills.* (See also Assertiveness Training and Social Skills Training in Chapter 5.)
- Collaborate with client's multidisciplinary team in development and implementation of a consistent plan that incorporates nursing, medical management, and nutritional rehabilitation; *a coordinated treatment approach reduces potential for client's attempt to replicate dysfunctional communication patterns used with his or her family and minimizes client's attempt to disrupt treatment plan.*
- Encourage client to prepare list of advantages and disadvantages for changing dietary patterns, interrupting binge–purge cycle; *this type of activity can serve as a starting point for client to begin to explore and gain insight into*

purpose of maladaptive behaviors, antecedents, and secondary gains.

- Collaborate with dietitian in the development of a dietary plan for gradual weight gain; ensure that dietitian discusses client's nutritional needs with him or her, emphasizing the importance of a well-balanced diet.
- Collaborate with client in the establishment of a weight goal and in the development of a contract that specifies the plan for dietary intake throughout the day, e.g., three food items at each meal, four nutritious snacks, no diet food; client will not ask dietary staff for changes. This contract might also include client's keeping a diary or daily journal of food intake and feelings associated with food intake (see also Contracting in Chapter 5). Emphasize that uncontrolled weight gain is not the goal, *to reduce fear of obesity.*
- Maintain a neutral, nonjudgmental position about client's weight gain or losses.
- Provide guidance and assistance for client's participation in development of weekly menu planning; *use these planning sessions to determine client's knowledge of calories; provide ongoing education as needed, incorporating relevant information about nutritional intake and estimated necessary weekly weight gain to achieve normal weight.*
- Inform client of plan for monitoring nutritional intake, elimination, vital signs, and electrolytes. Plan will likely include the following: client will void before being weighed and can expect random weighings; client will use bathroom only when accompanied by staff for 1 to 2 hours after eating *to prevent self-induced vomiting;* staff will provide close observation during period after mealtime *to prevent and extinguish emesis response because clients are less likely to vomit in presence of others.*
- Emphasize to client and family that the family is not permitted to bring food to client.
- Explore possible ambivalence client may have about plans to increase dietary intake and interrupt binge–purge cycle.
- Provide opportunity for client to experience social support after meal time and after weighing.
- Encourage client to talk with treatment team on ongoing basis about fears of possible weight gain, bingeing because

of feeling full, and lack of self-trust to control purging at the time that client is experiencing these feelings *to help client to reframe irrational thought processes to increase sense of self-control.*

- Encourage client to be candid and to disclose problems in adhering to contract *to help client reexamine vulnerable areas and to develop coping strategies for adhering to behaviors for goal achievement.*

- Facilitate client's preparation for discharge by having client practice menu selection with staff; go on therapeutic passes to arrange for and organize living arrangements, resuming employment, returning to school, and eating in restaurants *to help client begin to identify potential problematic, relapse-producing situations and to develop strategies for successful coping with perceived challenges.*

- Prior to client's discharge, collaborate with multidisciplinary team to meet with him or her for a mutual review (client and treatment team) of accomplishments and discussion of recommendations following discharge. (See also Discharge Planning in Chapter 5.)

Client With Bulimia Nervosa

NURSING DIAGNOSIS #2: *Body image disturbance related to dissatisfaction with self*

EXPECTED CLIENT OUTCOME

- The client will experience reintegration of body image as evidenced by developing a positive self/body image, maintaining a realistic and healthy weight, and establishing an appropriate exercise regimen.

NURSING INTERVENTIONS WITH RATIONALE

- Encourage client's description of perception of body image, e.g., aspects that are pleasing or not pleasing, perceived changes, perceived impact of attitudes and feelings of significant others.

- Determine possible origins for negative perceptions or appraisals, e.g. life crisis, influence of significant others.

- Provide ongoing opportunity for client to discuss fears, concerns about weight issues, body image, and perceptions of ability to change maladaptive behaviors. *Identifi-*

cation of client's attitudes about food, eating, body weight and shape, in addition to eating habits, are important components for achievement of change. Successful recovery requires changes in client's attitudes towards his or her shape and weight as well as a change in disturbed eating habits.

- Develop a teaching plan that provides factual information about nutrition, e.g., factors that increase likelihood of binge eating (maintaining low body weight, omitting meals, continual dieting) and the effects of chronic dieting on cognitive functioning *to provide a cognitive framework for client to understand own experiences.*

- Collaborate with treatment team in assessing need for antidepressant medication; *a significant number of clients with BN also have mood disturbances; antidepressant medication has been found to improve clients' mood and to reduce psychopathological symptoms that include preoccupation with shape and weight.*

- Collaborate with dietitian to develop a plan to coordinate increased activity schedule that is contingent on gradual controlled weight gain and/or maintenance.

- Use contracting to develop an exercise plan that is contingent on client's weight gain and weight maintenance (see also Contracting in Chapter 5).

- Collaborate with treatment team in the development of a plan that uses cognitive approaches *to reshape cognitive distortions by challenging and correcting client's irrational thinking about body image; cognitive behavioral therapy has been determined to be the treatment of choice for BN.* This plan could include strategies such as:
  - Client maintaining a food/feeling diary or journal that includes factual reports of eating, activity, feeling states about body image, and descriptions of specific difficulties that client is experiencing; *information from these written reports can be shared in individual or group discussion to challenge dysfunctional thinking.*
  - Group approach that incorporates psychoeducational component for addressing body image dissatisfaction, e.g., social-cultural emphasis on thinness, as well as other aspects of client's problems with BN
  - Body image therapy in individual or group setting, e.g., relaxation techniques, guided imagery, kinesthetic strategies

- ○ Role-playing techniques, using individual or group approach for client
- Encourage client to accept positive appraisals of self and to take pride in appearance.

NURSING DIAGNOSIS #3: *Constipation related to laxative dependence and abuse*

EXPECTED CLIENT OUTCOME

- The client will have a daily elimination of a normally formed stool without use of laxatives.

NURSING INTERVENTIONS WITH RATIONALE

- Obtain history of elimination pattern prior to initiation of laxative abuse.
- Obtain history of laxative use, including specific types of laxatives; *clients with BN often use non-prescription laxatives to lose weight, e.g., stimulant types such as Ex-Lax, Corrector, and Senekot are often used because of their rapid action and ability to produce watery diarrhea when taken in sufficient doses.*
- Inquire about history of constipation that has led to increase in dosage.
- Find out what other stimulus client may use for defecation, e.g., coffee, prune juice.
- Collaborate with the treatment team in gradually tapering excessive laxative use.
- Ensure that client has PRN provision of mild laxative, bulk agent, and/or stool softener.
- Collaborate with treatment team to obtain GI consultation for client whose course is severe or chronic or who has problems in weaning or significantly decreasing laxative dependence.
- Develop a teaching plan that includes normal physiology of elimination as well as negative health consequences and futility of laxative use for losing weight; this plan might include the following information:
  - ○ unwanted calories are not eliminated by laxatives because most of the ingested food that reaches colon will have already been absorbed
  - ○ negative effects of laxatives, e.g., relationship between use and reflex hypofunctioning of bowel

- ○ dangers of cathartic colon, a permanent impairment that can require colon resection
- ○ risk for gastrointestinal bleeding
- ○ possible complications from protein and fat losses, e.g., dehydration and electrolyte abnormalities
- ○ dietary education about high-fiber foods and adequate fluid intake
- ○ appropriate amount of exercise.

CHAPTER 17

Sleep Disorders

▌ Definition/Major Categories *

Sleep Disorders comprise four major categories based on etiology:

1. Primary Sleep Disorders
2. Sleep Disorder Related to Another Mental Disorder
3. Sleep Disorder Due to a General Medical Condition
4. Substance-Induced Sleep Disorder

▌ Definition/Major Symptoms of Selected Major Categories†

Primary Sleep Disorders

DYSSOMNIAS

These are abnormalities in the timing, quality, or amount of sleep that are not the result of another mental disorder, a substance such as a medication, or a medical condition. Types of dyssomnias include:

1. Primary Insomnia: a problem in initiating or maintaining sleep or of nonrestorative sleep that lasts at least 1 month, causing distress or impaired functioning in important life areas, such as occupational or social roles; daytime fatigue.
2. Primary Hypersomnia: prolonged sleep episodes or general daytime sleep episodes. This excessive sleepiness causes impaired functioning in important life areas and lasts at least 1 month.

*Reference 2
†References 2,14

3. Narcolepsy: daily attacks of sleep lasting at least 3 months, along with cataplexy (bilateral loss of muscle tone, often with severe emotion) or REM (rapid eye movement) sleep occurrences during the transition from sleep to wakefulness.
4. Breathing-Related Sleep Disorder: a sleep disruption resulting in sleepiness or insomnia due to a sleep-related breathing condition, e.g., obstructive sleep apnea syndrome, central sleep apnea syndrome.
5. Circadian Rhythm Sleep Disorder: a sleep disruption resulting in sleepiness or insomnia due to a mismatch between a person's circadian sleep–wake pattern and the demands of the environment.
6. Dyssomnia Not Otherwise Specified: dyssomnia that does not fit the above categories, e.g., sleepiness due to sleep deprivation.

PARASOMNIAS

These are abnormalities in behavioral or physiological events associated with sleep, sleep stages, or sleep-to-wakefulness transitions that are not due to another mental disorder, a substance such as a medication, or a medical condition. Types of Parasomnias include:

1. Nightmare Disorder: a sleep disturbance resulting from repeated awakenings, with recall of very frightening dreams, that affect functioning (i.e., social, occupational, and other role functioning).
2. Sleep Terror Disorder: an abrupt sleep awakening with intense fear, rapid pulse, and respirations that is unresponsive to efforts of comfort; lacks dream recall and impacts functioning
3. Sleepwalking Disorder: walking about during sleep, unresponsive to efforts at communication; lacks recall of the episode and affects functioning.
4. Parasomnia Not Otherwise Specified: parasomnia that does not fit above categories, e.g., REM sleep behavior disorder (violent motor activity during REM sleep).

Sleep Disorder Related to Another Disorder

This describes a sleep disturbance due to an actual mental disorder, e.g., Mood Disorders. Types include:

- Insomnia Related to Another Mental Disorder: difficulty falling or staying asleep that results in impaired functioning and that is related to a major disorder, e.g., Adjustment Disorder With Anxiety.
- Hypersomnia Related to Another Mental Disorder: excessive sleepiness lasting at least 1 month leading to impaired general daily functioning and related to a major mental disorder.

Sleep Disorder Due to a General Medical Condition

This is a sleep disturbance due to physiological effects of a medical condition. Subtypes include Insomnia Type, Hypersomnia Type, Parasomnia Type, and Mixed Type.

Substance-Induced Sleep Disorder

This is a sleep disturbance due to the effects of a substance, e.g., medications, or the recent discontinuation of a substance. Subtypes include Insomnia Type, Hypersomnia Type, Parasomnia Type, and Mixed Type; specifiers include With Onset During Intoxication and With Onset During Withdrawal.

■ Incidence*

Sleep disturbances and disorders are among the most common complaints, affecting about one third of the adults in the United States. Of these, insomnia is the most common.

- Primary Insomnia: Among the general population, 30% to 40% of adults suffer from insomnia in any given year, but the percentage of Primary Insomnia is unknown; in sleep clinics, 15% to 25% of persons with chronic insomnia are diagnosed with Primary Insomnia.
- Insomnia Related to Another Mental Disorder: In sleep clinics, 35% to 50% of persons with chronic insomnia receive this diagnosis.
- Primary Hypersomnia: In sleep clinics 5% to 10% of persons with daytime sleepiness conform to this diagnosis.
- Narcolepsy: In the adult population the rate of this disorder is low, only .02% to .16%.

*References 2,3,12,16,23,29,32,33,34,35

- Breathing-Related Sleep Disorder (e.g., obstructive or central sleep apnea syndrome): The rate of incidence is from 1% to 10% in adults, with a higher incidence in the elderly.
- Circadian Rhythm Sleep Disorders: Incidence rate varies, e.g., 60% of all night shift workers.
- Nightmare Disorder: The rate of occasional Nightmare Disorder may reach 50% in adults.
- Sleep Terror Disorder: The rate of Sleep Terror Disorder is about 1% in adults.
- Sleepwalking episodes range from 1% to 7% among adults.

Age-Related

- Difficulties in both falling asleep and staying asleep are common complaints in infancy and early childhood.
- Insomnia, night terrors, somniloquy, and somnambulism are common during late childhood and adolescence.
- Elderly persons have more difficulty falling asleep (may shift to earlier bedtimes and early rising) and maintaining sleep and have more shallow breathing during sleep than younger people.
- Elderly persons have decreased REM sleep; among clients with Dementia, REM sleep is even more disrupted and decreased.
- Elderly persons experience greater difficulty in maintaining daytime alertness.
- Elderly women experience greater sleep–wake pattern changes than men.

▌ Course*

General

- Sleep is described as a reversible behavioral state that is characterized by perceptual disengagement and unresponsiveness to the surrounding environment.
- Although the mechanisms and functions of sleep are not totally understood, most sleep experts define the function of sleep as restorative for the mind and body, needed to maintain health as well as energy, and affecting the quality of life and well-being of individuals.

*References 2,3,13–15,18–20,22,27,33,35,37

- Normal sleep is difficult to define because different people need different amounts of sleep: sleep becomes less efficient as one ages; men need less sleep; subjective complaints of insomnia can differ from objective assessment; and measures are highly variable and subjective in adults.
- Sleep stages include the following:
  - Stage I—transitory period in which the sleeper experiences a floating sensation; lasts about 5 minutes (2%–5% of sleep)
  - Stage II—slightly deeper sleep with EEG changes (45%–55% of sleep)
  - Stage III—slowing of pulse and respirations
  - Stage IV—deeper sleep with slowest pulse and respirations (13%–23% of sleep occurs in stages 3 and 4)
  - REM sleep—rapid side-to-side movement of the eyes, shallow breathing, and mixed-frequency brain waves (20%–25% of sleep)
- REM sleep is needed for maintaining the immune function and helping with memory functions.
- Growth hormones increase during sleep, so sleep may induce tissue anabolism.

Primary Insomnia

- The most common subjective reasons patients give for their sleeping difficulties include a decrease in the total amount of actual sleep, dissatisfaction with the quality of sleep, and difficulty falling asleep.
- Sleep disturbances can be manifested in a variety of ways, e.g., difficulty in falling asleep, waking up periodically and not being able to go back to sleep, waking up early in the morning and not being able to go back to sleep, and not feeling rested from a generally normal amount of sleep.
- Subjective estimates of sleep disturbance may exaggerate the actual sleep disturbance.
- Subjective reports of sleep disturbance can be supported to varying degrees by actual objective measures of sleep disturbance.
- The chronic state of insomnia is characterized by chronic fatigue; impaired concentration, thinking, and remember-

ing; dysphoria; decreased facial expression; apathy and feeling blue; muscle tremors or weakness; burning of eyes; and difficulty in working efficiently.

- Primary Insomnia can persist even after initial causative stressor(s) are eliminated.
- Primary Insomnia can be a lifetime disorder with a constitutional predisposition for fragmented sleep.
- Generally the disorder begins in early to middle adulthood.
- The disorder can persist from a couple of months to years.

▮ Contributing Factors*

Primary Insomnia

- Before a diagnosis of Primary Insomnia is made, other more specific etiologies must be ruled out. Chronic Primary Insomnia may be a result of neurochemical or structural disorders. The symptoms presented must also be differentiated from expected or usual problems the client has in sleeping.
- Stressors such as physical health, social problems (e.g., marital discord, parenting problems, excessive social demands), and psychological difficulties can be indicators of the onset of Primary Insomnia.
- Learned insomnia may be related to the irregular sleep patterns of newly widowed or retired persons.
- Emotional and social changes and problems experienced most intensely during middle adolescence contribute to the greater occurrence of sleep disturbance in middle compared with late adolescence.
- Sleep requirements may increase during times of stress, including times of illness and hospitalization.
- There may be negative associations with the usual place used to sleep (i.e., the bedroom).
- Increased arousal preventing sleep can be caused by fear of the inability to sleep, worry about the time it takes to go to sleep, or environmental cues such as a visible clock.
- Poor sleep hygiene practices include spending excessive time in bed, especially in nonsleep activities such as eating, watching television, and using the telephone; irregu-

*References 1,2,9,11,14,15,23,27,31,36,39,40

lar bedtime; irregular sleep hours; excessive caffeine intake; and daytime napping, although there is variable support for this, e.g., napping may not affect certain aspects of nighttime sleep such as sleep latency.[11]

- Other possible causes of insomnia include the following:
  ○ Hunger or excessive eating before bedtime
  ○ Drinking alcohol before bedtime, which fragments sleep and prevents deeper stages of sleep
  ○ Chronic use of tobacco
  ○ Discomfort or pain
  ○ Exercise close to bedtime
- The clinical care environment may be a factor when characterized by frequent disturbances or simply by its unfamiliarity.
- Environmental factors such as altitude, extreme temperature changes, undimmed lights, and noise can be contributing factors; if they are primary contributing factor, a diagnosis of Dyssomnia Not Otherwise Specified may be made.

▌ Laboratory and Physical Examination Findings[*]

Primary Insomnia

- Controversies surrounding this diagnostic term center on "(1) the extent to which Sleep Disorders, particularly those involving insomnia, can be classified into subtypes; (2) the feasibility and utility of more differentiated versus general classifications in the practice of psychiatry; and (3) the value and place of the sleep laboratory in the differential diagnosis of insomnia complaints."[20, p. 602; 31, p. 607]
- The client complains of fatigue.
- The presence of signs and symptoms of Primary Insomnia must be differentiated from the expected or usual problems the person has in sleeping.
- Polysomnography is considered the "gold standard" as a laboratory procedure to diagnose the physiological parameters of sleep. Polysomnographic evidence of sleep disturbance includes intermittent wakefulness, decreased sleep efficiency, increased muscle tension, and greater sleep latency.

[*]References 2,4,6,14,20,28,31

- Neuroimaging can be used to to evaluate sleep disturbance in neurologic illness.
- Psychophysiological tests can indicate a high arousal state.
- Personality inventories can indicate higher levels of anxiety or depression.
- Since insomnia is often associated with the use or abuse of substances (e.g., caffeine, sympathomimetics, methylphenidate, thyroid drugs, estrogen, antihistamines, opioids), the diagnosis of Substance-Induced Sleep Disorder must be ruled out.

▌ Special Assessment Considerations[*]

- Primary Insomnia must be differentiated from other Sleep Disorders such as Circadian Rhythm Sleep Disorder, Narcolepsy, Parasomnias, Breathing-Related Sleep Disorder, Insomnia Related to Another Mental Disorder, Sleep Disorder Due to a General Medical Condition/Insomnia Type, and Substance-Induced Sleep Disorder/Insomnia.
- Obtain a sleep history.
- Have the client keep a diary of his or her sleep activities for 2 weeks.
- With the client's permission, conduct an interview of his or her sleep partner.
- Use a 24-hour history as a tool to evaluate the client for Sleep Disorders.
- Psychometric/psychiatric and medical/neurological evaluations may be required.
- Polysomnography may be useful.

▌ Treatment[†]

Primary Insomnia

PSYCHOPHARMACOLOGIC/BIOLOGIC

- Aromatherapy (e.g., pre-mixed blend of oils of basil, lavender, juniper, marjoram) is a vaporization of oil and herbs into atmosphere that can be followed with a massage with the oils.[5]
- Pharmacotherapy is especially useful for short-term treatment, e.g., benzodiazepines as a sedative and hyp-

[*]References 2,40
[†]References 5,10,25,34

notic and nonbenzodiazepine hypnotics such as zolpidem, chloral hydrate.
- Tricyclic antidepressants are effective in treating insomnia related to Affective Disorders or chronic pain.
- Also available are over-the-counter sleep aids, most of which contain antihistamines that produce drowsiness.

PSYCHOTHERAPY
- Behavioral treatment is used to strengthen the association between sleep behaviors and related stimuli and to consolidate sleep over a shorter time.
- Biofeedback may be used.
- Autogenic training may be used, which engages the client in pleasant visual imagery along with relaxing sensations such as warmth.
- Cognitive therapy may help the client to reevaluate thoughts about the reasons for insomnia: faulty appraisal, misattributions, unrealistic expectations, cognitive errors.

OTHER APPROACHES
- Progressive relaxation may be used (see also Stress Management in Chapter 5).
- Repetitive, non-threatening noise (e.g., white noise such as ocean sounds) can provide distraction, enhance relaxing imagery, and enhance sleep.[10]
- Sleep hygiene education can change such elements as health practices and environmental influences.

▌ Commonly Occurring Nursing Diagnoses[*]

Altered role performance
Anticipatory grieving
Anxiety
Dysfunctional grieving
Fatigue
Hopelessness
Impaired social interaction
Ineffective individual coping
Rape trauma syndrome
Risk for activity intolerance
Sleep pattern disturbance

[*]References 15,17,26

▌ Selected Nursing Diagnoses, Outcome Criteria, and Nursing Interventions with Rationale*

DMS-IV Disorder: Primary Insomnia

NURSING DIAGNOSIS #1:   *Sleep pattern disturbance related to internal and external factors*

EXPECTED CLIENT OUTCOME

- Client will identify stressors and gain an understanding of factors contributing to sleep disturbance.

NURSING INTERVENTIONS WITH RATIONALE

- Assess client's perceived quality and quantity of sleep, difficulties in falling asleep and maintaining sleep, and premature awakening. Use assessment tools such as the Sleep Questionnaire[33] or the Insomnia Interview Scale,[25, pp. 195–198] Sleep Impairment Index,[25, p. 199–200] and Beliefs and Attitudes about Sleep Scale.[25, pp. 201–204]
- Ask client to describe his or her personal understanding of sleep and sleep difficulties. *"The meaning of sleep to an individual will affect his response to its disruption and must affect the approach of the nurse in effectively promoting sleep and rest."*[37, p. 255]
- Ask client to keep a sleep diary; aid from significant other may be helpful in keeping an accurate record. *Sleep state misperception can occur, e.g., client may report more nighttime awakenings than actually occurred.*
- Assess client's overall usual daily sleep–wake pattern. *Factors such as irregular bedtime, daytime napping, spending excessive time in bed, and physical exercise too close to bedtime can contribute to sleep disturbance.*
- Assess client's sleep-related habits, including activities and experience in preparing for sleep. *Negative conditioning such as fear of not being able to sleep or worrying about not being able to go to sleep can lead to arousal and difficulty in achieving sleep.*
- Assess the sleep environment; interview family members if necessary; have client describe his or her usual experience in preparing for sleep. *Environmental cues, e.g., a visible clock, can be linked to arousal at bedtime.*

*References 3,7–9,11,13,15,16,21,24,25,27,30,34,38,39

Environmental factors, e.g., extreme temperature changes, bright lights, and loud noise, can contribute to poor sleep.
- Determine the client's use of alcohol, caffeine, and tobacco, as well as eating patterns. *Drinking alcohol before bedtime, chronic use of tobacco, hunger, or excessive eating prior to bedtime can contribute to sleep disturbance.*
- Assess for presence of stressors experienced by client such as social problems, physical health, emotional problems, and tensions. *Stressors such as physical illness, social problems and psychological difficulties are related to the onset of Primary Insomnia. It is particularly important for clients to achieve satisfactory sleep during times of stress since sleep requirements may increase during such times.*
- Assess the effects of the client's sleep–wake pattern on social, occupational, and other role functioning. *Primary Insomnia can lead to impaired functioning in critical daily roles of the client.*
- Review and discuss assessment data with client *in order to assist client in identifying and understanding the most important internal and external factors that may be contributing to poor sleep.*

EXPECTED CLIENT OUTCOME

- Client will engage in sleep hygiene practices, manage factors contributing to poor sleep, and achieve more satisfactory sleep as evidenced by client verbalizing experiencing less distress and reporting improved daily functioning.

NURSING INTERVENTIONS WITH RATIONALE

- Assist client in decreasing levels of anxiety. (See also Chapter 11 for more specific nursing strategies to decrease anxiety.)
- Assist client in decreasing levels of depressed mood and hopelessness. (See also Chapters 5 and 10 for nursing interventions to counter hopelessness.)
- Collaborate with treatment team in developing plan and administering measures to control any pain experienced by client. *Because pain is often cited as a reason for poor sleep, pain control is a priority in intervening in sleep disturbance. Clients with chronic pain usually have sleep*

problems. In these clients, avoid use of opioids. Benzodi-azepines can be used to assist with self-management of pain, although pain cannot always be eliminated; attempting to eliminate all pain is futile.

- If client is hospitalized, reduce the number of disturbances during the night to a minimum, e.g., post "Do Not Disturb" sign. *Sources of disturbances include noise from other clients, nurses providing care to other clients, telephones and lights, and staff talking; these can all be disruptive to good nighttime sleep and must be controlled.*

- Use behavioral therapy strategies consisting of a combination of sleep restrictions and stimulus control strategies *in order to strengthen the association of the bedroom and sleep-related behaviors. Clients prone to conditioning can develop negative responses to bedtime-related sleep activities during periods of high stress that persist over time and contribute to ongoing poor sleep. The sleep environment, which was relaxing, is now associated with a state of insomnia. A maladaptive cycle of sleep disturbance, arousal, and further insomnia develops. Behavioral therapy strategies can be useful to break this cycle.* For example:
  - "Lie down only when sleepy and ready to sleep.
  - Use bedroom only for sleep (and relaxing intimacy).
  - If sleep does not occur within 10 minutes, get up, go elsewhere, read, or do something boring.
  - When sleepy, lie down again but not for longer than 10 minutes. Repeat as necessary.
  - Instruct client to set an alarm and get up at same time every morning regardless of the time that client goes to sleep.
  - No or little napping during the day."[34, p. 22] *Clients should monitor effects of napping on overall functioning and actual sleep.*

- Teach client progressive relaxation, autogenic training, and other stress management techniques (see Stress Management in Chapter 5). *Relaxation and stress management techniques focus on reducing somatic and cognitive arousal that interferes with sleep.*

- Encourage meditation or prayer as a supportive bedtime routine.

- Teach client to engage in health-promoting activities that also enhance the quality and quantity of sleep. For example, teach client to:

- Engage in a program of regular daily exercise; heavy exercise in late afternoon can enhance sleep.
- Drink alcohol in moderation, avoiding it near bedtime.
- Decrease or eliminate use of tobacco. Do not smoke tobacco close to bedtime or during awakenings.
- Avoid being hungry; a very light snack may be sleep enhancing, as is warm milk.
- Avoid caffeine intake for about 4 hours before bedtime.
- Avoid strenuous physical activity within 3 hours before sleep. *Adhering to these health-promoting activities can eliminate some of the factors that have been found to contribute to poor sleep.*
- Discuss with client and/or implement ways to manage environmental factors contributing to poor sleep *in order to promote a relaxing and comfortable environment conducive to quality sleep.* For example:
  - Control temperature and keep it at comfortable level.
  - Curtail loud noise.
  - Dim lights.
  - Use soft music or white noise.
  - Maintain adequate ventilation.
  - Sleep on a comfortable mattress and pillow.
- Use cognitive therapy strategies in order to alter and correct client's appraisal of his or her sleep experience. For example:
  - Assist client in correcting faulty appraisal. *Faulty appraisal can lead the client to view sleeplessness as loss of personal control instead of seeing it in relation to life stressors or circumstances faced. The former appraisal can lead to sleep performance anxiety and contribute to an ongoing pattern of poor sleep.*
  - Assist client in correcting misattributions. *Attributing the majority of daytime impairments to sleep difficulties can serve as a self-fulfilling prophecy.*
  - Assist client in altering unrealistic expectations. *Setting rigid standards for sleep can increase sleep performance anxiety and contribute to difficulties in falling asleep.*
  - Assist client in reducing cognitive errors. *Magnifying the degree of sleep disturbance and its effect on daytime functioning, for example, can be counterproductive.*
- In collaboration with physician, administer sedative-hypnotic medications, when necessary. For reasons of

efficacy and safety, benzodiazepines are generally the treatment of choice when sleep medication is needed for short-term management of insomnia; they have few side effects and a relatively low potential for addiction. Some experts are of the opinion, however, that trazodone is safer. Hypnotics with a rapid absorption rate are prescribed for sleep onset insomnia; hypnotics with slower action and longer duration are prescribed for sleep maintenance problems.

- Zolpidem is an alternative to benzodiazepines; it does not cause rebound insomnia or impair daytime alertness.
- Chloral hydrate is potentiated by the use of alcohol and has a high risk of lethal overdose.
- "Hypnotics should only be considered after making a thorough diagnostic assessment of secondary causes of insomnia, after improving sleep hygiene and after attempting behavioral treatments. If these approaches are unsuccessful, then hypnotics can be used, starting with very low doses and limiting use for short periods."[27, p. 839]
- Antidepressant medications may be used when a depressed mood is present; however, SSRI antidepressants may cause insomnia. Anxiolytics can be used for clients with high levels of anxiety.

Impulse Control Disorders Not Elsewhere Classified

▌ Definition/Major Symptoms*

The Impulse Control Disorders are a group of six mental disorders in which impulse control is the main concern. The client may have a coexisting mental disorder or Personality Disorder.

The major symptoms include:

- An impulse, or an irresistible urge to commit an act that may be harmful to self or others; the client lacks the ability to resist acting on the impulse.
- Tension that increases before the act.
- Pleasure and relief from tension during the act.
- Impulsivity does not occur between outbursts of behavior.

▌ Definition/Major Categories†

Intermittent Explosive Disorder

This is characterized by a loss of control accompanied by violence, mostly to property; only one or more incidents are needed to make this diagnosis. The client may have a poor work history, problems with the family and marriage, and a history of problems with the law. The client is not suffering from head trauma, Alzheimer's disease, drug

*References 1,5,13
†References 1,4,5,11,13

abuse, e.g., PCP, medication, or a manic episode and is not responding to a delusion or hallucination.

Kleptomania

This is characterized by loss of control over the impulse to steal. The client has no plan or need to steal and is able to pay for the object. There is increasing tension before taking the object and relief during the act. The client does not think about how to avoid arrest; if this occurs, the client may feel remorse, guilt, or depression but not display any feelings of revenge or anger. No other antisocial behavior is displayed. There are associated problems in interpersonal relationships. Most information about the disorder has been gained from shoplifters.

Pyromania

This is characterized by the planned, determined intent to set fires. The client is fascinated by fires, fire-fighting equipment, fire alarms, and related activities. The client may be seen at fires in the community, watching with intense interest. The client experiences increasing tension before setting the fires, during the activity, and watching the results. The client is unable to resist the impulse to set fires.

Fire-setting behavior has been observed in psychiatric inpatient treatment facilities and among the chronically mentally ill.

Pathological Gambling

This is characterized by a loss of control over the impulse to gamble and other maladaptive behaviors. These include borrowing money excessively, committing illegal acts, imperiling significant relations and/or employment, lying to cover up gambling, returning to gamble to regain loss, using gambling as way to deal with dysphoric mood, failing to stop gambling after several attempts, using more and more money to experience more excitement, and being constantly preoccupied by gambling. Behaviors that affect family, friends, and community include lying, cheating, forgery, breaking promises, fraud, failing at work, belonging to illegal groups, and being arrested and imprisoned.

Criteria for the disorder are similar to those for Substance Abuse Disorders.

Trichotillomania

This is characterized by loss of control over the impulse to pull out one's hair. The client experiences increasing tension before the act and relief while pulling out hair on the scalp, eyebrows, armpits, pubic area, etc. Specific changes in hair follicles occur, and the areas that lack hair can be biopsied to confirm the diagnosis. Clients may also place hair in the mouth, swallow it, or move it over the lips; this is called trichophagy.

Impulse Control Disorders Not Elsewhere Specified

These are characterized as a disorder not meeting criteria of other specific categories of Impulse Control Disorders. They include repeated self-mutilation, compulsive shopping, and compulsive sexual behavior.

■ Incidence[*]

- All these disorders are relatively rare except for Pathological Gambling, which is reported in 1% to 3% of the population of the U.S.
- Pathological Gambling is reported among 6% of clients admitted to psychiatric units of general hospitals.
- Intermittent Explosive Disorder is probably under-reported.
- Pyromania and Trichotillomania rates are unknown.
- Kleptomania rates range from 5% to 24% of shoplifters.

■ Course[†]

Intermittent Explosive Disorder

Onset usually occurs in adolescence to early adulthood, and symptoms decrease with age.

Kleptomania

This is a chronic condition. Few clients seek treatment, although the prognosis is good. Complications, e.g., Major

[*]References 1,5,13
[†]References 1,3,5,11,13

Depression, may follow when the client is caught stealing and arrested. This condition may be associated with Dementia.

Pyromania

Onset occurs in childhood; the prognosis is good if it is treated. Prognosis for the adult is questionable because the client may be alcohol dependent, use denial as a coping strategy, and lack insight.

Pathological Gambling

Onset for males occurs in adolescence and for females in adulthood. It is a chronic condition with a guarded outcome because the client tends not to stay in therapy. The following phases occur: (1) winning phase, in which client becomes fully entangled after profiting greatly; (2) progressive loss phase, in which the client becomes more involved to the point of organizing life around gambling; and (3) desperate phase, in which the client gambles with reckless abandonment using any means at hand, including breaking the law. Behaviors include suicidal ideation and attempts, alcohol abuse, and hopelessness. The client may be arrested; divorce is common. The client may not seek treatment until pressured by legal and family problems. Relapses are frequent.

Trichotillomania

Onset occurs primarily in childhood or adolescence to later in life. Most cases will resolve with no special treatment. Psychiatric referral is recommended for adolescents or adults when hair-pulling behaviors are present.

▌ Contributing Factors[*]

Intermittent Explosive Disorder

- Biological:
  - Evidence suggests that there is a decrease in serotonin synthesis or its activity that aids in inhibiting aggression.
  - Diseases and traumas originating in childhood, e.g., trauma at birth, seizures, head trauma, encephalitis, brain dysfunctions
- Sex: Male

[*]References 4,5,11–13

- Psychosocial: Childhood experiences in home with Alcohol Dependence, physical abuse, threats, and promiscuity.

Kleptomania

- Biological:
  - Postulates a disturbance in serotonin metabolism.
  - Associated with other disease, e.g., Mental Retardation, brain diseases, Dementia.
- Increased stress, trauma, e.g., loss, separation.
- Sex: Females appear to have a greater incidence.
- Increased association with other mental disorders, i.e., Mood Disorders, Obsessive Disorders, Bulimia Nervosa.
- Psychodynamic: A variety of reasons have been offered to explain impulsive acts: expression of infantile needs, aggression, sexual desire, attempts to restore mother–child relationship.

Pyromania

- Biological: Associated with Mild Mental Retardation, Alcohol Abuse.
- Psychodynamic: Suggests fire as symbolic of sex, power, rage, revenge. Absence of the father in the early years and the wish for his return to rescue the child may be associated with the disorder.

Pathological Gambling

- Biological:
  - Evidence suggests a catecholamine metabolism problem.
  - There may be a dysfunctional attention and impulse-control mechanism.
- Genetic: Both parents are frequently found to be alcohol dependent. First-degree relatives have a higher percentage of major affective disorders and Alcohol Abuse or Dependence.
- Sex: Male.
- Frequently associated with Major Depressive Disorder, Panic Disorder.
- Psychosocial factors: Loss of parent before the age of 15, inappropriately harsh discipline, accessibility to gam-

bling, family valuing materialism highly, lack of emphasis in family on budgeting, saving, and preparing for future.
- Psychodynamic: Postulates an unconscious need for punishment, release of sexual tension.

Trichotillomania

- Biological: Family history of alopecia.
- May be associated with Obsessive-Compulsive Disorder.
- Stress or trauma: Onset has been related to increased stress in a few cases.
- Sex: Female.
- Psychosocial factors: Problems in mother–child relationship, losses, and being left alone.

▌Laboratory and Physical Examination Findings[*]

- The Minnesota Multiphasic Personality Inventory (MMPI) gives some indication of the presence of impulsive behavior.
- Biopsy of hair follicles may be obtained to confirm diagnosis of Trichotillomania.

▌Special Assessment[†]

Intermittent Explosive Disorder

It has been noted that a client receiving a diagnosis of Intermittent Explosive Disorder may have evidence of other disorders, drug use, head trauma, Alcohol Abuse, abnormal EEG, neurological abnormality, and learning disability; prodromal symptoms may be reported. The client also should have psychological tests to rule out Antisocial or Borderline Personality Disorder.

Trichotillomania

Two observations may assist in diagnosis:

1. Nail biting may be noted, but changes in fingernails or toenails usually found in dermatological conditions are not present.

[*]References 5,13
[†]References 5,13

2. Hair will grow in bald areas when collodion is applied; hair growth is visible after 1 week.

■ Treatment*

There is no one specific treatment, drug, or psychotherapy modality of choice, although SSRIs are commonly used. The clinician continues to collect data and to treat the anxiety and depression as they occur.

Intermittent Explosive Disorder

- Pharmacological management of aggressive impulses. The following suggestions are made:
  - Ictal or seizure-like aggression and soft neurological signs, e.g., inability to touch finger to nose, to hop on one foot, nystagmus: Treat with anticonvulsant.
  - Violence associated with chronic medical conditions: Treat with beta blocker.
  - Violence associated with mood lability: Treat with mood stabilizer and/or lithium.
  - Violence with underlying depression: Treat with antidepressant.
  - Violence associated with criminal behavior with underlying epileptic base: Treat with primidone, Tegretol, phenytoin.
  - Violence associated with Obsessive-Compulsive Disorder: Treat with benzodiazepines.
  - Violence associated with Personality Disorder: Treat with lorazepam or alprazolam.
- The client needs to be compliant with the medication regimen because there is a risk of suicide with the noncompliant person, who may direct violence to self and thereby overdose.
- Teaching the client about the disinhibiting effects of alcohol, stimulants, and hallucinogens and the need to avoid their use.
- Psychotherapy is difficult because of the severity of the violence, problems in limit-setting, and counter-transference issues.

*References 2,4,5,8,10–13

- Physical restraint may be needed in managing violent behavior. Use antipsychotics, e.g., haloperidol or benzodiazepine (lorazepam).

Kleptomania

- Pharmacological: SSRIs, fluoxetine (Prozac) may be helpful.
- Psychotherapy: The client may hesitate to inform the clinician that the problem exists; this knowledge tends to be kept as a secret and be covered up by the family. Behavior therapy focuses on desensitization and aversive conditioning, with some success. Insight psychotherapy is successful when the client is motivated. Family therapy is recommended. The client causes problems in the community, resulting in other family members feeling guilty and ashamed.
- Self-treatment: Clients report refusing to shop as a way to deal with theft.
- Legal assistance

Pyromania

- There is no motivation for treatment; data in the treatment of Pyromania are lacking.
- Fire-setting behaviors may involve the use of court-mandated treatment until the client develops some degree of insight.
- If the client is in prison, behavior therapy can be provided with use of aversive or positive reinforcement techniques to manage impulses.

Pathological Gambling

- Gamblers Anonymous is an effective program and is based on AA principles.
- Psychotherapy includes behavior and/or cognitive psychotherapy and psychoanalysis. Insight psychotherapy is not recommended until the client has not gambled for 3 months.
- Issues that need to be explored in therapy include why the client gambles, how to deal with anxiety leading to gambling, and management of time and finances.

- Hospitalization is recommended for client experiencing suicidal ideation, several concurrent addictions, total exhaustion, or emotional decompensation.

Trichotillomania

- Pharmacological management includes treatment of skin with topical steroids, use of a variety of medications, such as an anxiolytic with histamine properties, use of antidepressants (if clinical picture is associated with obsessional features), monoamine oxidase inhibitors, clomipramine, amitriptyline, fluoxetine, lithium or chlorpromazine or antipsychotic drugs.
- Psychotherapy: Various forms, including insight, behavior, and family or marriage counseling.

■ Commonly Occurring Nursing Diagnoses

Anxiety
Coping, defensive
Coping ineffective, family
Coping ineffective, individual
Denial, ineffective
Hopelessness
Role performance, altered
Self-esteem, chronic low
Violence, risk for: self-directed or directed at others

■ Selected Nursing Diagnoses, Outcome Criteria, and Nursing Interventions With Rationale[*]

Example: Client With Undifferentiated Schizophrenia With Fire-Setting Behavior in the Community, Group Home

NURSING DIAGNOSIS #1: *Risk for violence: directed toward others: fire-setting behavior*

EXPECTED CLIENT OUTCOMES

- The client will have verbalized an increased awareness of cost to others and self when fire is set.
- The client will identify one effective way to stop self from setting a fire.

*References 5–10

NURSING INTERVENTIONS WITH RATIONALE

- Provide teaching regarding fire prevention and danger of fire and give informational material *to enable client to be more conscious of and responsible for his or her behavior and its consequences.*
  - Support client when he or she asks for and receives information from peers on how fire-setting affects them.
  - Discuss alternative living arrangements and ways to make group home a safer place to live, free from danger of fire.
  - Discuss client responsibilities as member of house to make it free from fire hazards.
- Provide behavior management *to control fire-setting behavior and promote safe use of matches and other ways to communicate with people.*
  - Model the safe handling of cigarettes.
  - Identify with the client and group home staff on a weekly basis the technique the client will use to stop his or her fire-setting behavior.
  - Provide support to group home staff to meet weekly with client to discuss his or her goals, needs, and behavior *to prevent the use of fire-setting behavior to communicate needs.*
  - If a fire is set, aid the client to recognize that the police will come and probably make an arrest. *Identification of consequences places responsibility for behavior on the client; the negative reinforcement of arrest may increase motivation to stop fire-setting behavior.*
  - Discuss other consequences of fire-setting, such as nightly search of possessions before bedtime, denial of permission to have matches in the group home, etc. *It is important for the client to be responsible for his or her choices; clarification of the consequences of a behavior assists in this process.*
  - Inform the client of the legal consequences of future fire-setting incidents.

Example: Client With Pathological Gambling Disorder in Hospital Setting With Risk for Suicide

NURSING DIAGNOSIS #1:   *Risk for violence: self-directed related to life crises and impending divorce*

EXPECTED CLIENT OUTCOMES

- The client will use socially approved ways to express anger instead of a threat of self harm to express feelings.
- The client will identify constructive ways to deal with loss of an important relationship.

NURSING INTERVENTIONS WITH RATIONALE

- Provide anger control assistance. *The nurse who is open and willing to hear feelings conveys an acceptance that the client can find useful in accepting his or her own angry feelings without defensiveness or the need to act.*
  - Validate feelings of anger and identify any other feelings experienced, e.g., hopelessness.
  - Discuss ways to express anger to others *so that support from others will not be cut off and further client's loss and despair* (see also Stress Management in Chapter 5).
  - Encourage client to write down feelings—those related to gambling and those related to the divorce—*to assist client in making a connection between feeling and actions.*
  - Schedule some form of physical activity twice daily *to reinforce adaptive ways of dealing with anger.*
- Provide grief-work facilitation regarding divorce. *Talking about grief and loss enables the client to find meaning, decrease anxiety, and examine behavior.*
  - Assist client to describe current adaptation to divorce and in dealing with stress.
  - Determine if suicide is still considered an option; if so, initiate change in nursing diagnosis and plan of care. (See also Protective Interventions: Observation for Suicide in Chapter 5.)
  - Listen to problems created by divorce and assist in identifying resources *to assist in resolving problems,* e.g., a lawyer for legal problems.
  - Give positive feedback regarding client's ability to manage the loss.

NURSING DIAGNOSIS #2: *Noncompliance with recommendation to attend Gamblers Anonymous (GA)*

EXPECTED CLIENT OUTCOME

- The client will participate in GA and verbalize understanding of the consequences of not being involved in a therapy program.

NURSING INTERVENTIONS WITH RATIONALE

- Provide emotional support and encouragement to become involved in GA. *A full discussion of client's situation leads to feeling of self-acceptance and the beginning of recognition of needs.*
  - Facilitate discussion of therapy, e.g., seeking help for gambling behavior versus avoidance of therapy.
  - Assist in identifying the reasons why help is definitely needed, e.g., problems of divorce, increasing indebtedness, lying, avoiding certain situations, feeling desperate, etc. *Increasing motivation for treatment will assist client in becoming involved.*
  - Ensure that client has access to information to contact available resources *to increase probability of client's use of the help available.*
  - Reinforce the positive benefits of being a member, e.g., social support, increasing self-respect *as an additional way of supporting client's efforts towards effective managing of gambling behavior.*
  - Provide referral for legal or financial counseling.

CHAPTER 19

Adjustment Disorders

▍ Definition/Major Symptoms*

Adjustment Disorders are characterized by significant emotional or behavioral symptoms manifested within 3 months of encountering a stressor(s). The symptoms are excessive with respect to expected responses, or they significantly affect occupational/academic or social functioning and relationships. Symptoms generally resolve within 6 months of the elimination of the stressor, but they may persist longer if the stressor is chronic or has prolonged consequences. Impairments and maladaptive reactions range from mild to severe (e.g., suicidal behavior). Symptom presentation is heterogeneous, containing subcategories of mixed symptom presentation. Symptoms do not represent normal bereavement or other normal/usual reactions to stressors. The level of psychopathology or symptom patterns do not meet the criteria set for other major DSM-IV disorders and are therefore classified as a residual category for stress-related maladaptive reactions or as a subthreshold disorder.

▍ Definition/Symptoms of Selected Major Categories†

Adjustment Disorder With Depressed Mood

Predominant symptoms are sadness, irritability, hopelessness, tearfulness, low self-esteem, and dysphoria.

*References 1,6,11,12,47
†References 1,2

Adjustment Disorder With Anxiety

Predominant symptoms are anxiety, worry, nervousness, palpitations, hyperventilation, e.g., anxiety regarding separation from a significant attachment figure.

Adjustment Disorder With Mixed Anxiety and Depressed Mood

Predominant symptoms are those of both depression and anxiety.

Adjustment Disorder With Disturbance of Conduct

Predominant symptoms are conduct disturbance, disregard for expected social norms, and disregard for the rights of others, e.g., reckless driving, inappropriate aggression.

Adjustment Disorder With Mixed Disturbance of Emotions and Conduct

Predominant symptoms are emotional ones, such as anxiety or depression, as well as conduct disturbances.

Adjustment Disorder Unspecified

Predominant symptoms are maladaption with symptoms that cannot be classified into one of the subtypes above, e.g., school problems, occupational difficulties.

▌ Incidence[*]

- Patients with these disorders represent 5% to 20% of outpatient mental health clients.
- They represent 11% to 21% of clients in the general hospital psychiatric consultation population.
- They account for 50% of older clients undergoing cardiac surgery.
- They represent 5% of psychiatric inpatients.
- They account for up to 70% of the children in psychiatric settings.

*References 1,2,4,11,24,39,42,43,47

- Clients with Adjustment Disorder are frequently seen in emergency departments.
- The disorder has a high prevalence in oncology clients.
- This is a common emotional problem for elderly clients facing visual loss.
- Children are especially vulnerable due to their dependency on their environment and limited coping skills.
- Among nonpsychiatric pediatric clients with changed health status resulting in Adjustment Disorder, there is increased vulnerability to later psychopathology.
- The diagnosis occurs more frequently in young persons, single persons, and females.
- The average age of a client with this disorder is the mid-20s.
- Adolescents have a higher incidence of conduct disturbance, whereas adults experience more symptoms of depressed mood or anxiety.
- There is a high risk among disadvantaged persons due to increased incidence of multiple stressors.
- The disorder entails an increased risk for suicide, e.g., in adolescents or young adults suicidal behavior may be a reaction to a stressor even though other mental disorders are not present.

■ Course*

- Symptoms and maladaptations manifest themselves within 3 months of the encounter with the stressor. Symptoms can last up to 6 months (acute presentation) after termination of the stressor, unless the stressor is chronic or there are long-term consequences from the stressor resulting in a longer manifestation of the Adjustment Disorder (chronic presentation).
- There is an increased risk for suicide.
- For adults the prognosis is favorable; in adolescents major psychiatric disorders may eventually occur, with behavioral symptoms and chronicity of major mental disorder.
- Adjustment Disorder (in which stressors vary in intensity, resulting in a range of different symptoms) differs from Post-Traumatic Stress Disorder (in which the stres-

*References 1,11,12,19,37,38,40

sor is severe, with a specific resulting pattern of symptoms including flashbacks, hypervigilance) and Acute Stress Disorder (in which the stressor is severe with another specific pattern of symptoms).

- In inpatients, a diagnosis of Adjustment Disorder is found to be associated with suicidality and Substance Abuse Disorders.
- The course of an Adjustment Disorder can be complicated by substance abuse.
- The stressor can occupy the client's dreams/fantasies or negatively affect him or her if the maladaptive reaction is not treated.

▌ Contributing Factors*

General

- An identifiable stressor is present, i.e., there is a stress-related etiology; stressors can be recurrent; multiple stressors can have additive effects.
- Models for explaining the relationship of stress to psychopathology include (1) victimization—the accumulation of stressors in life; (2) vulnerability—existing social and personal conditions moderate relationship between stressors in life and psychopathology; (3) additive burden—personal and social dispositions contribute to psychopathology; (4) chronic burden—stable personal and social conditions and personal dispositions alone lead to psychopathology; and (5) proneness—mental disorder leads to a stressful life event, which exacerbates the condition.
- Stressors are divided into two classes: (1) stressful life events (recent stressors and remote stressors) and (2) chronic strains (persistent stressful situations, role strain, social responses, community stresses).
- Stressors can be natural or manmade disasters and can affect whole communities.
- In adolescents, common stressors include academic problems, leaving home for school, unwanted pregnancy, death of a peer, rejection by a significant other, divorce of parents, family discord, interpersonal problems with peers, and alcohol problems.

*References 1,2,3,11,12,31,36,44,47,49

- In adults, common stressors include financial problems, job loss, parenting, housing problems, family discord/divorce, legal difficulties, and relocation.
- In the elderly, common stressors include financial problems, loss of job, loss of spouse, loss of a good friend, major illness, and a major operation.
- How a given person responds to a particular type of stressor is highly variable; response is based in part on vulnerability.
- The meaning of a stressor is modified by such personal attributes as individual perception and meaning of stressor, ego strength, and prior experience and successful coping with stressor.
- Cultural setting can play a role in how the stressor is perceived.

Neurobiological/Genetic

- A serious illness or general medical condition may cause symptoms via a psychological mechanism.
- Clients with Dementia and other Cognitive Disorders or Mental Retardation are at risk.
- Adrenaline/other neurotransmitters play a role in stress.

Psychological

- Presence of psychosocial stressor
- Certain stressors appear at various developmental stages, e.g., those experienced in adolescence.
- Maladaptive/underdeveloped coping skills for dealing with stressor(s) may exist.
- Maladaptive defense mechanisms may exist.
- Psychoanalytic theory considers early childhood trauma and retarded ego development as contributing factors.
- Interpersonal factors, e.g., lack of social skills, may be contributors.
- Personality traits, e.g., lack of flexibility, may be contributors.

Family/Social/Cultural/Environmental

- The situational context is very important in understanding the onset of the disorder (e.g., economic situation, occupational opportunities, community resources, social network, cultural/religious support groups).

- Disadvantaged individuals may be at high risk for Adjustment Disorder since numerous stressors may be encountered.
- Persons with traumatic childhood experiences are at high risk for Adjustment Disorders.
- Inadequate role modeling in dysfunctional families may be a factor.
- Sociocultural adjustments faced, e.g., upon immigration, are risk factors.
- Cultural differences in reaction to trauma

▌Laboratory and Physical Examination Findings

Screen for possible drug abuse.

Perform a careful initial and ongoing assessment of the client before making a diagnosis of Adjustment Disorder in order to differentiate this disorder from the possibility of other DSM-IV diagnoses, such as Mood Disorder.

▌Special Assessment Considerations*

- All aspects of the diagnostic construct for the Adjustment Disorder are difficult to assess and measure, e.g., the stressor(s), the maladaptive reaction, the mood and emotions, and time and relationship between stressor and response.
- Conduct serial and ongoing observations and assessments of the clinical course.
- The diagnosis of Adjustment Disorder can be used as a "working" or "temporary" psychiatric diagnosis that can be modified with subsequent evaluations over time. Be alert to changing mental symptoms.
- Assess for risk factors and problems/stressors in childhood.
- Carefully assess the cultural setting of the client to determine the meaning and response to stressors.
- Clients with a general medical condition should be assessed for the presence of Adjustment Disorders when

*References 1–3,9,37,38,43,47,48

certain complications occur, e.g., noncompliance with treatment regimen.

- Assess the nature of the stressor(s): type, number, timing, and degree of change brought on by stressor. Open with such questions as, "In the last three months has something happened to you that has been particularly worrisome?" "Is this situation extra difficult for you to handle?"
- Assess client's perception of the stressor and its specific meaning, his or her perception of control over the stressor, and the degree to which the event is desired or undesired.
- Assess the client's coping skills and other strengths, e.g., ego strengths, prior success coping with similar stressor, social support systems, and community resources.
- Assess the client's interpersonal strengths and difficulties (social withdrawal).
- Assess the client's mood and sense of hopelessness, as well as other aspects of mental status: memory, attention span, thought patterns, etc.
- Assess past and present suicidal ideation and the actual potential for suicide.
- Assess for patterns of violence, spousal abuse, or potential for an inappropriate expression of anger.
- Assess for high-risk behavior, e.g., substance abuse.

█ Treatment*

General

- Outpatient treatment is preferred unless hospitalization is needed to treat acute phase.
- Disorder can be treated in primary care.
- A complete medical evaluation is extremely important. The evaluation findings may indicate that the diagnosis of Adjustment Disorder should be altered along with the treatment plan.
- The treatment of these symptoms may prevent a more serious mental disorder or more severe impairment in psychosocial and occupational functioning.

*References 2,11,46,47,48

Psychopharmacologic/Biologic

Appropriate, generally small doses of anxiolytics, antidepressants, and hypnotics may be useful.

Psychotherapy/Psychosocial Treatment

- Psychotherapeutic treatment primarily focuses on reducing the stressor, increasing coping skills, and facilitating the establishment and use of social and community resources to assist the client's successful coping with stressor.
- Effective treatment characteristics are brevity, immediacy, centrality, expectance, proximity, and simplicity.[48]
- Psychosocial therapies that are useful include crisis intervention, counseling, medical crisis counseling, individual psychotherapy, cognitive therapy, behavioral interventions, assertiveness training, supportive psychotherapy, group therapy, and family therapy.
- Children's support groups that teach children coping skills in dealing with divorce of parents include Support and Skill Building Group and Support, Skill Building, Transfer, and Parent Training Procedures Group.[46]
- Supportive psychotherapy is useful in helping clients with medical illness cope.
- Use of adjunctive therapies, e.g., occupational therapy and recreational therapy, may help enhance self-esteem.

▌ Commonly Occurring Nursing Diagnoses*

Altered family processes
Altered health maintenance
Altered role performance
Anticipatory grieving
Anxiety
Dysfunctional grieving
Hopelessness
Impaired adjustment
Impaired social interaction
Ineffective individual coping
Ineffective individual management of therapeutic regimen
Noncompliance

*References 23,30,33

Powerlessness
Risk for violence, self directed
Risk for violence, directed at others
Relocation stress syndrome
Self-esteem disturbance
Situational crisis
Situational low self-esteem

▌ Selected Nursing Diagnoses, Outcome Criteria, and Nursing Interventions with Rationale*

DSM-IV Disorder: Adjustment Disorder With Mixed Anxiety and Depressed Mood

NURSING DIAGNOSIS #1: *Situational crisis related to being diagnosed with a medical disorder*

EXPECTED CLIENT OUTCOME

- Client will achieve lowered level of anxiety and other emotional states to function in a more goal-directed manner.

NURSING INTERVENTIONS WITH RATIONALE

- Establish rapport through a warm, empathic, supportive, caring, nonjudgmental approach *because these nurse attributes/attitudes are important in developing a therapeutic nurse–client rationale to assist client in clarifying concerns, coping skills, and resources and options.* (See also Chapter 2.)
- Assist client in recognizing and expressing anxiety and other emotions.
- Provide immediate supportive counseling *in order to reduce anxiety and other emotional states, to normalize client's feelings and fear of being labeled crazy, sick, stupid, or weak; to reduce behavioral disorganization, if present; and to begin the process of enhancing optimal resolution in the long term.* (See also Crisis Intervention in Chapter 5.)
- Assist client in identifying stressor(s) and offer input that is stated in a noncomplex manner *so that client can more easily understand what is being said and begins to identify and understand the nature of stressor(s) during*

*References 5,7–10,13–18,20–22,25,27–29,32, 34,35,37,38,41,45,48

the phase when anxiety and other emotions are still at high levels.

EXPECTED CLIENT OUTCOME

• Client will achieve realistic perception of stressor and subsequent experiences.

NURSING INTERVENTIONS WITH RATIONALE

• Assist the client to describe the stressor(s) and sequence of emotions, thoughts, and behaviors *in order to gain an understanding of the stressor(s) by discussing the effect of the stressor(s) and the link to subsequent thoughts, emotions, and behaviors.*

• Help client to clarify the experience by restating previously unconnected facts in a simple, readily understood manner *to facilitate client's comprehension because emotional states may not yet be at normal levels.*

• Offer hope that client will be able to identify coping strategies for solving the difficulty *in order to convey empowerment to client.* (See also Supportive Therapy: Offering Hope in Chapter 5.)

• Offer support *in order to convey to the client that difficulties can be understood, that others have undergone similar problems, and that client possesses personal coping resources that can be relied upon.*

• Use client input to outline target behaviors and goals for therapy *in order to facilitate resourcefulness, i.e., the ability for client to self-regulate internal responses so that the stressor(s) can be managed.*

EXPECTED CLIENT OUTCOME

• Client will use and increase his or her own repertoire of coping skills.

NURSING INTERVENTIONS WITH RATIONALE

• Teach the client how to monitor own emotional state and to anticipate changes (ups and downs) in emotions *so that client can recognize what helps and what interferes with problem solving.*

• Encourage the client to describe his or her own accomplishments in dealing with the same or similar stressors in the past *in order for client to begin to tap into existing problem-solving skills and to promote individual responsibility for problem solving and decision making.*

- Teach the client problem-solving skills *in order to enhance client's own knowledge base of the problem-solving process, when necessary,* by:
  - clearly defining the problem
  - generating potential solutions
  - describing projected consequences of proposed solutions
  - choosing alternatives
  - testing behavior or action
  - evaluating results
  - redefining problem, if necessary.
- Teach the client decision-making skills *in order to enhance client's own knowledge base since these skills can be very useful in coping with stressors.* (See also Decision-Making in Chapter 5.)
- Use stress-management techniques.
- Explore and examine alternative ways of managing stress. (See also Stress Management in Chapter 5.)
- Assist client to formulate a plan of action that uses situational supports and sources of social support; identifies and mobilizes client's own personal strengths, e.g., decision-making and problem-solving skills; and develops a number of options for action. *"Effective coping strategies are central to stress resistance. Under stressful demands, personality strengths and social support function as coping resources: coping, in turn, mediates between available redsources and subsequent health...chronic and acute stressors and social resources are dynamically interrelated."* [21, p. 232]
- Support the client in an emerging, more positive self-concept.

EXPECTED CLIENT OUTCOME

- The client will develop and use situational supports.

NURSING INTERVENTIONS WITH RATIONALE

- Explore resources known to the client.
- Offer information about community resources, make referrals, or assist the client in contacting agencies.
- Assist the client in recognizing and activating social supports.

- Assist the client in increasing his or her social sphere when necessary or appropriate.
- Encourage client's use of and reliance on community supports, social service agencies, or significant others.
- Encourage client's use of the phone as a communication link.
- *Coping successfully with stressors is influenced by social support, use of community resources, and adequate discharge planning. Developing a plan of action can itself help reduce stress level. The client is assisted by means of all of the above nursing interventions in lowering the level of psychological distress and regaining participation in normal activities of daily living and resuming social and occupational roles, within limitations posed by the actual physical disorder.*
- Discuss with client the preventive technique of anticipatory planning, tailored to the client's unique circumstances *so that client thinks through potential future crises and possible coping strategies to draw upon.* (See also Discharge Planning in Chapter 5.)

NURSING DIAGNOSIS #2:   *Dysfunctional grieving related to loss of a significant other*

EXPECTED CLIENT OUTCOME

- Client will resolve dysfunctional grieving as evidenced by demonstrating emotional reactions congruent with cultural and personal expectations.

NURSING INTERVENTIONS WITH RATIONALE

- Assess the client for the defining characteristics of dysfunctional grieving, e.g., lack of movement of symptoms and other aspects related to loss and grieving experience *in order to definitively establish the nursing diagnosis of Dysfunctional Grieving.*
- The defining characteristics of dysfunctional grieving include excessive time spent in any stage of normal grieving and excessive or distorted emotional reactions. They may present in the following ways:
  - prolonged or excessive denial
  - prolonged social isolation or withdrawal
  - behavior suggesting that loss occurred yesterday

- ○ developmental regression
- ○ extremely low self-esteem
- ○ severe feelings of identity loss
- ○ unabated searching behavior for lost person or object
- ○ excessive idealization of dead person
- ○ excessive guilt and self-blame
- ○ extreme or prolonged anger toward dead person
- ○ suicidal ideation, severe hopelessness
- ○ prolonged panic attacks
- ○ prolonged depressive mood (to what degree?)
- ○ somatic complaints
- ○ engaging in self-detrimental activities
- ○ delayed emotional reactions
- *It is important to gain baseline data since the exact nature of the grief reaction may vary from person to person. In dysfunctional grieving, the normal grieving process becomes stuck in one phase of grieving with the presence of excessive emotional reactions or excessive length of time in a phase. It is very important to recognize and resolve dysfunctional grieving.*
- What is the client's actual behavior between the occurrence of the loss and the present?
- What is the nature of the loss, e.g., when did it occur, how did the client perceive the loss, what is the special meaning of the person?
- What is the significance of loss in relation to client's perceived and real abilities to meet own needs?
- How has client coped with losses in the past? What strengths were demonstrated in coping with loss?
- What is the nature of the social network present? What are the significant others' reactions to client's response to loss? *Perception of social support facilitates normal grieving.*
- What cultural factors may influence client's perception of loss and the grieving process?
- Assist the client in getting through the phase in which client is stuck by:
  - ○ assessing present stage of grieving and the current facts
  - ○ encouraging use of relaxation techniques
  - ○ using genogram to assist in identification of unresolved losses
  - ○ considering a referral to brief psychotherapy

○ determining need for a evaluation for antidepressant or anxiolytic medications.

EXPECTED CLIENT OUTCOME

• The client will engage in normal grieving as evidenced by engaging in normal grief work, constructively restructuring and reordering his or her life, and developing new relationships and emotional investments.

NURSING INTERVENTIONS WITH RATIONALE

• Help client to understand any physical symptoms experienced. *Physical symptoms that do not last long frequently appear immediately after loss and can include sighing respirations, a choking sensation, an empty feeling in the stomach, digestive upsets, physical distress, and shortness of breath.*
• Assist the client in working through denial, e.g.:
  ○ Do not force client to focus on his or her denial behavior since that is a necessary protective defense mechanism; however, observe for ineffective denial and intervene as necessary.
  ○ Help the client understand that others may respond similarly when mourning a loss.
  ○ Be genuine, honest, and realistic about the loss.
  ○ Use a caring tone of voice.
  ○ Correct misinformation about the cause of the loss.
  ○ Clarify and offer missing factual information.
  ○ Permit visual and tactile contact with the body of the dead person when possible and if desired by the client.
• *During denial, the client avoids acceptance of loss, thereby developing a buffer against reality; acting as if the deceased is still present, the loss has not occurred, and engaging in searching behavior. Although a certain level and duration of denial are appropriate in normal grieving, successful grief resolution depends on the client's ability to eventually face the reality of the loss and cope with other tasks and emotions.*
• Assist client in working through feelings of anger:
  ○ demonstrate tolerance, patience, and empathy
  ○ permit appropriate expression of anger: do not become defensive
  ○ assist the client in understanding reasons for feelings of anger

- ○ if the client has difficulty in expressing anger, provide an opportunity to be with others who can express this feeling openly but appropriately
- ○ reassure the client that feelings of guilt are part of the normal grieving process and assist him or her in working through these feelings
- ○ encourage the client to work out any conflicting aspects of the relationship with the deceased person and work through any ambivalence.
- *Anger can be inappropriately directed by the client toward the deceased person, toward self, or toward other persons or objects. The client may also blame health professionals or may misinterpret what it said by them; thus, it is important to express anger appropriately and work through the anger. Verbalization of feelings can assist client in working through unresolved issues and other aspects of the normal grieving process.*
- Assist client in working through bargaining:
- ○ acknowledge the client's need to talk about the loss through active listening
- ○ permit expression of feelings and thoughts and gently point out the reality.
- *During bargaining the client makes a last attempt to postpone realization of the loss, which may include bargaining with a deity. Client attempts to negotiate for the change in reality.*
- Assist client through the realization of loss:
- ○ observe for and monitor for depressive mood and suicidal ideation (extremely important)
- ○ be physically present; offer support to enhance client's self-esteem
- ○ offer presence and hope[14]
- ○ offer acceptance and unconditional positive regard
- ○ reinforce past and present strengths in dealing with difficulty
- ○ through sympathetic understanding, show that crying is acceptable
- ○ encourage support for client from family members and friends
- ○ facilitate review of positive and negative aspects of the lost person
- ○ use touch to offer support, if appropriate.

- *During realization of loss, the client gains a full awareness of the loss, including the meaning and value of the person to self, awareness of lost or changed roles, and realization of new responsibilities and roles. Although the client may still be preoccupied with the loss, the intensity of the thoughts and feelings associated with the loss will eventually lessen.*
- Assist the client through acceptance of the loss:
  - explore the nature of the problems encountered that are linked to loss
  - raise questions regarding the next steps in coping
  - assist the client in thinking through adaptive coping strategies
  - assist the client in developing new or coordinating present resources to cope with the loss, to make readjustments in lifestyle, and to make new emotional investments[28]
  - support the client as new coping strategies are tried; use role playing techniques when possible
  - avoid suppression of symptoms of normal grieving with drugs such as benzodiazepines: rely on use of supportive interventions instead
  - answer questions directly and tactfully
  - orient the client to new aspects of the environment in a simple, clear way
  - foster an environment in which loss can be placed in a spiritual context by engaging the client in religious or spiritual rituals and practices
  - be cognizant of the possibility of different stages of grieving occurring among family member, e.g., help the client and family members communicate with one another, offer special assistance to children (e.g., structured programs) to help them resolve their grief.[20,32]
- *During acceptance and reintegration, problem-solving behavior is initiated relative to the loss and concomitant problems and change. Restructuring and reordering of life is achieved and client again engages fully in social and occupational roles.*

CHAPTER 20

Personality Disorders

▌ Definition/Major Symptoms*

The Personality Disorders are a group of behaviors and traits that form life-long patterns that become maladaptive in early adulthood in school, work, and intimate relationships. When the traits become increasingly inflexible and maladaptive and cause marked impairment in functioning and/or distress to the client, the label Personality Disorder is used. The client does not understand that his or her behavior is the problem, nor does client experience increased anxiety about his or her own behavior. A medical condition does not cause the presenting behaviors.

These disorders are coded on Axis II, which consists of the identified Personality Disorder and may state the presence of a frequently used mental mechanism. Axis II permits further description of the manifestation of the mental disorder.

Clinicians may achieve stability of the major mental disorder on Axis I and then be confronted with management problems arising from the personality disorder on Axis II, the physical disorder on Axis III, the psychosocial and environmental problems on Axis IV, and/or the prior level of functioning, Axis V. Features of Personality Disorders frequently exist with other major mental disorders.

The Personality Disorders are divided into three clusters, identifying an overall picture of the major behaviors.

- Cluster A: Odd or eccentric behaviors; includes Paranoid, Schizoid, Schizotypal Personality Disorders.

*References 1,13,21,34,40

- Cluster B: Dramatic, emotional, or erratic behaviors; includes Borderline, Histrionic, Narcissistic Personality Disorders.
- Cluster C: Anxious, fearful behaviors; includes Avoidant, Dependent, Obsessive-Compulsive Personality Disorders

▌ Definition/Major Symptoms of Selected Major Categories*

Cluster A

PARANOID PERSONALITY DISORDER

This disorder is characterized by long-standing mistrust and suspicion of others, whom the client believes wish to cause harm or suffering to him or her. The client exhibits five of the following traits: perceives others as causing harm, "doing him in," being disloyal or unfaithful, being threatening or disrespecting, attacking the client's reputation, or being an unfaithful spouse or lover. The client does not admit concerns, believing it will be held against him or her, and does not apologize or forgive others. The client reacts to others in an irritable, attacking manner, especially when questioned. He or she is forever searching for hidden messages and special meanings. Ideas of reference, illusions, and restricted mood are frequently present. Socially the client appears effective, efficient, and practical. Others may fear the client, and in general conflict and turmoil surround him or her. He or she is attentive to relative positions of power, especially to those persons in authority.

SCHIZOID PERSONALITY DISORDER

This disorder is characterized by long-standing withdrawal from social interaction and limited expression of emotions. The client exhibits the following traits/behaviors: does not exhibit much warmth or affection towards others; lacks interest in sexual relationships or participation in groups or family; prefers to do things alone; has few friends other than family; demonstrates little pleasure in things or activities; and is not usually affected by criticism and praise. The client is susceptible to anything that triggers fears of abandonment. The defense mechanism predominantly

*References 1,5,12,13,20,21,26,31,35–38,40,41

used is withdrawal. During an interview the client exhibits fear, poor eye contact, lack of spontaneous interaction, and shortness and directness in answers to questions. In interactions with others he or she appears aloof, cold, and indifferent, and may participate in an activity or group that has little personal demands, e.g., study of stars, care of animals, health fads. The client may be very effective and creative at work.

SCHIZOTYPAL PERSONALITY DISORDER

This is characterized by long-standing peculiarities of thinking, perceiving, behaving, and communicating and by distress in relationships. The client exhibits ideas of reference, magical thinking, illusions, suspiciousness, increased anxiety related to paranoid fears, and disturbances of affect; has odd ways of expressing self in speech, dress, and/or general manner; and has few friends other than family. Symptoms closely resemble Schizophrenia. Abandonment fear often acts as a trigger for increasing the odd behaviors. The defense mechanism used predominantly is projection. Socially the client is peculiar and has difficulty forming relationships because of odd ways of talking, dressing, and behaving.

Cluster B

ANTISOCIAL PERSONALITY DISORDER

This disorder is characterized by a history of disregarding social rules, committing criminal acts, manipulating others, and dishonesty. The client has a history and continuous pattern of disrespectfulness of the law, even when arrested; dishonesty; desire for personal gain; impulsivity with no thought of the future; aggressiveness; irresponsibility at work; lack of following through on agreements made with others; disregard for safety of others as well as for self; and lack of remorse for an act done to another. No effort is made to rationalize or justify his or her actions. These patterns have been in place before 15 years of age, and there is a history of Conduct Disorder in childhood. Socially and at work the client is charming, smooth, and has the ability to handle social situations with ease—a "con man." He or she may be highly somatic, that is, report or endorse multiple symptoms during a review of body systems. The client may have problems holding a job, be involved in money-making schemes, may engage in illegal activities, and be arrested and incarcerated.

BORDERLINE PERSONALITY DISORDER

This disorder is characterized by a history of instability in relationships, in affect, in views of self, and by impulsivity. The client exhibits suicidal behaviors, intense affect to deal with real or imagined abandonment, idealization and then devaluation of the same person, impulsive participation in self-damaging activities (e.g., promiscuity), instability of affect, feelings of loneliness, instability in sense of self, problems in anger control, paranoid thinking or dissociative symptoms (e.g., amnesia, forgetting), and anxiety intolerance. The client experiences affect dysregulation, shifting from extreme dysphoria to irritability and then to anxiety in a rapid manner. Socially and at work the client is often involved in self-created conflict and turmoil because his or her allegiance shifts from one person or group to another. The defense mechanism predominantly used is that of splitting, an unconscious process that divides ambivalently viewed people into categories that are all good and all bad, e.g., incompetent or highly skilled, sensitive and caring or punitive and uncaring. When the process plays out in group settings, there is confusion and chaos in interpersonal relationships. If the client has a relationship, it is a dependent one. It lasts until a situation occurs in which needs are not met, resulting in the expression of intense anger. The relationship is lost; the client quickly identifies another person to become involved with to assuage the loneliness.

HISTRIONIC PERSONALITY DISORDER

This disorder is characterized by a history of very dramatic displays of emotions, seduction, and attention-seeking behaviors. The client exhibits discomfort when not the focus of attention, uses dress style to call attention to self, and talks in a colorful manner. He or she displays lability and shallowness of emotions and may dramatize and exaggerate emotions. The client displays sexually provocative behaviors and exaggerates intimacy in relationships. He or she does not give detailed descriptions of events and is highly suggestible. The client is cooperative, dramatic, and anxious to please during an interview. He or she denies the presence of anger, depression, or sexual desires and may not be able to recall situations or facts that evoke many emotions. Problems exist in maintaining relationships over time.

NARCISSISTIC PERSONALITY DISORDER

This disorder is characterized by an exaggerated sense of self-importance and uniqueness, a need for special attention, and little awareness or concern for others. The client perceives self as very talented but actually has few talents, as very special and therefore deserving of high-status associates, and as being entitled to special treatment and considerations. He or she has fantasies of being successful, brilliant, beautiful; of being the ideal, perfect model; and of having power and control. The client demands admiration; demonstrates an arrogant, better-than-you attitude; is envious of others; uses others for personal gain; and is disrespectful, uncaring, and unconcerned about others. He or she experiences loss and rejection in social and work relationships. His or her policies and procedures are to be followed; criticism by others and others' success are difficult to tolerate.

Cluster C

AVOIDANT PERSONALITY DISORDER

This disorder is characterized by a history of hypersensitivity to rejection, low self-confidence (inferiority complex), and a desire for uncritical acceptance. The client exhibits a self-perception of inferiority, unattractiveness, and clumsiness in social situations; avoids situations without assurance of approval; avoids involvement in individual or group settings because of fear of ridicule or shame; is unwilling to take a chance or do something new; is uncertain in new situations and/or overconcerned with critical or nonaccepting remarks; and is involved in activities requiring little interpersonal contact. He or she ingratiates self with another as a way to avoid rejection and disapproval. The client is viewed as hard working and wanting to please those in authority. Job promotions are not sought; management positions may be avoided.

DEPENDENT PERSONALITY DISORDER

This disorder is characterized by subordination of one's own needs, deferring to others' decisions, and close, clinging attachments to others. The client exhibits fear and worry about being left alone to care for self, feels helpless when left alone, and has problems in doing things by himself or herself. He or she seeks assurance and advice in many aspects of everyday living; has a need for someone else to be responsible; seldom expresses any disagreement; goes to great lengths to obtain care and be noticed; and quickly seeks a new close relationship when another one ends. At work or socially the client avoids positions of responsibility and may do another's work better than his or her own work. He or she does not want to be alone, seeks involvement with other(s), and will remain in abusive situations for long periods of time.

OBSESSIVE-COMPULSIVE PERSONALITY DISORDER

This is characterized by a long history of perfectionism and rigid conformity to principle. The client exhibits involvement in details, organization, and schedules; inflexibility; concern about morals, ethics, or values; willingness to work overtime without pay or despite interference with family and social life; problems in completing a task until the job is perfect; difficulty in delegating work because he or she needs it to be done in a certain way; an inability to throw away useless, worn-out things that have no value; and tight control over money and its use by others. Defense mechanisms used are rationalization, isolation, intellectualization, undoing, and reaction formation. The client is eager to please those in authority at work; carries out instructions well and is considered a good employee; and is vulnerable to change in routines, downsizing, and new ideas.

PERSONALITY DISORDERS NOT OTHERWISE SPECIFIED

This category is used for disorders not described in another category, those containing features of several categories, or those causing significant distress or impairment in functioning. Examples follow:

- Passive-aggressive personality disorder or negativistic disorder is characterized by a history of procrastination, obstinacy, ineffectiveness, and impeding progress.
- Depressive personality is characterized by a history of the traits associated with depression, of being non-assertive, responsible and disciplined, critical of others and of self, pessimistic, and preoccupied with many worries and feelings of inadequacy.

■ Incidence*

Cluster A

PARANOID PERSONALITY DISORDER

- Found in 0.5% to 2.5% of the population.
- Found more frequently in refugees, prisoners, elderly, and hearing-impaired.

SCHIZOID PERSONALITY DISORDER

- Not known but may be as much as 7.5% of the population.

SCHIZOTYPAL PERSONALITY DISORDER

- Found in 3% of the population.

Cluster B

ANTISOCIAL PERSONALITY DISORDER

- Found in 3% of men and 1% of women.
- Found in 50% of persons in prison.

BORDERLINE PERSONALITY DISORDER

- Found in 2% to 3% of the population.
- Found in 11% of persons in outpatient settings.

HISTRIONIC PERSONALITY DISORDER

- Found in 2% to 3% of the population.

NARCISSISTIC PERSONALITY DISORDER

- Found in 1% of the population.

Cluster C

AVOIDANT PERSONALITY DISORDER

- Found in 1% to 10% of the population.

*References 1,8,10,13

DEPENDENT PERSONALITY DISORDER

- Found in 1% of the population.
- May be more common in women.
- It is the most common personality diagnosis in mental health clinics.

OBSESSIVE-COMPULSIVE PERSONALITY DISORDER

- Unknown or may be found in 2% of the population.
- More common in men and in oldest siblings.

▌ Course*

Onset occurs in adolescence, with behaviors already apparent in childhood and lasting through life. Conditions and complications that may occur are discussed under the appropriate Personality Disorder.

Cluster A

PARANOID PERSONALITY DISORDER

- Some clients may develop Delusional Disorder or Schizophrenia.
- Problems in work and marriage are frequent.
- Some clients may mature and exhibit more concern for others.
- Prognosis is poor; the individual seldom seeks treatment.

SCHIZOID PERSONALITY DISORDER

- Some clients may develop Schizophrenia.

SCHIZOTYPAL PERSONALITY DISORDER

- It is believed to be the premorbid personality of the schizophrenic client; 10% to 20% develop Schizophrenia later.
- Risk for suicide: 10% of clients commit suicide.
- There is an increased risk for Agoraphobia, Obsessive-Compulsive Disorder, and Alcohol and Substance Abuse or dependence.
- If treatment is sought, it is because of related symptoms or problems.

*References 1,2,7,10,13,21,26,35,37,38,40

Cluster B

ANTISOCIAL PERSONALITY DISORDER

- This is associated with mental disorders such as Somatization Disorder, Major Depressive Disorder, Alcohol Use Disorders, Substance Abuse Disorders, and Generalized Anxiety Disorders.
- Problems and complications include criminal behaviors and serving jail time, abuse of spouses and children, promiscuity, variable employment, alcohol and substance abuse, and various related activities.

BORDERLINE PERSONALITY DISORDER

- This entails a high incidence of Depressive Disorder episodes.
- High risk of self-mutilation to obtain help, to express feelings of anger, or to deal with overwhelming anxiety.
- Risk for suicide is greater when client experiences isolation and disconnectedness. The suicide rate may be as high as 10%. Frequently associated with sexual abuse.

HISTRIONIC PERSONALITY DISORDER

- Symptoms decrease with age.
- Frequently associated with Somatization Disorder and Dissociative Disorder.
- Suicide may be attempted.
- Problems with the law include substance abuse and public expressions of promiscuity.

NARCISSISTIC PERSONALITY DISORDER

- Frequently perceives insults at work or at home, causing increased distress and discomfort, because of client's exaggerated sense of self. May experience depression.
- Stress increases with age as the client has more problems in competing, is less beautiful or handsome, has lost youth, etc. May experience depression.

Cluster C

AVOIDANT PERSONALITY DISORDER

- Social Phobia may develop.

- If the social support system fails to provide stable environment, the client experiences anxiety, depression, and anger.

DEPENDENT PERSONALITY DISORDER
- May develop a Shared Psychotic Disorder.

OBSESSIVE-COMPULSIVE PERSONALITY DISORDER
- May develop Schizophrenic Disorder, Obsessive-Compulsive Disorder, or Major Depressive Disorder.

▌ Contributing Factors*

- Genetic: Some evidence of a genetic factor has been found in studies of twins and biological relatives with other mental disorders.
- Biological: The following may contribute to development of Personality Disorders:
  - Central nervous system deficit or brain damage
  - Increased levels of testosterone/estrogen
  - Low platelet monoamine oxidase
  - Neurotransmitter dysfunction, e.g., low levels of serotonin
  - Changes in electroencephalogram (EEG)
- Severe stress, e.g., death, separation from parental figures, abuse, divorce, may contribute to the development of Personality Disorders.
- Childhood sexual abuse is found in Borderline Personality Disorder.
- Cultural/socioeconomic:
  - Support of aggressive behaviors by a culture
  - Environmental restrictiveness, e.g, limits on room to play, explore
  - Traumatic school environment
  - Lower socioeconomic class
  - Poverty
  - Exposure to criminal behaviors and substance abuse

Psychoanalytic Theory

- Freud postulates that stages of psychosexual development exist during which certain traits may become fixed (see also Chapter 1).

*References 5,8,13,16,18,20–22,27,31,34,39,40,42

- Reich postulates that a defensive style determines an individual's unique personality. Emotional states may or may not cause distress since the person depends on the effectiveness of the defenses to manage anxiety. When they are effective, the client is able to manage anxiety and other emotions and is not motivated to enter treatment. However, the use of the defense can be devastating to others and cause disturbed relationships, e.g., projection.
- Postulates that a pattern of relating to others develops by the introjection of a parental figure or object into the self as part of the self. During life the person seeks to relate to others in ways he or she did as child; more comfort is experienced in that type of relationship.
- Common defenses associated with Personality Disorders include projection, splitting, dissociation, fantasy, acting out, undoing, and passive aggression.

PARANOID PERSONALITY DISORDER

Postulates a development of splitting as a major defense mechanism that serves to split off the "bad" impulses of the self and project them onto another. Relationships in the developing years were not experienced as trusting and predictable; as a consequence, the person experiences others as hurtful and unpredictable. The client converts his or her own experiences into fact and does not question them or seek other data. He or she attempts to protect self from the "bad" others through the pathological creation of obligations and subservience of others to the client. Persons around the client experience this as his or her need for control. The low self-esteem of the client is projected in terms of grandiosity about self; he or she is finely tuned into people in power or those having higher rank.

SCHIZOID AND SCHIZOTYPAL PERSONALITY DISORDERS

Postulates an early splitting of representations of self that are not integrated into self. A failure of mothering results in needs that cannot be satisfied; it is so great that the infant fears that the mother may be devoured or driven away. The self will be left alone. There is a continuous fear of being abandoned.

ANTISOCIAL PERSONALITY DISORDER

Postulates a profound absence of a soothing mother before the separation–individuation phase of development. There was no one there to soothe and care for infant; he or she experienced neglect and abuse. As a result, two processes are present: (1) the child detaches from all relationships and emotional experiences and (2) the child tries to bond to another, using his or her power even to the point of being destructive. In withdrawing from others, the infant does not perceive the other as separate from the self or as having feelings. The child does not develop the ability to become depressed or to feel guilty for hurting another. There is a constant search for the ever-lurking danger.

BORDERLINE PERSONALITY DISORDER

Postulates a crisis in early infant development, the rapprochement subphase of separation and individuation (16 to 30 months of age), which involves abandonment by the mother forever. The child experiences little object constancy (mother); he or she is, therefore, unable to separate self from the mother, including good aspects as well as bad aspects. There are more bad self introjects; they are projected outward and the person feels persecuted—a victim. If the bad self introjects are re-introjected, the person feels unworthy or bad. Frequently there has been a history of sexual abuse or physical trauma by a parent or substitute. Much anger is present. The client acts as if growing up and developing emotionally will cause the loss of all love and support, so the choice is to remain dependent. If separation and individuation begin, the person will experience abandonment depression.

HISTRIONIC PERSONALITY DISORDER

Postulates that the female client experienced deprivation during the oral and oedipal stages of development. There is a lack of mothering that fosters a turning to the father for satisfaction of dependency needs. Dramatic acts, flirting, and other ways to draw attention to self are used to be "father's girl." The child defends against detachment from the father by becoming competitive with men, by selecting inappropriate male attachments, or by becoming more attached to the mother and hyperfeminine. The child may become a victim of incest. The male client also experiences deprivation and looks to the father for nurturance, consequently becoming more passive, woman-like, celibate, or hypermasculine, e.g., "woman chaser," body builder.

NARCISSISTIC PERSONALITY DISORDER

- One view postulates an early arrest in the development of the self. Specific necessary responses to the infant are not available. The developing self cannot be mirrored and admired by another, and yet be separate. The significant other is perceived as a source of needs; thus, a sense of self is not developed. The need to be admired, validated, and identified with another is defended against by isolation, grandiose fantasies, and shame.
- Another view postulates a defensive organization of the ego because of the lack of care by a loving person. Unacceptable self-images are projected to others, while a grandiose self-image is formed to protect against dependency needs. The aloofness and separation from others are understood as a defense against the anger, rage, and envy experienced.

AVOIDANT PERSONALITY DISORDER

Postulates that the disorder begins when the infant becomes aware of stranger danger, at about 8 months. The feelings of being different, of not living up to an expectation, or of having a shortcoming are reinforced during bowel and bladder training accidents and on other occasions. Shame is experienced repeatedly. The avoidance behavior defends against feelings of failure and rejection.

DEPENDENT PERSONALITY DISORDER

Postulates that during early development, the mother is overinvolved and very intrusive, generating a perception that independence is dangerous and a belief that a person must be loyal to parents and family. Dependency on the parents is reinforced throughout the growing years. Aggressive feelings may be hidden by the dependent behavior. Dependent behavior also can be a defense against reliving a traumatic experience.

OBSESSIVE-COMPULSIVE PERSONALITY DISORDER

Postulates an early developmental lack of parental availability; thus the person longs to be dependent on another and experiences rage when that is not possible. Both of these feelings are denied and defended against by reaction formation. For example, the client becomes very independent, appearing to need no one; however, he or she experiences a fear that at any time relationships that are present will disappear, that he or she will experience disapproval, and that things will not be right. Rationalization, intellectualization, undoing, displacement, regression, and isolation of affect are also used effectively to avoid anxiety.

Psychobiological Theory

This theory postulates four dimensions of abnormalities leading to development of traits, defenses, and coping styles.[34]

1. Cognitive/perceptual dimension: Problems are found in the attention/selection processes that help a person organize, evaluate, and relate to the environment. It is associated with Schizophrenia, Cluster A, particular biological indexes, traits of disorganization, and defenses of social isolation, detachment, and guardedness.
2. Impulsivity/aggression dimension: Problems are found in understanding the effects of behavior, in learning from undesirable consequences of past behavior, and in inhibiting or delaying action in the present. It is associated with impulse disorders, Borderline and Antisocial Personality Disorders, particular biological indexes, traits of readiness for action and irritability/aggression, and defenses of externalization, dissociation, and enactment regression.
3. Affective instability dimension: Problems are related to a high level of sensitivity to environmental events, e.g., separation, criticism, frustration. It is associated with major affective disorders, Borderline and Histrionic Personality Disorders, particular biological indexes, traits of transient affective states that are sensitive to environment, and the defenses of splitting, manipulation, and exaggerated affectivity.
4. Anxiety/inhibition dimension: Problems exist in managing anxiety and perhaps an increased sensitivity to punishment. It is associated with Anxiety Disorders, Cluster

C personality disorders, particular biological indexes, traits of autonomic arousal, fearfulness, and inhibition, and defenses of avoidant, compulsive, and dependent behaviors.

Integrative Theory

This postulates a developmental process in the formulation of personality. Environmental forces and biogenic-psychogenic factors interact in a complex process, reciprocally, circularly, and sequentially over the life span. Three sensitive neuropsychological stages are postulated that are basic to all other stages of development.[27]

1. Sensory-attachment stage—birth to 18 months. Necessary neurological development for sensory processes occurs, and the infant becomes attached to and dependent on mother figure. Stimulus impoverishment results in deficits in sensory capabilities and a sensitiveness toward others. Excessive stimulus may result in overdependency, stimulus-seeking behaviors, and hypersensitivities.
2. Sensorimotor-autonomy—12 months to 6 years. Motor skills are coordinated with sensory skills so that the child can walk, run, manipulate, and speak. Stimulus impoverishment results in deficits in exploratory behavior, lack of competitiveness, timidity, and submissiveness. Excessive stimulus results in uncontrolled self-expression, irresponsibility, and narcissism.
3. Intracortical-initiative—4 years through adolescence. Cortical centers enabling child to reflect, plan, and act are developed. Integration completed at an earlier stage is reorganized during puberty. Stimulus impoverishment results in identity confusion and inability to direct one's own energy, skill, and impulses. Excessive stimulus results in lack of spontaneity, creativity, and flexibility.

Over the years a particular pattern of dealing with the environment emerges. Coping strategies are described as (1) methods used by the person seeking positive reinforcement, (2) being within the self or in others, and (3) descriptions of active or passive use. The individual has internal defense patterns that are functional or dysfunctional within a particular social context, e.g., interpersonal, familial, etc.

Eight basic coping strategies are proposed:

1. Passive-dependent: Person looks to others for security, affection, and direction.
2. Active-dependent: Person looks continuously and indiscriminately for stimulation and affection.
3. Passive-independent: Person expects others to recognize his or her specialness and uses others to his or her own advantage.
4. Active-independent: Person mistrusts others and seeks autonomy and retribution for all injustices done.
5. Passive-ambivalent: Person's behavior is overly conforming, based on conflict over hostility towards others and fear of disapproval.
6. Active-ambivalent: Person's behavior—stubborn and angry, full of guilt or shame—is based on conflict over hostility toward others and fear of disapproval that is frequently acted out.
7. Action-detached: Person is constantly living in fear and mistrust of others.
8. Passive-detached: Person remains apart from relationships as an observer.

Three other coping strategies identified by Millon[27] are more dysfunctional: cycloid (changing intense moods), paranoid, and schizoid personalities.

▌ Laboratory and Physical Examination Findings*

- No test is diagnostic.
- Longitudinal data or history is needed to make diagnosis; school and legal records may be important.
- The Minnesota Multiphasic Personality Inventory (MMPI) may be helpful because it identifies specific personality traits in ten categories; interpretation of results requires an experienced clinician.
- EEG (electroencephalograph) may be indicated to rule out head injury, epilepsy, etc., that may contribute to the behavior noted.
- Specific blood and urine tests to rule out the presence of drugs and/or alcohol may be ordered.

*References 1,13,38,40

▌ Treatment[*]

- Establishment of a therapeutic relationship. Psychodynamic therapy is based on providing a relationship in which the client can experience empathy, positive self-regard, and acceptance. The client having any of the Personality Disorders described is fearful of the therapeutic encounter. Development of a client–therapist relationship proceeds at a slow pace. It requires the clinician to have knowledge of self and to manage the transference–countertransference issues that arise. The client relates to the therapist as if he or she were the significant person(s) in the client's life. The therapist may interpret behavior and events in the life of the client using various techniques. The experience of relating to the therapist over time offers another way of relating to others, new views of reality, and understanding of self. (See also Chapter 2.)
- Family therapy focuses on assisting parents to adjust their expectations of the adolescent, to dealing with ongoing problems in the relationships that may enhance and/or prevent development or stability in the family, and to develop new strategies for dealing with anxiety-provoking situations in daily life.
- Pharmacotherapy targets symptoms of anxiety, depression, mood swings, and somatic complaints with appropriate antipsychotic, antidepressant, and anxiolytic medications.

Cluster A

PARANOID PERSONALITY DISORDER

- Psychodynamic therapy focuses on changing the client's perception of problem from an external cause to his or her own internal one. Feeling states are labeled and distinguished from true facts and emotions; any gaps in knowledge are identified and help is given to fill in the gaps; the client is encouraged to be a questioner. The client will become in touch with feelings of weakness, insecurity, vulnerability, and inadequacy. Turmoil will be expressed, as client recognizes self as a victim or aggressor. At this point the client begins to deal with mourning for the loss of earlier attachments.

[*]References 3,5,6,9–13,16,17,19,21,23–25,28,31–33,37–40

There is a risk of the client becoming aggressive. The following interventions are suggested to prevent violence: assisting the client to save face in a particular situation, e.g., for the moment accepting and not encouraging a feeling; maintaining predictability by not making overly friendly remarks, touching the client to make a point, or making fast or surprising moves; assisting the client to maintain sense of control, e.g., taking medications, mutually changing subject, or taking time out; always encouraging the client to talk about feelings rather than acting on them; and maintaining an appropriate distance, e.g., not moving into personal space.

- Pharmacotherapy: Antipsychotic drugs may assist in managing anger, outbursts, agitation, and dysfunctional thinking.

SCHIZOID AND SCHIZOTYPAL PERSONALITY DISORDERS

- Psychodynamic therapy focuses on providing a relationship in the face of non-relatedness. Much patience is required. Long periods of silence are accepted and not interpreted as resistance. The use of fantasies and other defensive mechanisms against the feelings of ineffectiveness and low self-esteem is explored. Perceived beliefs and expectations of the therapist, as well as other people in daily life, are discussed and gradually become more realistic. Improvement may be noted in the ability to test reality or to make better judgments, but not necessarily in the ability to relate to others.
- Short-term/brief psychotherapy focuses on increasing the capacity to tolerate the feelings of aloneness or other affective states or making the solitary life more satisfying.
- Supportive/educational theory focuses on listening, giving information, problem solving, advising, and providing relatedness to another. Social skills training may be useful. This treatment approach is most frequently used.
- Cognitive-behavioral theory focuses on substituting negative assumptions, e.g., "I do not fit anywhere, people are too complicated, I'm better off keeping a low profile."
- Group therapy uses a supportive or dynamic group orientation to help the client deal with negative assumptions or strange thoughts, to learn how to make small

talk or pleasantries, and to learn about the thoughts and behaviors of others.

- Pharmacotherapy: Schizotypal client may experience anxiety, ideas of reference, paranoid ideation, depression, and intense anger. Anxiolytics, antidepressants, and antipsychotics may be used for a brief time.
- Residential treatment settings: Day treatment program, crisis bed, or half-way house may be indicated at times when the client is particularly isolated or experiencing increased stress.

Cluster B

ANTISOCIAL PERSONALITY DISORDER

- Treatment is not sought but clinicians become involved in treating the client for other mental disorders or when client is in a special program, e.g., jail, prison, drug program.
- Treatment is focused on treatable aspects, e.g., substance abuse, Major Depression Disorder, anger management, or on situational factors that can be eliminated.
- Pharmacotherapy targets symptoms of anxiety and depression with anxiolytics, antipsychotics, and antidepressants. Medications are prescribed with care because the client also may be using alcohol and/or drugs.
- Psychotherapy is undertaken only after the client has demonstrated some capacity to develop an attachment, evidenced the presence of superego, and shown that the experience can be safe for the client and psychiatrist. Treatment is difficult and generally not effective. Those clients who are more severely affected and who do not benefit from treatment are described as unable to experience pain, not responsive to aversive consequences (jail time), unable to determine a consequence of an act, and unable to apply past experiences to the present.
- Hospitalization may be necessary to control violence towards others or to treat Major Depression Disorder. Having the client on a general hospital unit or psychiatric unit can be very disruptive. The client steals, sexually acts out, and uses others to benefit self. Therapy focuses on limiting self-destructive behaviors, accepting responsibility for self, dealing with loss, and fear of intimacy. Suicidal thoughts are related to rage and anger

and *not* hopelessness. The length of stay is short; admission should not be used as a means to avoid consequences of action.

- Milieu/residential/special program: Some type of external structure is needed to target more specific behaviors or for the client to deal with therapy. Motivation for treatment increases in specialized settings offering a homogeneous peer group who are more confrontational.
- Cognitive-behavior therapy focuses specifically on strengthening the external and internal factors to control antisocial behaviors. Clients are taught the trigger effects of alcohol, drugs, other stimulants, guns, knives, and other means for damaging objects or persons, and of the presence of person(s) who are perceived as victim(s). The internal factors of thoughts, perceptions, feelings, wishes, and fantasies contributing to the immediate, intense response are identified. Focus is maintained on the here and now and denial of any antisocial act is confronted consistently.

  Interventions in the milieu focus on faulty thought processes. The client is not a "victim"; he is responsible. The client is assisted to identify the failure to think about the consequence of an act. The therapy also focuses on assisting the client to think before acting and asking self what can be expected if a certain thing is done.
- Family therapy focuses on assisting families to manage their feelings about being manipulated, which range from hate, dislike, and anger to guilt.

BORDERLINE PERSONALITY DISORDER

Psychoanalysis is generally considered inappropriate because the client develops an inappropriate transference with the psychiatrist and acts out in disorganized and uncontrollable manners.

- Psychodynamic therapy focuses on resolving the failure of the attachment experience in early childhood that results in inadequate sense of self, on making connections among feelings, motivations, and actions in the present, and on decreasing the gratification experienced in self-destructive behaviors.
- Supportive psychotherapy focuses on the problems of everyday living and improving relationships. Areas of

exploration are managing relationships to avoid distortions, reducing self-destructive responses and impulsivity, resolving problems in relationships by being more tolerant towards others, and learning strategies to lessen dysphoria.

- Group supportive therapy provides a modeling of social roles, uses group peer pressure to manage impulsivity, teaches ways of providing a structure in a small environment, and confronts maladaptive behavior. It is another way of providing support to the client in addition to the individual therapy; the 12-step approach may be used.
- Short-term/brief psychotherapy focuses on specific relationship problems in certain situations, thereby reducing the risk for regression. Since it is time-limited, clients who drop out of longer-term therapies may remain involved and then later have additional short-term therapy sessions.
- Family therapy: Overinvolvement, neglect, and abuse are frequently noted in the family, necessitating the family's involvement in therapy. Overinvolved families support and gratify the client's dependency needs when he or she is trying to become a differentiated person. Other families may neglect the client; they do not consider the needs of or are seldom responsive to him or her; the client would benefit from their support. Families with a history of abuse or knowledge of it seek to maintain the secret, and the client does not have the opportunity to clarify perceptions. Family therapy focuses on lessening the parents' fears of separating from client, the client's fear of abandonment by the parents, providing education on the process of therapy for the disorder, supporting client, and helping the client feel safe from abusive situations through the family's acknowledgment of abuse. A full reconciliation with the family following physical abuse may not be possible.
- Cognitive-behavioral therapy: Two approaches have been developed and used in groups of clients. One focuses on identifying the pathological cognitions of the world as unsafe and desiring that evil will occur, and of the self as powerless, weak, and intrinsically unacceptable. The other approach focuses on teaching the client how to deal with the dysregulation of emotions and the resulting behaviors. The strategies are pursued in order, targeting the most difficult or self-destructive behaviors first as follows: (1) suicidal behaviors; (2) behaviors that interfere with treatment, e.g., stopping treatment, non-

compliance; (3) behaviors that interfere with daily activities; (4) post-traumatic stress behaviors; and (5) self-respect behaviors with outcomes of improvement in interpersonal functioning.

- Pharmacotherapy targets symptoms of brief psychotic states, depression, intense anger, impulsivity, and anxiety, using antipsychotics, antidepressants (especially monoamine oxidase inhibitors), lithium, and SSRIs (drugs that increase serotonin), e.g., fluoxetine. Benzodiazepines do not alleviate anxiety but may lead to impulsive behavior.

  Involvement of client in the medication regimen is extremely important because medications may exacerbate feelings of powerlessness and increase noncompliance or lead to suicide attempt.

- Hospitalization is indicated if the client becomes self-destructive, self-mutilating, or more impulsive in response to a crisis or increased inner conflict with regressive behaviors. In addition to management of crises and self-destructive behaviors, the hospitalization assists in further diagnostic evaluation (if needed), management of medications, individual therapy, treatment planning and consultation, and engaging the family in therapeutic process. A program of full activities provides structure to assist the client in identifying and maintaining perception of self. The hospitalization should be brief to avoid regression and struggle with ward rules and routines. Several brief hospitalizations may be more beneficial than longer stays with regression. The client can participate in making the decision to be discharged.

  The client needs to learn (1) what precipitated the crisis, e.g., problems in managing intense emotion and anger or strong dependency needs; (2) to delay the expression of feeling in impulsive, self-destructive ways by seeking an alternative; (3) to anticipate or foresee the consequences of an action; and (4) to think about behavior before acting and thus become more responsible for his or her own behavior.

  Staff members in the hospitalized setting are involved in the therapeutic regimen since they help to prevent regressive behaviors such as angry outbursts and demands for attention and care. They need knowledge about the disorder and support to focus on the maladaptive interpersonal patterns. The client may easily involve the staff in splitting. The client projects his or her good objects towards staff that are more caring and nurturing and projects his or her bad objects to those who are more inflexible and less accepting. Staff members easily become immersed in the transference–countertransference process and experience frustration in dealing with the client. Staff members become split, seeing the client as "bad news, trouble, not treatable" or as "helpless, being mistreated"; interactions can deteriorate and conflicts erupt. Other signs of splitting are punitiveness, indulgence, protectiveness towards the client, and expressions of the belief that no one understands the client.

Meetings to discuss the views of all involved with the client are sometimes indicated to help all become more realistic and the negative feelings and remarks more reasonable. The client also learns that feelings can be controlled without a disaster.

HISTRIONIC PERSONALITY DISORDER

- Psychodynamic therapy focuses on stabilizing the intense emotions (emotional storms), unresolved dependency needs, and anger, which threaten to overwhelm; on dealing with avoiding or control processes; on the use of sexual displays to have the opposite sex become a substitute mother; on modifying internal beliefs and processes, e.g., avoiding conflicts by premature closure, providing many topics, stereotyping behavior of others, by "not knowing"; on developing new patterns for relating to others and increasing the stability of relationships. The client needs to learn to think and reflect on a feeling or an idea and not just say it; to identify what he or she thinks, wants, or feels; to identify his or her role pattern in relating, and to interrupt it and change the way of relating.
- Marital therapy focuses on assisting the couple as the client with the disorder becomes more assertive and less passive and dependent on the spouse. The other spouse may have some emotional needs that are met by being in control and feel threatened with the loss of control. The therapist acts to decrease the level of anxiety and/or depression in both persons.

- Group therapy is used in addition to individual therapy to foster ways to handle different situations and to give feedback about one's behavior.
- Brief or short-term therapy may be helpful in a crisis situation to problem solve the situation, to deal with self-image, and to manage the excessive emotional display, but not to change overall behavior patterns.

NARCISSISTIC PERSONALITY DISORDER

- Psychodynamic therapy utilizes two approaches. One approach focuses on the goal of developing a structure of the self by allowing the client to be like the therapist. This approach assists the client in understanding these protective devices, in experiencing security and protection, and in learning the misinterpretation that leads to defensive behavior and feelings of rage. Another approach focuses on the defensive structure of the ego, the grandiose self. The idealization of the therapist is interpreted as pathological. The view of the therapist as a perfect, all-loving person is analyzed as a defense, a projection of anger, rage, and envy because of a lack or unavailability of love. The goal is to work through the feelings and behaviors to perceive the self and others as more independent, separate selves.
- Supportive therapy: The disorder is difficult to treat because the client alternately idealizes and disparages the therapist. Short-term therapy is often used, focusing on lessening anxiety in relating with the other, examining social withdrawal, and promoting connectedness to others, e.g., managing conflict.

Cluster C

AVOIDANT PERSONALITY DISORDER

- Psychodynamic therapy focuses on uncovering the meaning of the anxiety as it relates to fears of losing control of self, being criticized, and then feeling rejected or ashamed. The client is taught how to handle causes of avoidance, to identify the outcomes of distancing behaviors, and to become more action focused.
- Behavior/exposure therapy: focuses on presenting social situations associated with shame to reduce the emotional reactions by use of flooding or gradual exposure.

- Behavior-cognitive therapy focuses on identifying cognition and correcting the distortions of self-worth ("I am a failure"), the expectation of negative feedback and rejection, and the belief that an unpleasant thought or interaction cannot be endured. Strategies are developed to handle the anxiety, identify avoidance behavior, and discuss the consequence of distancing from others. Teaching includes emphasizing action, recognizing that avoidance occurs as anxiety increases or the expectations of self are too high; learning ways to become less defensive, the importance of thinking of ways to be helpful to others to decrease fear, and valuing the various motivations of people for behaving in certain ways. Social skill training, particularly assertiveness and avoidance reduction, is useful.
- Supportive therapy focuses on overcoming fear and rejection and on teaching the client to be more assertive.
- Group therapy focuses on providing support to deal with new social situations, increasing social skills, and decreasing feelings of embarrassment.
- Pharmacotherapy: MAOIs and benzodiazepines may be useful in alleviating emotional pain and cognitive misinterpretations.

DEPENDENT PERSONALITY DISORDER

- Psychotherapy focuses on the anxiety associated with being independent through the development of a trusting, dependent relationship with the therapist. The client will seek advice and direction and will expect the situation to be handled by the therapist. The therapist, however, seeks to work through the defense of protecting the self from abandonment and separation and to help the client make his or her own plans, become knowledgeable about potential effects of goals/actions, become more realistic in demands on others, manage the separation anxiety, frustration, and conflicts involved in decision making, and be more responsible for himself or herself. Therapy may require 2 years or more.
- Cognitive-behavior therapy focuses on identifying the maladaptive dichotomous thinking, e.g., "I cannot make it in school...at work, I am incapable, I cannot do it." Such thinking is questioned by providing situations that are anxiety producing and helping the client to more accu-

rately appraise self and capabilities. Assertiveness skills, social skills, and relaxation techniques offer additional avenues for the client to develop more independence and sense of self.
• Group therapy has been reported as a successful modality.

OBSESSIVE-COMPULSIVE PERSONALITY DISORDER

This is the only personality disorder for which the client frequently seeks help.

• Psychodynamic therapy may focus on the defensive pattern of control to deal with unacceptable aggressive impulses, on the developmental arrest that occurred when the child sought autonomy and acceptance from the mother, and on problems with feelings of tenderness. The client desires to be the best or perfect patient and will use all the defenses to be so; however, he or she needs to learn to be human, not perfect. The client is difficult to deal with because of the use of many techniques to maintain control, e.g., intellectualizing (will have reasons for being late), questioning (will ask clarification of what is said), distracting (will expand a minor issue), evading (will add detail after detail that do not clarify), colluding (will appear to agree with the point being made or add so much to it that it is useless); the therapy may become nonproductive. The client needs to learn to manage anxiety, moderate the superego effect on his or her behavior, and resolve conflicts of dependency/interdependence, anger/rage, and sexuality.
• Cognitive-behavior therapy focuses on the misinterpretation of situations and the client's role that result in feelings of distress and on strategies to manage anxiety. The client may perceive a situation as more dangerous than necessary. This approach is frequently used.

▌ Commonly Occurring Nursing Diagnoses

Anxiety
Body image disturbance
Caregiver role strain
Coping, defensive

Coping, ineffective family
Coping, ineffective individual
Denial, ineffective
Family processes, altered
Hopelessness
Injury, risk for
Personal identity disturbance
Role performance, altered
Self-esteem, chronic low, situational low
Self-mutilation, risk for
Sexual pattern, altered
Social interaction, impaired
Social isolation
Thought processes, altered
Violence, risk for: self directed or directed at others

▍ Selected Nursing Diagnoses, Outcome Criteria, and Nursing Interventions with Rationale*

Example: Client With Dependent Personality Disorder in General Hospital With Fractured Hip and Multiple Bruises

NURSING DIAGNOSIS #1: *Ineffective individual coping related to focus on overwhelming emotional need to be taken care of and abuse by spouse*

EXPECTED CLIENT OUTCOME

- The client will identify a plan to protect self in the abusive situation.

NURSING INTERVENTIONS WITH RATIONALE

- Provide coping enhancement *to assist client in recognizing the emotional and cognitive aspects of coping with stress, so that more appropriate strategies can be developed*
  - Discuss how emotions interfere with objectivity and problem solving *to assist in client's understanding of the overwhelming feelings. Intense emotional states interfere with thinking through problems; focus is constricted. A person is ready to fight or flee or may be immobilized.*
  - Discuss importance of safety as well as security needs *to increase knowledge about human behavior and needs*

*References 3–8,10,13,14,16,17,19,22,26,28–33,35,36,38–40

and to develop a way to view own needs. Note: There is danger to life itself.

○ Encourage client to identify one or two things making it difficult to plan ahead, then begin to specify actions to take *to encourage more effective coping for self.* (See also Abuse Protection, Decision Making in Chapter 5.)

NURSING DIAGNOSIS #2: *Self-esteem disturbance related to dependency needs and fear of independence*

EXPECTED CLIENT OUTCOME

• The client will demonstrate the ability to make a decision about daily care and express less concern about being alone, e.g., frequent use of call light, making numerous requests.

NURSING INTERVENTIONS WITH RATIONALE

• Provide self-care assistance by *encouraging client's participation in own care and by helping client to see the results of this effort in contributing to maintaining self-esteem.*
   ○ Schedule daily care and amount of assistance needed with client.
   ○ Identify expectations of client for each task *to prevent becoming enmeshed with client in meeting the needs expressed.*
• Provide self-esteem enhancement *to increase perceptions of self as a manager and as having worth.*
   ○ Encourage client to accept the task of planning care, e.g., marking own menu, determining time and choice of reading material.
   ○ Give approval for tasks well done and actions done independently *to promote feelings of approval and acceptance.*
   ○ Provide an opportunity to talk about asking for help and having to make choices *because discussion offers chances to question misperceptions and mistaken beliefs about dependency.*

NURSING DIAGNOSIS #3: *Defensive Coping: anger related to inability to meet the need to be cared for and protected, life style of depressive behaviors*

EXPECTED CLIENT OUTCOME

- The client will schedule a psychotherapy session before leaving the hospital.

NURSING INTERVENTIONS WITH RATIONALE

- Assist in identifying reason for seeking professional help *to provide minimum support to begin therapy.*
  - Validate the abuse problem and the long duration of a problem of low self-esteem.
  - Make a list of behaviors and feelings to be explored in therapy sessions. *Fear can be reduced when a concrete idea of what to expect is identified.*
  - Discuss ways to encourage client to stay in therapy, because dropping out is common.
  - Discuss how anger and fear may interfere with therapy *so that if therapy is discontinued, the failure and anger will not be reinforced.*
- Coordinate referral process as necessary.

Example: Client With Borderline Personality Disorder in Hospital Setting

NURSING DIAGNOSIS #1: *Risk for violence towards self: self-mutilation*

EXPECTED CLIENT OUTCOMES

- The client will not injure self during hospitalization.
- The client will identify when he or she begins to feel numb or not connected to self.

NURSING INTERVENTIONS WITH RATIONALE

- Provide surveillance *to prevent harmful acts towards self and to maintain safety for client.*
  - Maintain continuous around-the-clock observation for violence to self.
  - Assess for the presence of hopelessness, inability to experience pleasure, agitation, and a safety plan; also assess the client's ability to interrupt thoughts about harming self.
  - Take action as necessary to stop act of mutilation.

- ○ Ask what problem client is trying to resolve by self-destructive acts, e.g., burning self, cutting hair, etc. Remove potential hazards from environment.
- ○ Provide emotional support to identify feelings, e.g., numbness, a sense of nonbeing, or thoughts that are troublesome and lead to the mutilation act. *This is an important way to prevent an act.*
- ○ Instruct client to write, draw, or pantomime placing thoughts and feelings in a box or room or on paper to *assist in making the thought or feeling more concrete, connected, and containable.*
- ○ Assist in finding words to describe the experience.
- ○ Validate thoughts or feelings whenever possible *to assist in making connections from feeling to acts.*
- Teach ways to maintain sense of connectedness to self and *thus assist in preventing acts of self-mutilation.*
  - ○ Assist client in maintaining an external boundary by having a plan for the day, going to a place that is perceived as safe, having an image of a safe area, wrapping self in a sheet or blanket, bathing, or applying lotion. *These are concrete ways to feel, touch, see self as having a boundary and being safe and secure.*
  - ○ Assist client in maintaining an internal boundary by setting time for tasks, recreation, schoolwork, etc. *Internal boundaries become more stable in a structured environment.*
  - ○ Request feedback on effectiveness of different strategies.

References

Chapter 1

1. American Psychiatric Association: Diagnostic and Statistical Manual of Mental Disorders, DSM-IV, 4th ed. Washington, DC: American Psychiatric Association, 1994
2. Beck AT, Freeman A: Cognitive Therapy and Personality Disorders. New York, Guilford Press, 1990
3. Beck AT: Cognitive Therapy and the Emotional Disorders. New York: NAL-Dutton, 1988
4. Bion WR: Experiences in Groups: And Other Papers. New York: Routledge, 1991
5. Bion WR: Learning from Experience. Northvale, NJ: Jason Aronson, 1994
6. Bloom B: Health Psychology: A Psychosocial Perspective. Englewood Cliffs, NJ: Prentice Hall, 1988
7. Bloom Bernard: Planned Short-Term Psychotherapy: A Clinical Handbook. Needham Heights, NY: Allyn & Bacon, 1991
8. Bootzin RR, Acocella JR: Abnormal Psychology: Current Perspectives, 6th ed. New York: McGraw-Hill, 1993
9. Bowen M: Family Therapy in Clinical Practice. New York: Jason Aronson, 1978
10. Cartwright D, Zander A: Group Dynamics: Research and Theory. New York: Harper & Row, 1968
11. Corsini RJ, Wedding D: Current Psychotherapies, 4th ed. Itasca, IL: FE Peacock, 1989
12. Department of Health and Human Services: Healthy People 2000. Washington, DC: DHHS, 1990
13. Dumas RG: Psychiatric nursing in an era of change. Journal of Psychosocial Nursing and Mental Health Care Services 32(1):11–14, 1994
14. Ellis A, Dryden W: Rational-emotive therapy: An excellent counseling theory for NPs. Nurse Pract 12(7):16–37, 1987
15. Erikson E: Childhood and Society. New York: WW Norton, 1993
16. Erikson E: Identity and the Life Cycle. New York: WW Norton, 1994
17. Erikson E: Identity: Youth and Crisis. New York: WW Norton, 1994
18. Erikson E: Insight and Responsibility. New York: WW Norton, 1964
19. Erikson E: The Life Cycle Completed: A Review. New York: WW Norton, 1985
20. Frankl V: Man's Search for Meaning: An Introduction to Logotherapy. Boston: Beacon Press, 1992

21. Frankl V: The Doctor and the Soul: From Psychotherapy to Logotherapy. New York: Random House, 1986

22. Frankl VE: Man's Search for Meaning. Cutchogue, NY: Buccaneer Books, 1993

23. Giffin RB: Managed Care and National Health Care Reform: Nurses Can Make It Work: Working Paper. Washington, DC: American Academy of Nursing, 1993

24. Grob G, ed: Jahoda Marie Current Concepts in Positive Mental Health. Salem, NH: Ayer, 1979

25. Gurman AS, ed: Casebook of Marital Therapy. New York: Guilford Press, 1985

26. Gurman AS, Kniskern DP, eds: Handbook of Family Therapy, Vol. II. New York: Brunner-Mazel, 1991

27. Gurman AS, Kniskern DR: Handbook of Family Therapy, Vol. 1. New York: Brunner-Mazel, 1981

28. Haber J, Billings CV: Primary mental health care: A model for psychiatric-mental health nursing 1(5):154–163, 1995

29. Hales RE, et al, eds: American Psychiatric Press Textbook of Psychiatry, 2nd ed. Washington, DC: American Psychiatric Press, 1994

30. Haley J, Hoffman L: Techniques of Family Therapy. Northvale, NJ: Jason Aronson, 1994

31. Haley J: Problem-Solving Therapy, 2nd ed. San Francisco: Jossey-Bass, 1991

32. Haley J: Problem-Solving Therapy: New Strategies for Effective Family Therapy. San Francisco: Jossey-Bass, 1994

33. Harrington C, Feetham SL, Moccia PA, Smith GR: Health Care Access Problems and Policy Recommendations: Working Paper. Washington, DC: American Academy of Nursing, 1993

34. Hellwig K: Psychiatric home care nursing: Managing patients in the community setting. Journal of Psychosocial Nursing and Mental Health Care Services 31(12):21–24, 1993

35. Hicks LL, Stallmeyer JM, Coleman JR: Role of the Nurse in Managed Care. Washington, DC: American Nurses Association, 1994

36. Kaplan HI, Sadock B: Comprehensive Textbook of Psychiatry, 6th ed. Baltimore: Williams & Wilkins, 1995

37. Kaplan HI, Sadock BJ, eds: Comprehensive Group Psychotherapy, 3rd ed. Baltimore: Williams & Wilkins, 1993

38. Kaplan HI, Sadock BJ: Synopsis of Psychiatry, 7th ed. Baltimore: Williams & Wilkins, 1994

39. Keltner NL: Introduction to psychiatric nursing. In Keltner NL, Schwecke LH, Bostrom CE: Psychiatric Nursing. St. Louis: Mosby, 1995

40. Kneisl CR: One thing psychiatric nurses need to do to thrive in the decade of the brain. Capsules and Comments in Psychiatric Nursing 2(4):247–248, 1996

41. Krauss JB: Health Care Reform: Essential Mental Health Services. Washington, DC: American Nurses Publishing, 1993

42. Maslow AH: The Farther Reaches of Human Nature. New York: Viking Penguin, 1993

43. McCrone SH: The impact of the evolution of biological psychiatry on psychiatric nursing. Journal of Psychosocial Nursing and Mental Health Services 34(1):38–46, 1996

44. Minuchin S, Nichols MP: Family Healing: Tales of Hope and Renewal from Family Therapy. Free Press, 1992

45. Minuchin S: Families and Family Therapy. Cambridge, MA: Harvard University Press, 1974
46. Mohr WK: Values, ideologies and dilemmas: Professional and occupational contradictions. Journal of Psychosocial Nursing and Mental Health Care Services 33(1):29–34, 1995
47. Reamer FG: The contemporary mental health system: Facilities, services, personnel and finances. In Rochefort DA, ed: Handbook on Mental Health Policy in U.S. New York: Greenwood Press, 1989
48. Rogers CR: Client Centered Therapy. Boston: Houghton Mifflin, 1951
49. Rogers CR: Freedom to Learn for the Eighties. New York: Macmillan, 1983
50. Rogers CR: On Becoming a Person, Boston: Houghton Mifflin, 1972
51. Rogers CR: The Therapeutic Relationship and Its Impact. Westport, CT: Greenwood, 1976
52. Rowland LP, ed: Merritt's Textbook of Neurology, 8th ed. Baltimore: Williams & Wilkins, 1989
53. Sarason IG, Sarason BR: Abnormal psychology. The problem of Maladaptive Behavior, 7th ed. Englewood Cliffs, NJ: Prentice-Hall, 1993
54. Satir VM: Conjoint Family Therapy, 3rd ed. Palo Alto, CA: Science & Behavior Books, 1983
55. Scahill L: Toward the National Plan for Research in Child and Adolescent Mental Health Disorders: Midterm Report Card. JCAPN 8(4):31–32, 1995
56. Shea CA: Mental health care reform: A historic town meeting of psychiatric nurses. Journal of Psychosocial Nursing and Mental Health Care Services 31(8):30–33, 1993
57. Shea CA: Moving into the mainstream. Journal of Psychosocial Nursing 31(3):5–7, 1993
58. Siegel GJ, et al, eds: Basic Neurochemistry: Molecular, Cellular, and Medical Aspects, 5th ed. New York: Raven, 1994
59. Slater P: Microcosm, Structural, Psychological and Religious Evolution in Groups. New York: John Wiley & Sons, 1966
60. Smith GB: Hospital case management for psychiatric diagnoses: focusing on quality and cost outcomes. Journal of Psychosocial Nursing and Mental Health Care Services 32(2):3–4, 1994
61. Subcommittee of the Joint Commission on Public Affairs. A Psychiatric Glossary, 5th ed. Washington, DC: APA, 1984
62 Sudarsky L: Pathophysiology of the Nervous System. Boston: Little, Brown, 1990
63. Sullivan HS: Clinical Studies in Psychiatry. New York: WW Norton, 1973
64. Sullivan HS: Conceptions of Modern Psychiatry. New York: WW Norton, 1966
65. Sullivan HS: The Interpersonal Theory of Psychiatry. New York: WW Norton, 1968
66. Thompson J, Strand K: Psychiatric nursing in a psychosocial setting. Journal of Psychosocial Nursing and Mental Health Care Services 32(2):25–29, 1994
67. Vaillant GE: Adaptation to Life. Boston: Little, Brown, 1978
68. Vaillant GE: Ego Mechanisms of Defense: A Guide for Clinicians & Researchers. Washington, DC: American Psychiatric Press, 1992
69. World Health Organization: World Health Statistical Manual. Geneva: WHO, 1986

70. Yalom I: Inpatient Group Psychotherapy. New York: Basic Books, 1983
71. Yudofsky S, Hales R, eds: Synopsis of Neuropsychiatry. Washington, DC: American Psychiatric Press, 1994
72. Yudofsky S, Hales R, eds: The American Psychiatric Press Textbook of Neuropsychiatry, 2nd ed. Washington, DC: American Psychiatric Press, 1992

Chapter 2

1. Abdullah SN: Towards an individualized client's care: Implication for education: The transcultural approach. J Advanced Nursing 22:715–720, 1995
2. Alonso A: The quiet profession: Supervisors of psychotherapy. New York: Macmillan, 1985
3. American Nurses Association Council on Psychiatric and Mental Health Nursing, American Psychiatric Nurses Association, Association of Child and Adolescent Psychiatric Nurses, Society for Education and Research in Psychiatric-Mental Health Nursing: Statement on Psychiatric-Mental Health Clinical Nursing Practice and Standards of Psychiatric-Mental Health Clinical Nursing Practice. Washington, DC: American Nurses Publishing, 1994
4. Armstrong ME, Kelly AE: Enhancing staff nurses' interpersonal skills: Theory to practice. Clinical Nurse Specialist 7(6):313–317, 1993
5. Arnold E: Developing therapeutic communication skills. In Arnold E, Boggs KU: Interpersonal Relationships: Professional Communication Skills for Nurses, 2nd ed. Philadelphia: WB Saunders, 1995
6. Banks L: Counseling. In Bulechek GM, McCloskey JC: Nursing Interventions: Essential Nursing Treatments, 2nd ed. Philadelphia: WB Saunders, 1992
7. Bischoff MM, Tracey TJG: Client resistance as predicted by therapist behavior: A study of sequential dependence. J Counseling Psychology 42(4):487–495, 1995
8. Boggs K: Communication styles. In Arnold E, Boggs KU: Interpersonal Relationships: Professional Communication Skills for Nurses, 2nd ed. Philadelphia: WB Saunders, 1995.
9. Carson VB: Losses and endings in the nurse–client relationship. In Arnold E, Boggs KU: Interpersonal Relationships: Professional Communication Skills for Nurses, 2nd ed. Philadelphia: WB Saunders, 1995
10. Chapman AH: The Treatment Techniques of Harry Stack Sullivan. New York: Brunner/Mazel, 1978
11. Charonko CV. Cultural influences in "non-compliant" behavior and decision-making. Holistic Nursing Practice 6(3):73–78, 1992
12. Devereaux D: The issue of race and the client–therapist assignment. Issues Mental Health Nursing 12(3):283–290,1991
13. Dombeck MT, Brody SL: Clinical supervision: A three-way mirror. Archives Psychiatric Nursing IX(1):3–10, 1995
14. Farkas-Cameron MM: Clinical supervision in psychiatric nursing: A self-actualizing process. J Psychosocial Nursing and Mental Health Services 33(2):31–37,1995
15. Field WF: The Psychotherapy of Hildegard E. Peplau. New Braunfels, Texas: PSF Productions, 1979

16. Forchuk C: Development of nurse–client relationships: What helps? J Amer Psychiatric Nurses Association 1(5):146–153, 1995

17. Forchuk C: The orientation phase of the nurse–client relationship: How long does it take? Perspectives Psychiatric Care 28(4):7–10, 1992

18. Forchuk C, Brown B: Establishing a nurse–client relationship. J Psychosoc Nurs Ment Health Serv 27(2):30–34,1989

19. Greipp ME: Culture and ethics: A tool for analysing the effects of biases in the nurse-patient relationship. Nursing Ethics 2(3):211–221, 1995

20. Hale SL, Richardson JH: Terminating the nurse-patient relationship. Am J Nurs 63(9):116–119,1963

21. Hays JS, Larson K: Interacting with Patients: Communications for General and Psychiatric Nurses. New York: Macmillan, 1963

22. Heim E: Coping-based intervention strategies. Patient Education and Counseling 26:145–151, 1995

23. Jones SL: Editorial: More on confidentiality. Archives Psychiatric Nursing 7(3):123–124,1993

24. Kramer P: Empathic immersion. In Spiro EM, Curnen MGM, Peschel E, St James D, eds. Empathy and the Practice of Medicine: Beyond Pills and the Scalpel. New Haven, Yale University Press, 1995

25. Krouse HJ, Roberts SJ: Nurse–patient interactive styles: Power, control, and satisfaction. West J Nurs Res 11(6):717–725,1989

26. McCloskey JC, Bulechek GM (eds): Nursing Interventions Classification (NIC), 2nd ed. St. Louis: Mosby, 1996

27. Miles MW: The evolution of countertransference and its applicability to nursing. Perspectives Psychiatric Care 29(4):13–20, 1993

28. Nachinski C: The communication process. In McFarland GK, Thomas MD. Psychiatric Mental Health Nursing. Philadelphia: JB Lippincott, 1991

29. Olsen JK: Relation between nurse-expressed empathy, patient perceived empathy and patient distress. Image: J Nursing Scholarship 27(4):317–322, 1995

30. O'Toole AW, Welt SR (eds): Interpersonal Theory in Nursing Practice: Selected Works of Hildegard E. Peplau. New York: Springer, 1989

31. Peplau HE: Interpersonal Relations in Nursing: A Conceptual Frame of Reference for Psychodynamic Nursing. New York: Springer, 1991 (originally published 1952)

32. Peplau HE: Basic Principles of Patient Counseling: Extracts from Two Clinical Nursing Workshops in Psychiatric Hospitals. Philadelphia, Smith Kline & French Laboratories, 1964

33. Peplau HE: Talking with patients. Am J Nurs 60(7):964–966, 1960

34. Pesut DJ, Williams CA: The nature of clinical supervision in psychiatric nursing: A survey of clinical specialists. Arch Psychiatric Nurs IV(3):188–194,1990

35. Pilette PC, Berck CB, Achber LC: Therapeutic management of helping boundaries. J Psychosoc Nurs Ment Health Services 33(1):40–47, 1995

36. Rankin DJ: Therapy supervision: The phenomena and the need. Clinical Nurse Specialist 3(4):204–208,1989

37. Ryden M: Active Listening. In Snyder M: Independent Nursing Interventions, 2nd ed. Minneapolis: Delmar Publishers Inc, 1992

38. Sullivan V: Bridges and barriers in the therapeutic relationship. In Boggs KU: Interpersonal Relationships: Professional Communication Skills for Nurses, 2nd ed. Philadelphia: WB Saunders, 1995

39. Sutherland JA: Historical concept of empathy. Issues Mental Health Nursing 16:555–566, 1995
40. Thomas MD: Cultural concepts and psychiatric mental health nursing. In McFarland GK, Thomas MD. Psychiatric Mental Health Nursing: Application of the Nursing Process. Philadelphia: JB Lippincott, 1991
41. Thomas MD: Therapeutic relationships with clients. In McFarland GK, Thomas MD. Psychiatric Mental Health Nursing. Philadelphia: JB Lippincott, 1991
42. Thompson L: Peplau's theory: An application to short-term individual therapy. J Psychosoc Nurs Ment Health Serv 24(8):26–31,1986
43. Wheeler K: A nursing science approach to understanding empathy. Arch Psychiatric Nurs II(2):95–102, 1988
44. Young JC: Rationale for clinician self-disclosure and research agenda. Image: J Nurs Scholarship 20(4):196–199, 1988

Chapter 3

1. American Nurses Association: Statement on Psychiatric-Mental Health Clinical Nursing Practice and Standards of Psychiatric-Mental Health Clinical Nursing Practice. Washington, DC: American Nurses Publishing, 1994
2. American Psychiatric Association: Diagnostic and Statistical Manual of Mental Disorders, 4th ed. Washington, DC: American Psychiatric Association, 1994
3. Andreasen, NC, Black, DW: Introductory Textbook of Psychiatry, 2nd ed. Washington DC: American Psychiatric Press, 1995.
4. Breitner JC, Welsk KA: Diagnosis and management of memory loss and cognitive disorders among elderly persons. Psychiatric Services 46 (1):29–30, 1994
5. Cardell R, Horton-Deutsch S: A model for assessment of inpatient suicide potential. Archives Psychiatric Nursing 8(6):366–372, 1994
6. Clarkin, JF, Hurt SW, Mattis S: Psychological and neuropsychological assessment. In Hales RE, Yudofsky SC, Talbott JA (eds): The American Psychiatric Press Textbook of Psychiatry, 2nd ed. Washington, DC: American Psychiatric Press, 1994
7. Elliott, DM: Assessing adult victims of interpersonal violence. In Briere J (ed): Assessing and Treating Victims of Violence: New Directions for Mental Health Services. San Francisco: Jossey-Bass Inc, 1994
8. Faber R: Neuropsychiatric assessment. In Coffey CE, Cummings JL (eds): The American Psychiatric Press Textbook of Geriatric Neuropsychiatry. Washington, DC: American Psychiatric Press, 1994
9. Hersen, M, Turner SM (eds): Diagnostic Interviewing, 2nd ed. New York: Plenum Press, 1994
10. Jerrell JM, Ridgely MS: Evaluating changes in symptoms and functioning of dually diagnosed clients in specialized treatment. Psychiatric Services 46(3):233–238, 1995
11. McFarland GK, Butcher HK: Assessment of the psychiatric mental health client. In McFarland GK, Thomas MD: Psychiatric Mental Health Nursing. Philadelphia: JB Lippincott, 1991
12. Morihisia JM, Rosse RB, Cross CD: Laboratory and other diagnostic tests in psychiatry. In Hales RE, Yudofsky SC, Talbott JA (eds); The American Psychiatric Press Textbook of Psychiatry, 2nd ed. Washington DC: American Psychiatric Press, 1994

13. Mueller J, Kiernan RJ, Langston JW: The mental status examination. In Goldman HH: Review of General Psychiatry. Norwalk: Appleton and Lange, 1995
14. North American Nursing Diagnosis Association: NANDA Nursing Diagnoses: Definitions and Classifications 1995–1996. Philadelphia: North American Nursing Diagnosis Association, 1994
15. Othmer E, Othmer SC: The Clinical Interview Using DSM-IV, Vol. 1: Fundamentals. Washington, DC: American Psychiatric Press, 1994
16. Othmer E, Othmer SC: The Clinical Interview Using DSM-IV, Vol. 2: The Difficult Patient. Washington, DC: American Psychiatric Press, 1994
17. Pinegar C: Screening for dissociative disorders in children and adolescents. JCAPN 8(1):5–14, 1995
18. Richards HN, Maletta GJ: History and mental status examination. In Copeland JRM, Abou-Saleh MT, Blazer DG (eds): Principles and Practice of Geriatric Psychiatry. New York: John Wiley and Sons, 1994
19. Robins L, Helzer JE: The half-life of a structured interview: The NIMH Diagnostic Interview Schedule (DIS). Special issue: A ten-year retrospective on the NIMH Epidemiologic Catchment Area (ECA) Program. International Journal of Methods in Psychiatric Research 4(2):95–102, 1994
20. Roy-Byrne P, Dagadakis C, Reis R, et al: A psychiatrist-rated battery of measures for assessing the clinical status of psychiatric inpatients. Psychiatric Services 46(4):347–352, 1995
21. Scheiber SC: The psychiatric interview, psychiatric history, and mental status examination. In Hales RE, Yudofsky SC, Talbott JA (eds): The American Psychiatric Press Textbook of Psychiatry. Washington, DC: American Psychiatric Press, 1994
22. Smith SL, Sherril KA, Colenda CC: Assessing and treating anxiety in elderly persons. Psychiatric Services 46(1):36–42, 1995
23. Sultzer DL: Mental status examination. In Coffey CE, Cummings JL: The American Psychiatric Press Textbook of Geriatric Neuropsychiatry. Washington, DC: American Psychiatric Press, 1994
24. Worthington C: An examination of factors influencing the diagnosis and treatment of black patients in the mental health system. Archives Psychiatric Nursing 6(3):195–204, 1992

Chapter 4

1. American Psychiatric Association: Diagnostic and Statistical Manual of Mental Disorders, 4th ed. Washington, DC: American Psychiatric Association, 1994
2. Ballinger BR: New drugs: Hypnotics and anxiolytics. Br Med J 300(6722):456–58, 1990
3. Ballenger JC: Benzodiazepines. In Schatzberg AF, Nemeroff CB, eds: The American Psychiatric Press Textbook of Psychopharmacology. Washington, DC: American Psychiatric Press, 1995
4. Barrett N, Ormiston S, Molyneux V: Clozapine: A new drug for schizophrenia. J Psychosoc Nurs Ment Health Serv 28(2):24–28, 1990
5. Bowden C, et al.: Efficacy of divalproex vs lithium and placebo in the treatment of mania. JAMA 271:918–924, 1994
6. Bressler R, Katz M: Drug therapy for geriatric depression. Drugs and Aging 3(3):195–329, 1993

7. Caley C, Weber S: Paroxetine: A selective serotonin reuptake inhibiting antidepressant. Ann Pharmacother 27:1212–1222, 1993

8. Callahan A, Fava M, Rosenbaum J: Drug interactions in psychopharmacology. Psychiatric Clinics North America 16:647–671, 1993

9. Casey D. Neuroleptic-induced acute extrapyramidal syndromes and tardive dyskinesia. Psychiatric Clinics North America 16:589–610, 1993

10. Castillo E, Rubin RT, Holsboer-Trachsler E: Clinical differentiation between lethal catatonia and neuroleptic malignant syndrome. Am J Psychiatry 146(3):324–328, 1989

11. Chutka D: Cardiovascular effects of the antidepressants: Recognition and control. Geriatrics 45:55–67, 1990

12. Cohen L: Risperidone. Pharmacotherapy 14(3):253–265, 1994

13. Cole J, Yonkers K: Nonbenzodiazepine anxiolytics. In Schatzberg AF, Nemeroff CB, eds: The American Psychiatric Press Textbook of Psychopharmacology. Washington, DC: American Psychiatric Press, 1995

14. Dave M: Two cases of risperidone-induced neuroleptic malignant syndrome. Am J Psychiatry 142(8):1233–1234,1995

15. Ellingrod V, Perry P: Venlafaxine: A heterocyclic antidepressant. Am J Hosp Pharm 51:3033–3046, 1994

16. DeVane C: Brief comparison of the pharmacokinetics and pharmacodynamics of the traditional and newer antipsychotic drugs. Am J Health-Syst Pharm 52(Suppl 1):S15–18, 1995

17. Dillon N: A screening system for tardive dyskinesia: Development and implementation. J Psychosoc Nursing 30(10):3–7, 1992

18. Garner EM, Kelly M, Thompson: Tricyclic antidepressant withdrawal syndrome. Ann Pharmacother 27:1068–1072, 1993

19. Gerner R: Treatment of acute mania. Psychiatric Clinics North America 16:443–460, 1993

20. Goldberg R, Posner D: Anxiety in the medically ill. In Stoudemire A, Fogel B, eds: Psychiatric Care of the Medical Patient. New York: Oxford University Press, 1993

21. Grubb B. et al: Fluoxetine hydrochloride for the treatment of severe refractory orthostatic hypotension. Am J Med 97:366–368, 1994

22. Guttmacher L: Concise Guide To Psychopharmacology and Electroconvulsive Therapy. Washington, DC: American Psychiatric Press, 1994

23. Guy W: ECDEU Assessment Manual for Psychopharmacology, revised 1976. Washington, DC: U.S. Government Printing Office, 1976

24. Hansten PD, Horn JR: Drug Interactions and Updates. Vancouver, WA: Applied Therapeutics, 1993

25. Hayes P, Kirkwood C: Anxiety disorders. In Dipiro J, et al, eds: Pharmacotherapy: A Pathophysiologic Approach, 2nd ed. Norwalk, CT: Appleton & Lange, 1993

26. Hollander E, Simeon D, Gorman J: Anxiety disorders. In Hales RE, ed: The American Psychiatric Press Textbook of Psychiatry, 2nd ed. Washington, DC: American Psychiatric Press, 1994

27. Holliday SM, Plosker GL: Paroxetine. Drugs and Aging 3:278–299, 1993

28. Jackson C: Obsessive-compulsive disorder in elderly patients. Drugs and Aging 7:438–448, 1995

29. Kaplan H, Sadock B, Grebb J: Anxiety disorders. In Kaplan and Sadock's Synopsis of Psychiatry, 7th ed. Baltimore: Williams & Wilkins, 1994

30. Keltner N: Serotonin syndrome: A case of fatal SSRI/MAOI interaction. Perspectives in Psychiatric Care 30:26–31, 1994

31. Krishnan KRR: Monoamine oxidase inhibitors. In Schatzberg AF, Nemeroff CB, eds: The American Psychiatric Press Textbook of Psychopharmacology. Washington, DC: American Psychiatric Press, 1995
32. Lahti A, Tamminga C: Recent developments in the neuropharmacology of schizophrenia. Am J Health-Syst Pharm 52(Suppl 1):S5–8, 1995
33. Lee H, Ryan J, et al: Neuroleptic malignant syndrome associated with the use of risperidone, an atypical antipsychotic agent. Human Psychopharmacology 9:303–305, 1994
34. Lenox R, Manji H: Lithium. In Schatzberg, AF, Nemeroff CB, eds: The American Psychiatric Press Textbook of Psychopharmacology. Washington, DC: American Psychiatric Press, 1995
35. Levinson ML, Lipsy RJ, Fuller DK: Adverse effects and drug interactions associated with fluoxetine therapy. DICP Ann Pharmacother 1991; 25:657–661
36. Lin K, Anderson D, Poland R: Ethnicity and psychopharmacology. Psychiatric Clinics North America 18:635–647, 1995
37. Lohr M: Psychopharmacology. In McFarland GK, Thomas MD: Psychiatric Mental Health Nursing. Philadelphia: JB Lippincott, 1991
38. Malseed RT: Pharmacology. In Drug Therapy and Nursing Considerations, 3rd ed. Philadelphia: JB Lippincott, 1990
39. Marder S, et al: Schizophrenia. Psychiatric Clinics North America 16:567–587, 1993
40. Marshall R, Klein D: Pharmacotherapy in the treatment of posttraumatic stress disorder. Psychiatric Annals 25:588–594, 1995
41. Martin L, et al: Recognition and management of anxiety and depression in elderly patients. Mayo Clin Proc 70:999–1006, 1995
42. McElroy S, Keckk P: Antiepileptic Drugs. In Schatzberg AF, Nemeroff CB, eds: The American Psychiatric Press Textbook of Psychopharmacology. Washington, DC: American Psychiatric Press, 1995
43. McEvoy G, ed: American Hospital Formulary Service Drug Information. Bethesda, MD: American Society of Health-Systems Pharmacists, 1996
44. Meltzer H: New drugs for the treatment of schizophrenia. Psychiatric Clinics North America 16:365–385, 1993
45. Middlemiss MA, Beeber LS: Issues in the use of depot antipsychotics. J Psychosoc Nurs Ment Health Serv 27(6):36–37, 1989
46. Murray S, Haller E: Risperidone and NMS? Psychiatric Services 46(9):951, 1995
47. Najara JE, Enikeev ID: Risperidone and neuroleptic malignant syndrome: A case report. J Clin Psychiatry 56(11):534–535, 1995
48. Naranjo CA, et al: Recent advances in geriatric psychopharmacology. Drugs and Aging 7:184–202,1995
49. Nelson M, Dunner D: Treatment resistance in unipolar depression and other disorders. Psychiatric Clinics North America 16:541–566, 1993
50. Noyes R, Holt C: Anxiety disorders. In Winokur G, Clayton P, eds: The Medical Basis of Psychiatry, 2nd ed. Philadelphia: WB Saunders, 1994.
51. Potter WZ, et al: Tricyclics and tetracyclics. In Schatzberg AF, Nemeroff CB, eds: The American Psychiatric Press Textbook of Psychopharmacology. Washington, DC: American Psychiatric Press, 1995
52. Preskorn S, Burke M, Fast G: Therapeutic drug monitoring. Psychiatric Clinics North America 16:611–645, 1993
53. Raitasuo V, et al: Risperidone-induced neuroleptic malignant syndrome in young patient. Lancet 344:1705, 1994

54. Remington G: Clinical considerations in the use of risperidone. Can J Psychiatry 38 (Suppl 3):S96–100, 1993

55. Richelson E: Treatment of acute depression. Psychiatric Clinics North America 16:461–478, 1993

56. Riesenman C: Antidepressant drug interactions and the cytochrome P450 system: A critical appraisal. Pharmacotherapy 15 (6 Pt 2):84S–99S, 1995

57. Rifkin A: Pharmacologic strategies in the treatment of schizophrenia. Psychiatric Clinics North America 16:351–363, 1993

58. Salzman C: Pharmacologic treatment of depression in the elderly. J Clin Psychiatry 54 (Suppl 2):23–28, 1993

59. Sheikh JI: Anxiety disorders and their treatment. Clinics in Geriatric Medicine 8:411-426, 1992

60. Shaughnessy R: Psychopharmacotherapy of neuropsychiatric disorders. Psychiatric Annals 25:634–640, 1995

61. Singer S, et al.: Two cases of risperidone-induced neuroleptic malignant syndrome. Am J Psychiatry 15(8):1234, 1995

62. Smith M, Buckwalter K: Medication management, antidepressant drugs, and the elderly: An overview. J Psychosoc Nursing 30(10):30–36, 1992

63. Solomon D, Bauer M: Continuation and maintenance pharmacotherapy for unipolar and bipolar mood disorders. Psychiatric Clinics North America 16:515–540, 1993

64. Sullivan G, Luckoff D: Sexual side effects of antipsychotic medication: Evaluation and interventions. Hosp Community Psychiatry 41(11):1238–1241, 1990

65. Sutherland SM, Davidson J: Pharmacotherapy for posttraumatic stress disorder. Psychiatric Clinics North America 17:409–423, 1994

66. Swartz JT, Brotman AW: A clinical guide to antipsychotic drugs. Drugs 44:981–992, 1992

67. Taylor CB: Treatment of anxiety disorders. In Schatzberg AF, Nemeroff CB, eds: The American Psychiatric Press Textbook of Psychopharmacology. Washington, DC: American Psychiatric Press, 1995

68. Tollefson GD: Selective serotonin reuptake inhibitors. In Schatzberg AF, Nemeroff CB, eds: The American Psychiatric Press Textbook of Psychopharmacology. Washington, DC: American Psychiatric Press, 1995

69. Tonda ME, Guthrie SK: Treatment of acute neuroleptic-induced movement disorders. Pharmacotherapy 14:543–560, 1994

70. U.S. Department of Health and Human Services: Depression in Primary Care. Clinical Practice Guideline. Rockville, MD: Agency for Health Care Policy and Research, 1993

71. Webster P, Wijeratne C: Risperidone-induced neuroleptic malignant syndrome. Lancet 344:1228–1229, 1994

72. Wells B, Hayes P: Obsessive-compulsive disorder. In Dipiro J, et al, eds: Pharmacotherapy: A Pathophysiologic Approach, 2nd ed. Norwalk, CT: Appleton & Lange, 1993

73. Wells B, ed: Special Report: Therapeutic Options in the Treatment of Depression. Washington, DC: American Pharmaceutical Association, 1994

74. Wells B, ed: Special Report: Fluvoxamine. Washington, DC: American Pharmaceutical Association, 1995

75. Winokur MZ: Restful sleep. The pharmacotherapy of insomnia. US Pharmacist 5:1–16, 1993

76. Young LY, Koda-Kimble MA, eds: Applied Therapeutics: The Clinical Use of Drugs, 6th ed. Vancouver, WA: Applied Therapeutics, 1994
77. Zind R, Furlong C, Stebbins M: Educating patients about missed medication doses. J PsychosocNursing 30(7):10–14, 1992

Chapter 5

1. Abdullah SN: Towards an individualized client's care: Implication for education: The transcultural approach. J Adv Nurs 22(4):715–720, 1995
2. Aguilera DC, Messick JM: Crisis intervention: Theory and Methodology, 7th ed. St Louis: Mosby, 1994
3. Ahmed M, Goldman JA: Cognitive rehabilitation of adults with severe and persistent illness: A group model. Commun Ment Health J 30(4):385–394, 1994
4. Alexander DI: Aggression (mild, moderate, extreme/violence). In McFarland GK, Thomas MD: Psychiatric Mental Health Nursing. Philadelphia: JB Lippincott, 1991
5. Altholz JAS: Group psychotherapy. In Burnside I, Schmidt MG, eds: Working with Older Adults: Group Process and Techniques. Boston: Jones and Bartlett, 1994
6. American Nurses Association Council on Psychiatric and Mental Health Nursing, American Psychiatric Nurses Association, Association of Child and Adolescent Psychiatric Nurses, Society for Education and Research in Psychiatric-Mental Health Nursing: Statement on Psychiatric-Mental Health Clinical Nursing Practice and Standards of Psychiatric-Mental Health Clinical Nursing Practice. Washington, DC: American Nurses Publishing, 1994
7. Amundson MJ: Family crisis care: A home-based intervention program for child abuse. Issues Ment Health Nurs 10:285–296, 1989
8. Anonymous: Social competence. Occup Ther Ment Health 9(4):73–88, 1989
9. Antai-Ontong D: Concerns of the hospitalized and community psychiatric client. Nurs Clin North Am 24(3):665–673,1989
10. Armstrong ML: Orchestrating the process of patient education: Methods and approaches. Nurs Clin North Am 24(3):597–604, 1989
11. Arnold E: Communicating with clients in crisis. In Arnold E, Boggs KU: Interpersonal Relationships: Professional Communication Skills for Nurses, 2nd ed. Philadelphia: WB Saunders, 1995
12. Arnold E: Communicating in groups. In Arnold E, Boggs KU: Interpersonal Relationships: Professional Communication Skills for Nurses, 2nd ed. Philadelphia: WB Saunders, 1995
13. Arnold E: Health promotion and client learning needs. In Arnold E, Boggs KU: Interpersonal Relationships: Professional Communication Skills for Nurses, 2nd ed. Philadelphia: WB Saunders, 1995
14. Arnold E: Health teaching in the nurse–client relationship. In Arnold E, Boggs KU: Interpersonal Relationships: Professional Communication Skills for Nurses, 2nd ed. Philadelphia: WB Saunders, 1995
15. Aschen SR: Restraints: Does position make a difference? Issues Ment Health Nurs 16:87–92, 1995

16. Azim HF: Group psychotherapy in the day hospital. In Kaplan HI, Sadock BJ: Comprehensive Group Psychotherapy, 3rd ed. Baltimore: Williams & Wilkins, 1993

17. Baskerville BH: Milieu therapy. In McFarland GK, Thomas MD: Psychiatric Mental Health Nursing. Philadelphia: JB Lippincott, 1991

18. Baughcum DR: Abused persons. In McFarland GK, Thomas MD. Psychiatric Mental Health Nursing. Philadelphia: JB Lippincott, 1991

19. Baumann A: Decision making during a crisis state. In Baumann A, Johnston NE, Antai-Otong D: Decision Making in Psychiatric and Psychosocial Nursing. Toronto/Philadelphia: BC Decker, 1990

20. Beck AT, Steer RA, Kovacs M, Garrison B: Hopelessness and eventual suicide: A 10-year prospective study of patients hospitalized with suicidal ideation. Am J Psychiatry 142(5):559–563,1985

21. Bellack AS, Turner SM, Hersen M, Luber RF: An examination of the efficacy of social skills training for chronic schizophrenic patients. Hosp Commun Psychiatry 35(10):1023–1028,1984

22. Bennett C: Sexually abused boys: Awareness, assessment and intervention. J Adolesc Psychiatr Nurs 6(2):29–35, 1993

23. Bennett C: Expanding the mind-body connection: Working women and stress. Capsules & Comments Psychiatric Nurs 2(4)249–254, 1996

24. Birns D, Cascardi M, Meyer, SL: Sex-role socialization: Developmental influences on wife abuse. Am J Orthopsychiatry 64(1):50–59, 1994

25. Bishai M: Visualization and guided imagery. In Baumann A, Johnston NE, Antai-Otong D: Decision Making in Psychiatric and Psychosocial Nursing. Toronto/Philadelphia: BC Decker, 1990

26. Bloch D: Words That Heal: Affirmations and Meditations for Daily Living. New York: Bantam, 1990

27. Boehm S: Patient contracting. In Bulechek GM, McCloskey JC: Nursing Interventions: Essential Nursing Treatments, 2nd ed. Philadelphia: WB Saunders, 1992

28. Borelli MD, DeLuca E: Physical health promotion in psychiatric day treatment. J Psychosoc Nurs Ment Health Serv 31(3):15–18, 1993

29. Brabender V: Inpatient group psychotherapy. In Kaplan HI, Sadock BJ: Comprehensive Group Psychotherapy, 3rd ed. Baltimore: Williams & Wilkins, 1993

30. Brady JP: Social skills training for psychiatric patients, I: Concepts, methods and clinical results. Am J Psychiatry 141(3):333–340,1984

31. Brady JP: Social skills training for psychiatric patients, II: Clinical outcome studies. Am J Psychiatry 141(4):491–498,1984

32. Briefing: Treatment competence study. J Am Psychiatric Nurs Assoc 1(4):125–127, 1995

33. Brown GT, Carmichael K: Assertiveness training for clients with a psychiatric illness: A pilot study. British J Occupational Therapy 55(4):137–40, 1992

34. Buchanan, CR, Huffman C, Barbour VM: Smoking health risk: Counseling of psychiatric patients. J Psychosoc Nurs Ment Health Serv 32(1):27–32, 1994

35. Buckwalter KC, Abraham IL: Alleviating the discharge crisis: the effects of a cognitive-behavioral nursing intervention for depressed patients and their families. Arch Psychiatr Nurs 1(5):350–358, 1987

36. Burnside I: History and overview of group work. In Burnside I, Schmidt MG, eds: Working with Older Adults: Group Process and Techniques. Boston: Jones and Bartlett, 1994

37. Burnside I: Membership Selection and criteria. In Burnside I, Schmidt MG, eds: Working with Older Adults: Group Process and Techniques. Boston: Jones and Bartlett, 1994

38. Burnside I: Leadership and co-leadership issues. In Burnside I, Schmidt MG, eds: Working with Older Adults: Group Process and Techniques. Boston: Jones and Bartlett, 1994

39. Burnside I: Reminiscence group therapy. In Burnside I, Schmidt MG, eds: Working with Older Adults: Group Process and Techniques. Boston: Jones and Bartlett, 1994

40. Campbell VG: Neurologic system. In Thompson JM, McFarland GK, Hirsch JE, Tucker SM: Mosby's Clinical Nursing, 3rd ed. St. Louis: Mosby, 1993

41. Cardell R, Horton-Deutsch S: A model for assessment of inpatient suicide potential. Arch Psychiatric Nurs VIII(6): 366–372, 1994

42. Carmen E, Brady SM: AIDS risk and prevention for the chronic mentally ill. Hosp Commun Psychiatry 41(6):652–657, 1990

43. Cascardi M, O'Leary KD, Lawrence EE, Schlee KA: Characteristics of women physically abused by their spouses and who seek treatment regarding marital conflict J Consult Clin Psychol 63(4):616–623, 1995

44. Chachkes E, Christ G: Cross cultural issues in patient education. Patient Education and Counseling (27)13–21, 1996

45. Charonko CV: Cultural influences in "noncompliant" behavior and decision making. Holistic Nurs Pract 6(3):73–78, 1992

46a. Chesla C: Parents' illness models of schizophrenia. Arch Psychiatric Nurs III(4):218–225, 1989

46b. Chiles JA, Strosahl K: The Suicidal Patient: Principles of Assessment, Treatment and Case Management. Washington DC: American Psychiatric Press, 1995

47. Collins AH, Goodman B: Innovative group methods in the general hospital setting: Psychiatric liaison groups and groups for medically ill patients. In Kaplan HI, Sadock BJ: Comprehensive Group Psychotherapy, 3rd ed. Baltimore: Williams & Wilkins, 1993

48. Connelly CE, Dilonardo JD: Self-care issues with chronically ill psychotic clients. Perspect Psychiatric Care 29(4):31–35, 1993

49. Corrigan PW, Liberman RP, Engel JD: From noncompliance to collaboration in the treatment of schizophrenia. Hosp Commun Psychiatry 41(11):1203–1211, 1990

50. Cotton NS: Seclusion as therapeutic management: An invited commentary. Am J Orthopsychiat 65(2):245–244, 1995

51. Courtright P, Johnson S, Baumgartner MA, et al: Dinner music: Does it affect the behavior of psychiatric inpatients. J Psychosoc Nurs Ment Health Serv 28(3):37–40,1990

52. Cousins N: Head First: The Biology of Hope. New York: EP Dutton, 1989

53. Coverdale JH, Bayer TL, McCullough LB, Chervenak FA: Sexually transmitted disease prevention services for female chronically mentally ill patients. Commun Ment Health J 31(4):303–315, 1995

54. Craig C, Ray F, Hix C: Seclusion and restraint: Decreasing the discomfort. J Psychosoc Nurs Ment Health Serv 27(7):17–19, 1989

55. Cunningham JM: Crisis intervention. In McFarland GK, Thomas MD: Psychiatric Mental Health Nursing. Philadelphia: JB Lippincott, 1991

56. Davidhizar R, Boonstra C, Lutz K, Poston P: Teaching safer sex in a long-term psychiatric setting. Perspect Psychiatric Care 27(1):25–29, 1991

57. Dingman CW, McGlashan TH. Characteristics of patients with serious suicidal intentions who ultimately commit suicide. Hosp Commun Psychiatry 39(3):295–299,1988

58. Dixon E., Park R: Do patients understand written health information? Nurs Outlook 38(6):278–281,1990

59. Dodge VH: Relaxation training: A nursing intervention for substance abusers. Arch Psychiatric Nurs V(2):99–104, 1991

60. Donner LL, Kopytko EE, McFolling SD, et al: Increasing psychiatric inpatients' community adjustment through therapeutic passes. Arch Psychiatric Nurs IV(2):93–98, 1990

61. Doughtery C: Surveillance. In Bulechek GM, McCloskey JC: Nursing Interventions: Essential Nursing Treatments, 2nd ed. Philadelphia: WB Saunders, 1992

62. Drysdale AE, Nelson CR, Wineman NM: Families need help too: Group treatment for families of nursing home residents. Clinical Nurse Spec 7(3):130–134, 1993

63. Dunn B: Growing up with a psychotic mother: A retrospective study. Am J Orthopsychiatry 63(2):117–189, 1993

64. Earle KA, Forquer SL: Use of seclusion with children and adolescents in public psychiatric hospitals. Am J Orthopsychiatry 65(2):238–244, 1995

65. Ehrensaft D: Preschool child sex abuse: The aftermath of the Presidio case. Am J Orthopsychiatry 62(2): 234–244, 1992

66. Ekland ES: Hopelessness. In McFarland GK, Thomas MD: Psychiatric Mental Health Nursing. Philadelphia: JB Lippincott, 1991

67. Eraker SA, Politser P: How decisions are reached: Physician and patient. In Dowie J, Elstein A, eds: Professional Judgment: A Reader in Clinical Decision Making. New York: Cambridge University Press, 1988

68. Falloon IRH, Boyd JL, McGill CW: Family Care of Schizophrenia: A Problem-Solving Approach to the Treatment of Mental Illness. New York: Guilford Press, 1984

69. Falloon IRH, Laporta M, Fadden G, Graham-Hole V: Managing Stress in Families. New York: Routledge, 1993

70. Falvo DR: Effective Patient Education: A Guide to Increased Compliance, 2nd ed. Gaithersburg, MD: Aspen Pub Inc, 1994

71. Farran CJ, Popovich JM: Hope: A relevant concept of geriatric psychiatry. Arch Psychiatr Nurs IV(2):124–130, 1990

72. Farran CJ, Salloway JC, Clark DC: Measurement of hope in a community-based population. Western J Nurs Res 12(1):42–59, 1990

73. Feshbach ND: The construct of empathy and the phenomenon of physical maltreatment of children. In Cicchetti D, Carlson V, eds: Child Maltreatment: Theory and Research on the Causes and Consequences of Child Abuse and Neglect. New York: Cambridge University Press, 1990

74. Fishel AH: A community-based program for emotionally disturbed children and youth. J Child Adolesc Psychiatr Ment Health Nurs 3(4):128–133, 1990

75. Fisher WA: Restraint and seclusion: A review of the literature. Am J Psychiatry 151(11):1584–1591, 1994

76. Fishwick N: Getting to the heart of the matter: Nursing assessment and intervention with battered women in psychiatric mental health settings. J Am Psychiatric Nurses Assoc 1(2):48–54, 1995

77. Foster SW: The pragmatics of culture: The rhetoric of difference in psychiatric nursing. Arch Psychiatric Nurs 4(5):292–297,1990

78. Fowler SB: Hope: Implication for neuroscience nursing. J Neuroscience Nursing 27(5):298–304, 1995

79. Fulmer TT: Mistreatment of elders: Assessment, diagnosis, and intervention. Nurs Clin North Am 24(3):707–716, 1989

80. Gallop R, McCay E, Esplen MJ: The conceptualization of impulsivity for psychiatric nursing practice. Arch Psychiatric Nurs VI(6):366–373, 1992

81. Gantt AB, Goldstein G, Pinsky S: Family understanding of psychiatric illness. Community Ment Health J 25(2):101–108, 1989

82. Gaudin JM, et al: Loneliness, depression stress, and social supports in neglectful families. Am J Orthopsychiatry 63(4):597–605, 1993

83. Gentilin J: Room restriction: A therapeutic prescription. J Psychosoc Nurs Ment Health Serv 25(7):12–16, 1987

84. Gessner BA: Adult education: The cornerstone of patient teaching. Nurs Clin North Am 24(3):589–595, 1989

85. Ghosh TB, Victor BS: Suicide. In Hales RE, Yudofsky SC, Talbott JA: The American Psychiatric Press Textbook of Psychiatry, 2nd ed. Washington, DC: American Psychiatric Press, 1994

86. Godbey KL, Courage MM: Stress-management program: Intervention in nursing student performance anxiety. Arch Psychiatric Nurs VIII(3):190–199, 1994

87. Goddaer J, Abraham IL: Effects of relaxing music on agitation during meals among nursing home residents with severe cognitive impairment. Arch Psychiatric Nursing VIII(3):150–158, 1994

88. Goldwyn RM: Educating the patient and family about depression. Med Clin North Am 72(4):887–896, 1988

89. Graham O, Naveau I, Cummings C: A model for ambulatory care of patients with epilepsy and other neurological disorders. J Neurosci Nurs 21(2):108–112, 1989

90. Gummit RJ: The Epilepsy Handbook: The Practical Management of Seizures, 2nd Ed. New York: Raven Press, 1994

91. Haddock KS: Collaborative discharge planning: Nursing and social services. Clin Nurse Spec 8(5):248–252, 1994

92. Hansen PA, Rhode JM, Wolf-Wilets V: Stress management. In McFarland GK, Thomas MD: Psychiatric Mental Health Nursing. Philadelphia: JB Lippincott, 1991

93. Hayes RL, Halford WK, Varghese FN: Generalization of the effects of activity therapy and social skills training on the social behavior of low functioning schizophrenic patients. Occup Ther Ment Health 11(4):3–20, 1991

94. Herman R, Kaplan M, Satriano J, et al: HIV prevention with people with serious mental illness: Staff training and institutional attitudes. Psychosoc Rehabil J 17(4):97–103, 1994

95. Herth K: Relationship of hope, coping styles, concurrent losses and setting to grief resolution in the elderly widow(er). Res Nurs Health 13(2):10—9-117,1990

96. Herth K: Engendering hope in the chronically and terminally ill: Nursing interventions. Am J Hosp Palliat Care 12(5):31–39, 1995

97. Hindmarsh DJ: Control in the psychiatric setting—children and adolescents. In Hersen M, Ammerman RT, Sisson LA, eds: Handbook of Aggressive and Destructive Behavior in Psychiatric Patients. New York: Plenum Press, 1994

98. Hogarth CR: Intervention strategies for adolescent psychiatric nurses: An overview. In Hogarth CR: Adolescent Psychiatric Nursing. St. Louis: Mosby Year Book, 1991

99. Hogarth CR: Strategies for Crisis Intervention. In Hogarth CR: Adolescent Psychiatric Nursing. St. Louis:, Mosby Year Book, 1991

100. Holmes H, Ziemba J, Evans T, Williams CA: Nursing model of psychoeducation for the seriously mentally ill patient. Issues Ment Health Nurs 15(1):85–104, 1994

101. Holnsteiner MG: Elopement, potential for. In McFarland GK, Thomas MD. Psychiatric Mental Health Nursing. Philadelphia: JB Lippincott, 1991

102. Hughes HM, Fantuzzo JW: Family violence—child. In Hersen M, Ammerman RT, Sisson LA: Handbook of Aggressive and Destructive Behavior in Psychiatric Patients. New York: Plenum Press, 1994

103. Huxley P, Warner R: Primary prevention of parenting dysfunction in high-risk cases. Am J Orthopsychiatry 63(4):582–588, 1993

104. Hyman RB, Feldman HR, Harris RB, et al: The effects of relaxation training on clinical symptoms: A meta-analysis. Nurs Res 38(4):216–220, 1989

105. Jiwani GN: Problem solving. In Baumann A, Johnston NE, Antai-Otong D: Decision Making in Psychiatric and Psychosocial Nursing. Toronto/Philadelphia: BC Decker, 1990

106. Johnson SW, McSweeney M, Webster RE: Leisure: How to promote inpatient motivation after discharge. J Psychosoc Nurs Ment Health Serv 27(9):29–33,1989

107. Jones R, O'Brien P: Unique interventions for child inpatient psychiatry. J Psychosoc Nurs Ment Health Serv 28(7):29–31, 1990

108. Kane CF, DiMartino E, Jimenez M: A comparison of short-term psychoeducational and support groups for relatives coping with chronic schizophrenia. Arch Psychiatr Nurs 4(6):343–353, 1990

109. Kashka MS, Keyser PK: Ethical issues in informed consent and ECT. Perspect Psychiatr Care 31(2):15–21, 1995

110. Kaufman J, Zigler E: The intergenerational transmission of child abuse. In Cicchetti D, Carlson, V, eds: Child Maltreatment: Theory and Research on the Causes and Consequences of Child Abuse and Neglect. New York: Cambridge University Press, 1990

111. Kelly KC, McClelland E, Daly JM: Discharge planning. In Bulechek GM, McCloskey JM. Nursing Interventions: Essential Nursing Treatments. Philadelphia: WB Saunders, 1992

112. Kennedy BR, Williams CA, Pesut DJ: Hallucinatory experiences of psychiatric patients in seclusion. Arch Psychiatr Nurs VIII(3):169–176, 1994

113. Kinney CK, Mannetter R, Carpenter MA: Support Groups. In Bulechek GM, McCloskey JC: Nursing Interventions: Essential Nursing Treatments, 2nd ed. Philadelphia: WB Saunders, 1992

114. Kirkpatrick H. A descriptive study of seclusion: The unit environment, patient behavior, and nursing interventions. Arch Psychiatr Nurs III(1):3–9,1989

115. Kirkpatrick H, Landeen J, Byrne C, et al: Hope and schizophrenia: Clinicians identify hope-instilling strategies. J Psychosoc Nurs Ment Health Serv 33(6):15–19, 40–41, 1995

116. Konker C: Rethinking child sexual abuse: An anthropological perspective. Am J Orthopsychiatry 62(1):147–153, 1992

117. Kus RJ: Crisis intervention. In Bulechek GM, McCloskey JC: Nursing Interventions: Essential Nursing Treatments, 2nd ed. Philadelphia: WB Saunders, 1992

118. Landenburger K: A process of entrapment in and recovery from an abusive relationship. Issues Ment Health Nurs 10:209–227, 1989

119. Liberman RP, DeRisi WJ, Mueser KT: Social Skills Training for Psychiatric Patients. New York: Pergamon Press, 1989

120. Lieberman MA: Self-help groups. In Kaplan HI, Sadock BJ: Comprehensive Group Psychotherapy, 3rd ed. Baltimore: Williams & Wilkins, 1993

121. Limandri BJ: The therapeutic relationship with abused women. J Psychosoc Nurs Ment Health Serv 25(2):8–16, 34, 35, 1987

122. Littrell KH, Freeman LY: Maximizing psychosocial interventions. J Am Psychiatric Nurses Assoc 1(6):214–218, 1995

123. Loring MT, Smith RW: Health care barriers and interventions for battered women. Public Health Reports 109(3):328–338, 1994

124. Lowenstein AJ, Hoff PS: Discharge planning: A study of nursing staff involvement. J Nurs Adm 24(4):45–50, 1994

125. Madden JF. Calming the storms of alcohol withdrawal. Emergency Medicine 22(7):22–24, 27, 28, 1990

126. Maier G, Van Rybroek GJ: A report on staff injuries and ambulatory restraints: Dealing with patient aggression. J Psychosoc Ment Health Nurs 32(11):23–29, 1994

127. Manderino MA, Bzdek VM: Social skill building with chronic patients. J Psychosoc Nurs Ment Health Serv 25(9):18–23, 1987

128. Mannion E, Mueser K, Solomon, P: Designing psychoeducation services for spouses of persons with serious mental illness. Comm Ment Health J 30(2):177–199, 1994

129. Maynard C: Psychoeducational approach to depression in women. J Psychosoc Nurs Ment Health Serv 31(12):9–14, 34–35, 1993

130. Mazza D, Dannerstein L, Ryan V: Physical, sexual and emotional violence against women: A general practice-based prevention study. Melbourne J Australia 164:14–17, 1996

131. McCloskey JC, Bulechek GM, eds: Nursing Interventions Classification (NIC), 2nd ed. St. Louis: Mosby, 1996

132. McFarlane WR, Lukens E, Link B, et al: Multiple-family groups and psychoeducation in the treatment of schizophrenia. Arch Gen Psychiatry 52(8):679–687, 1995

133. McGihon NN: Health care reform: Clinical implications for inpatient psychiatric nursing. J Psychosoc Nurs Ment Health Serv 32(11):31-33,42–43, 1994

134. McGrew, JH, Bond GR, Dietzen L, McKasson M, Miller LD: A multisite study of client outcomes in assertive community treatment. Psychiatric Services 46(7):696–701, 1995

135. McIntosh J, Worley N: Beyond discharge: Telephone follow-up and aftercare. J Psychosoc Nurs Ment Health Serv 32(10):21–27, 1994

136. Meadow R: The history of Munchausen Syndrome by Proxy. In Levin AV, Sheridan MS, eds: Munchausen Syndrome by Proxy: Issues in Diagnosis and Treatment. New York: Lexington Books, 1995

137. Miller JF: Analysis of coping with illness. In Miller JF: Coping with Chronic Illness: Overcoming Powerlessness, 2nd ed. Philadelphia: FA Davis, 1992

138. Miller JF: Inspiring hope. In Miller JF: Coping with Chronic Illness: Overcoming Powerlessness, 2nd ed. Philadelphia: FA Davis, 1992

139. Miller JF: Middlescent obese women: Overcoming powerlessness. In Miller JF: Coping with Chronic Illness: Overcoming Powerlessness, 2nd ed. Philadelphia: FA Davis, 1992

140. Mohr WK: A nurse-led educational program in psychiatric setting: developing a curriculum. J Psychosoc Nurs Ment Health Serv 31(3):34–38, 46, 1993

141. Montgomery CL, Webster D: Caring, curing and brief therapy: A model for nurse-psychotherapy. Arch Psychiatr Nurs VIII(5):291–297, 1994

142a. Monti PM, Abrams DB, Kadden RM, Cooney NL: Treating Alcohol Dependence: A Coping Skills Training Guide. New York: Guilford Press, 1989

142b. Monti PM, Rohsenow DJ, Colby SM, Abrams DB: Coping and social skills training. In Hester R, Miller W, eds: Handbook of Alcoholism Treatment Approaches: Effective Alternatives. Needham Heights, MA: Allyn & Bacon, 1995

143. Morrison EF: Toward a better understanding of violence in psychiatric settings: Debunking the myths. Arch Psychiatr Nurs 7(6):328–335, 1993

144. Morse JM, Doberneck B: Delineating the concept of hope. Image: J Nurs Scholarship 27(4):277–285, 1995

145. Mueser KT, Levine S, Bellack AS, et al: Social skills training for acute psychiatric inpatients. Hosp Commun Psychiatry 41(11):1249–1251, 1990

146. Newberger CM, Gremy IM, Watermaux CM, Newberger EH: Mothers of sexually abused children: Trauma and repair in longitudinal perspective. Am J Orthopsychiat 63(1):92–102, 1993

147. Nigro A, Maggio J: A neglected need: Health education for the mentally ill. J Psychosoc Nurs Ment Health Serv 28(7):15–19, 1990

148. Nikkel RE: Areas of skill training for persons with mental illness and substance use disorders: Building skills for successful community living. Commun Ment Health J 30(1):61–72, 1994

149. Norris J: Chronically mentally ill patients. In McFarland GK, Thomas MD: Psychiatric Mental Health Nursing. Philadelphia: JB Lippincott, 1991

150. O'Connor AM, D'Amico MJ: Decisional conflict. In McFarland GK, Thomas MD: Psychiatric Mental Health Nursing. Philadelphia: JB Lippincott, 1991

151. Olds DL, Henderson CR: The prevention of maltreatment. In: Cicchetti D, Carlson V, eds: Child Maltreatment: Theory and Research on the Causes and Consequences of Child Abuse and Neglect. New York: Cambridge University Press, 1990

152. Outlaw FH, Lowery BJ: An attributional study of seclusion and restraint of psychiatric patients. Arch Psychiatr Nurs VIII(2):69–77, 1994

153. Pape JM: The role of child abuse: Agencies and foster care. In Levin AV, Sheridan MS, eds: Munchausen Syndrome by Proxy: Issues in Diagnosis and Treatment. New York: Lexington Books, 1995

154. Peternelj-Taylor CA, Hartley VL: Living with mental illness: Professional/family collaboration. J Psychosoc Nurs Ment Health Serv 31(3):23–28, 40–41, 1993

155. Piranger P: A model for the development and implementation of a patient support group in a medical-surgical setting. Holistic Nurs Practice 8(1):16–26, 1993

156. Plante TG: Social skills training: A program to help schizophrenic clients cope. J Psychosoc Nurs Ment Health Serv 27(3):6–10, 1989

157. Posner CM, Wilson KG, Fral MJ, et al: Family psychoeducational support groups in schizophrenia. Am J Orthopsychiatry 62(2):206–218, 1992

158. Raybuck JA: Support groups for caregivers of persons with Alzheimer's disease: Implication for practice and research. American J Alzheimer's Care and Related Disorders & Research 10(1):26–31,1995

159. Redman BK, Thomas SA: Patient teaching. In Bulechek GM, McCloskey JC: Nursing Interventions: Essential Nursing Treatments, 2nd ed. Philadelphia: WB Saunders, 1992

160. Redman BK: The Process of Patient Education, 7th ed. St. Louis: Mosby Year Book, 1993

161. Rickelman BL, Houfek JF: Toward an interactional model of suicidal behaviors: Cognitive rigidity, attributional style, stress, hopelessness, and depression. Arch Psychiatr Nurs IX(3):158–168, 1995

162. Rose SR: Cognitive behavioral group psychotherapy. In Kaplan HI, Sadock BJ: Comprehensive Group Psychotherapy, 3rd ed. Baltimore: Williams & Wilkins, 1993

163. Rosenberg D: From lying to homicide: The spectrum of munchausen syndrome by proxy. In Levin AV, Sheridan MS, eds: Munchausen Syndrome by Proxy: Issues in Diagnosis and Treatment. New York: Lexington Books, 1995

164. Rothner AD: Epilepsy. In Kaufman DM, Solomon GE, Pfeffer CR: Child and Adolescent Neurology for Psychiatrists. Baltimore: Williams & Wilkins, 1992

165. Rudd MD, Rajab MH, Dahm PF: Problem-solving appraisal in suicide ideators and attempters. Am J Orthopsychiatry 64(1):136–149, 1994

166. Ruttan JS, Stone WN: Psychodynamic Group Psychotherapy, 2nd ed. New York: Guilford Press, 1993

167. Sadler AG: Assertiveness training. In Bulechek GM, McCloskey JC: Nursing Interventions: Treatments for Nursing Diagnoses. Philadelphia: WB Saunders, 1985

168. Samuels M, Samuels N: Healing with the Mind's Eye: A Guide for Using Imagery and Visions for Personal Growth and Healing. New York: Summit Books, 1990

169. Sambandham M, Schirm V: Music as a nursing intervention for residents with Alzheimer's disease in long-term care. Geriatr Nurs 16(2): 79–83, 1995

170. Sapp M: The effects of guided imagery on reducing the worry and emotionality components of test anxiety. J Mental Imagery 18(3-4): 165–179, 1994

171. Sanchez-Gallegos, Viens DC: When the client is armed or dangerous: Management of violent and difficult patients in primary care. Nurs Pract 20(6):26–32, 1995

172. Saveman B, Norberg A: Cases of elder abuse, intervention and hopes for the future, as reported by home service personnel. Scandinavian J Caring Sciences 7(1):21–28, 1993

173. Scandrett-Hibdon S: Cognitive reappraisal. In Bulechek GM, McCloskey JC: Nursing Interventions: Essential Nursing Treatments, 2nd ed. Philadelphia: WB Saunders, 1992

174. Scandrett-Hibdon S, Uecker S: Relaxation training. In Bulechek GM, McCloskey JC: Nursing Interventions; Essential Nursing Treatments, 2nd ed. Philadelphia: WB Saunders, 1992

175. Schmidt MG: Ethical issues in group work. In Burnside I, Schmidt MG, eds: Working with Older Adults: Group Process and Techniques. Boston: Jones and Bartlett, 1994

176. Schneider JK: Clinical nurse specialist: Role definition as discharge planning coordinator. Clin Nurse Spec 6(1):36–39,1992

177. Schweitzer PB, Nesse RM, Fantone RF, Curtis GC: Outcomes of group cognitive behavioral training in the treatment of panic disorder and agoraphobia. J Am Psychiatr Nurses Assoc 1(3):83–91, 1995

178. Segal UA: Child abuse by the middle class? A study of professionals in India. Child Abuse Negl 19(2):217–231, 1995

179. Shagle SC, Barber BK: A socio-ecological analysis of adolescent suicidal ideation. Am J Orthopsychiatry 65(1):114–124, 1995

180. Shugar G, Smith IJ, Katz G: Transfer of psychiatric inpatient: The family perspective. Am J Orthopsychiatry 62(2):303–308, 1992

181. Sigal M, Altmark: Adult victims. In Levin AV, Sheridan MS eds: Munchausen Syndrome by Proxy: Issues in Diagnosis and Treatment. New York: Lexington Books, 1995

182. Slusher MP, Anderson CA: Belief perseverance and self-defeating behavior. In Curtiss R, ed: Self-Defeating Behaviors: Experimental Research, Clinical Impressions and Practical Implications. New York: Plenum Press, 1989

183. Smith-Bell M, Winslade WJ: Privacy, confidentiality and privilege in psychotherapeutic relationships. Am J Orthopsychiatry 64(2):180–193, 1994

184. Smith SB: Restraints: Retraumatization for rape victims? J Psychosoc Nurs Ment Health Serv 33(7)23–28, 1995

185. Snyder M: Independent Nursing Interventions, 2nd ed. Albany: Delmar Publishers, 1992

186. Sodergren KM: Guided imagery. In Snyder M: Independent Nursing Interventions, 2nd ed. Albany: Delmar Publishers, 1992

187. Spillers GM. Suicide potential. In McFarland GK, Thomas MD: Psychiatric Nursing. Philadelphia: JB Lippincott, 1991

188. Stading PJ, Boros SJ: Nursing care and responsibilities. In Levin AV, Sheridan MS, eds: Munchausen Syndrome by Proxy: Issues in Diagnosis and Treatment. New York: Lexington Books, 1995

189. Starkey D, Deleone H, Flannery RB: Stress management for psychiatric patients in a state hospital setting. Amer J Orthopsychiatry 65(3):446–450, 1995

190. Steele NF, Sterling YM: Application of the case study design: Nursing interventions for discharge readiness. Clin Nurs Spec 6(2):79–84, 1992

191. Steele RL: Staff attitudes toward seclusion and restraint: Anything new? Perspect Psychiatric Care 29(3): 23–28, 1993

192. Stein CH, Cislo DA, Ward M: Collaboration in the college classroom: Evaluation of a social network and social skills program for undergraduates and people with serious mental illness. Psychosoc Rehab J 18(1):130–133, 1994

193. Stelzer J, Elliott CA: A continuous-care model of crisis intervention for children and adolescents. Hosp Commun Psychiatry 41(5):562–564, 1990

194. Stephens R: Imagery: A strategic intervention to empower clients: Part I—review of research literature. Clin Nurse Spec 7(4):170–174, 1993

195. Stephens R: Imagery: A strategic intervention to empower clients: Part II—a practical guide. Clin Nurse Spec 7(5):235–240, 1993

196. Sussman N: Integrating psychopharmacology and group psychotherapy. In Kaplan HI, Sadock BJ: Comprehensive Group Psychotherapy, 3rd ed. Baltimore: Williams & Wilkins, 1993

197. Sutorius D: The transforming force of laughter, with the focus on the laughing meditation. Patient Ed Counseling 26:367–371, 1995

198. Swearingen L: Transitional day treatment: An individualized goal-oriented approach: Short-term psychiatric care. Arch Psychiatric Nurs. I(2):104–110, 1987

199. Tabloski PA, McKinnon-Howe L, Remington R: Effects of calming music on the level of agitation in cognitively impaired nursing home residents. Am J Alzheimer's Care Related Disorders & Research 10(1):10–15, 1995

200. Tardiff K: Management of the violent patient an emergency situation. Psychiatr Clin North Am 11(4):539–549,1988

201. Tardiff K: Concise Guide to Assessment and Management of Violent Patients. Washington, DC: American Psychiatric Press, 1989

202. Tardiff, K: Violence In: Hales RE, Yudofsky SC, Talbott JA, eds: The American Psychiatric Press Textbook of Psychiatry, 2nd ed. Washington, DC: American Psychiatric Press, 1994

203. Teare JF, Peterson RW, Furst D, et al: Treatment implementation in a short-term emergency shelter program. Child Welfare 73(3):271–281, 1994

204. Temple S, Robson P: The effect of assertiveness training on self-esteem. British J Occupational Ther 54(9):329–332, 1991

205. Ulrich YC: What helped most in leaving spouse abuse: Implications for interventions. AWHONNS Cinical Issues in Perinat Womens Health Nurs 4(3):385–390, 1993

206. van Servellen G, Nyamathi AM, Mannion W: Coping with a crisis: Evaluating psychological risks of patients with AIDS. J Psychosoc Nurs Ment Health Serv 27(12):16–21, 30, 31, 1989

207. van Servellen G, Poster EC, Ryan J, Allen J Randell B: Methodological concerns in evaluating psychiatric nursing care modalities and a proposed standard group protocol format for nurse-led groups. Arch Psychiatr Nurs VI(2):117–124, 1992

208. Ventura MR, Lenz S, Rizzo J: Developing an appropriateness-of-care monitor to manage patients in seclusion or seclusion/ restraints. J Nurs Care Qual; (Spec Rep):44–48, 1992

209. Vinogradov S, Yalom ID: Group therapy. In Hales RE, Yudofsky SC, Talbott JA, eds: The American Psychiatric Press Textbook of Psychiatry, 2nd ed. Washington, DC: American Psychiatric Press, 1994

210. Warnken WJ, Rosenbaum A: Family violence—adult. In Hersen M, Ammerman RT, Sisson LA: Handbook of Aggressive and Destructive Behavior in Psychiatric Patients. New York: Plenum Press, 1994

211. Wieland V, Cummings S: Group Psychotherapy. In Bulechek GM, McCloskey JC: Nursing Interventions: Essential Nursing Treatments, 2nd ed. Philadelphia: WB Saunders,1992

212. Weiler K, Buckwalter KC: Geriatric mental health: Abuse among rural mentally ill. J Psychosoc Nurs Ment Health Serv 30(9):32–36, 38, 39, 1992

213. Wilberding JZ: Values clarification. In Bulechek GM, McCloskey JC: Nursing Interventions: Essential Nursing Treatments, 2nd ed. Philadelphia: WB Saunders, 1992

214. Williams-Burgess C, Kimball MJ: The Neglected elder: A family systems approach. J Psychosoc Ment Health Nurs 30(10):21–25, 38, 39, 1992

215. Wilson JH, Hobbs H: Therapeutic partnership: A model for clinical practice. J Psychosoc Nurs Ment Health Serv 33(2):27–30, 1995

216. Winkler GE: Assessing and responding to suicidal jail inmates. Community Ment Health J 28(4):317–326, 1992

217. Wood A, Seymour LM: Psychodynamic group therapy for older adults: The life experiences group. J Psychosoc Ment Health Nurs 32(7):19–24, 1994

218. Worley NK, Albanese N. Independent living for the chronically mentally ill. J Psychosoc Nurs Ment Health Serv 27(9):18–23, 1989

219. Yalom ID: The Theory and Practice of Group Psychotherapy, 4th ed. New York: Basic Books, 1995

220. Zambelli GC, DeRosa AP: Bereavement support groups for school-age children: Theory, intervention and case example. Am J Orthopsychiatry 62(4): 484–493, 1992

221. Zappe C, Epstein D: Assertive training. J Psychosoc Nurs Ment Health Serv 25(8):23–26, 1987

222. Ziel SE, Pesut DJ: Schizophrenia, neuroleptics and tardive dyskinesia: Issues to consider in client decision making. Capsules and Comments in Psychiatric Nursing 1(3):4–9, 1994

223. Zuravin SJ, Benedict M, Somerfield M: Child maltreatment in family foster care. Am J Orthopsychiatry 63(4):589–596, 1993

Chapter 6

1. American Psychiatric Association: Diagnostic and Statistical Manual of Mental Disorders, DSM-IV, 4th ed. Washington, DC: American Psychiatric Association, 1994

2. Andreasen NC, Black DW: Introductory Textbook of Psychiatry, 2nd ed. Washington, DC: American Psychiatric Press, 1995

3. Beck C, Heacock P, Mercer S, Walton CG, Shook J: Dressing for success. Promoting independence among cognitively impaired elderly. Journal of Psychosocial Nursing and Mental Health Services 29(7):30–35, 1991

4. Blazer D: Geriatric psychiatry. In Hales RE, Yudofsky SC, Talbott JA, eds: The American Psychiatric Press Textbook of Psychiatry, 2nd ed. Washington, DC: American Psychiatric Press, 1994

5. Bolger JP, Carpenter BD, Strauss ME: Behavior and affect in Alzheimer's disease. Clinics in Geriatric Medicine 10(2):315–337, 1994

6. Breitner JCS, Welsh KA: Diagnosis and management of memory loss and cognitive disorders among elderly persons. Psychiatric Services 46(1):29–34, 1995

7. Burnside I: Reminiscence: An independent nursing intervention for the elderly. Issues in Mental Health Nursing 11:33–48, 1990

8. Byrne EJ: Confusional States in Older People. Boston: Little, Brown, 1994

9. Clark LW, Witte K: Nature and efficacy of communication management in Alzheimer's disease. In Lubinski R: Dementia and Communication. San Diego: Singular Publishing Group, 1995

10. Cohen-Mansfield J, Werner P: Environmental influences on agitation: An integrative summary of an observational study. American Journal of Alzheimer's Care and Related Disorders and Research 10(12):32–39, 1995

11. Davis C, Drew L, Nida A, Showalter P, Wilken C: A Caregiver's Guide for Alzheimer's and Related Disorders. Topeka, KA: Kansas Department on Aging, 1991

12. Edwards AJ: Dementia. New York: Plenum Press, 1992

13. Edwards AJ: When Memory Fails: Helping the Alzheimer's and Dementia Patient. New York: Plenum Press, 1994

14. Evans CA, Kenny PJ, Rizzuto C: Caring for the confused geriatric surgical patient. Geriatric Nursing 14(5):237–241, 1993

15. Farrell KR, Ganzini L: Misdiagnosing delirium as depression in medically ill elderly patients. Arch Intern Med 155:2459–2464, 1995

16. Foreman MD: Complexities of acute confusion. Geriatric Nurs 11(3):136–139, 1990

17. Frances A, First MB, Pincus HA: DSM-IV Guidebook. Washington, DC: American Psychiatric Press, 1995

18. French M, McWhorter K: Impaired memory. In Kim MJ, McFarland GK, McLane AL: Pocket Guide to Nursing Diagnoses, 6th ed. St. Louis: Mosby Year Book, 1995

19. Gerety EK: Acute confusion. In Kim MJ, McFarland GK, McLane AL: Pocket Guide to Nursing Diagnoses, 6th ed. St. Louis: Mosby, 1995

20. Giacometti AR, Davis PC, Alazraki NP, Malko JA: Anatomic and physiologic imaging of Alzheimer's disease. Clinics in Geriatric Medicine 10(2):277–293, 1994

21. Goldsmith SM, Hoeffer B, Rader J: Problematic wandering behavior in the cognitively impaired elderly. Journal of Psychosocial Nursing 33(2):6–12, 1995

22. Goldstein M, Haltzman SD: Intensive care. In Stoudemire A, Fogel BS, eds: Psychiatric Care of the Medical Patient. New York: Oxford University Press, 1993

23. Hall GR, Gerdner L, Zwygart-Stauffacher M, Buckwalter KC: Principles of nonpharmacological management: Caring for people with Alzheimer's Disease using a conceptual model. Psychiatric Annals 25(7):432–440, 1995

24. Hamdy RC, Turnbull JM, Clark W, Lancaster MM: Alzheimer's Disease: A Handbook for Caregivers. St. Louis: Mosby, 1994

25. Hogan S: Care for the caregiver: Social policies to ease their burden. Journal of Gerontological Nursing 16(5):12–17, 1990

26. Hopkins RW, Rindlisbacher P: Some clinical consequences of the rest and activity disturbance in Alzheimer's disease. American Journal of Alzheimer's Care and Related Disorders and Research 10(1):16–25, 1995

27. Hornbostel R: Legal and financial decision making in dementia care. In Whitehouse PJ (Ed.): Dementia. Philadelphia: FA Davis, 1993

28. Hunter S: Adult Day Care: Promoting quality of life for the elderly. Journal of Gerontological Nursing 18(2):17–20, 1992

29. Inaba-Roland KE, Maricle RA: Assessing delirium in the acute care setting. Heart and Lung 21(1):48–55, 1992

30. Inouye SK, et al: A predictive model for delirium in hospitalized elderly medical patients based on admission characteristics. Ann Intern Med 119:474–481, 1993

31. Joyce EM: Dementia associated with alcohol. In Burns A, Levy R, eds: Dementia. London: Chapman & Hall Medical, 1994

32. Kim E, Rovner BW: Depression in dementia. Psychiatric Annals 24(4):173–177, 1994

33. Kim MJ, McFarland GK, McLane AM: Pocket Guide to Nursing Diagnoses, 6th ed. St. Louis: Mosby Year Book, 1995
34. Kishi Y et al: Delirium in critical care unit patients admitted through an emergency room. Gen Hosp Psychiatry 17:371–379, 1995
35. Koss E: Neuropsychology and Alzheimer's disease. Clinics in Geriatric Medicine 10(2):299–313, 1994
36. Lipowski ZJ: Delirium: Acute Confusional States. New York: Oxford University Press, 1990
37. Maas ML, Swanson E, Buckwalter KC: Alzheimer's Special Care Units. Nursing Clinics of North America 29(1):173–194, 1994
38. Mace NL, Rabins PV: The 36 Hour Day. Baltimore: Johns Hopkins University Press, 1981
39. Mann DMA, Neary D, Testa H: Color Atlas and Text of Adult Dementias. London: Mosby-Wolfe, 1994
40. McDougall GJ: A critical review of research on cognitive function/impairment in older adults. Archives of Psychiatric Nursing IX(1):22–33, 1995
41. McFarland GK, Wasli E, Gerety E: Nursing Diagnoses and Process in Psychiatric Mental Health Nursing, 2nd ed. Philadelphia: Lippincott, 1992
42. McLane AM: Caregiver role strain. In Kim MJ, McFarland GK, McLane AL: Pocket Guide to Nursing Diagnoses, 6th ed. St. Louis: Mosby Year Book, 1995
43. McWhorter K, French M: Chronic confusion. In Kim MJ, McFarland GK, McLane AL: Pocket Guide to Nursing Diagnoses, 6th Ed. St. Louis: Mosby Year Book, 1995
44. Mobily PR, Maas ML, Buckwalter KC: Staff stress on an Alzheimer's unit. Journal of Psychosocial Nursing and Mental Health Services 30(9):25–31, 1992
45. Morency CR: Mental status change in the elderly: Recognizing and treating delirium. J Professional Nurs 6(6):356–365, 1990
46. Morris JC: Differential diagnosis of Alzheimer's disease. Clinics in Geriatric Medicine 10(2):257–276, 1994
47. Nicholas LM, Lindsey BA: Delirium presenting with symptoms of depression. Psychosomatics 36(5):471–479, 1995
48. North American Nursing Diagnoses Association: NANDA Nursing Diagnoses: Definitions and Classification 1995–1996. Philadelphia: NANDA, 1994
49. Patterson C, Clarfield AM: Diagnostic procedures for dementia. In Emery VOB: Dementia Presentations, Differential Diagnosis, and Nosology. Baltimore: Johns Hopkins University Press, 1994
50. Post SG: Alzheimer's disease. Ethics and the progression of dementia. Clinics in Geriatric Medicine 10(2):379–394, 1994
51. Ripich DN: Differential diagnosis and assessment. In Lubinski R: Dementia and Communication. San Diego: Singular Publishing Group, 1995
52. Rummans TA, et al: Delirium in elderly patients: Evaluation and management. Mayo Clin Proc 70:989–998, 1995
53. Saul RW, Keltner NL: Cognitive disorders. In Keltner NL, Schwecke LH, Bostrom CE: Psychiatric Nursing. St. Louis: Mosby, 1995
54. Scanland SG, Emershaw LE: Reality orientation and validation therapy: Dementia, depression, and functional status. Journal of Gerontological Nursing 19(6):7–11, 1993
55. Shua-Haim JR, Burnstein L, Gross JS: C-ADAT: Caregiver-Alzheimer's disease assessment tool. American Journal of Alzheimer's Care and Related Disorders and Research 10(1):2–5, 1995

56. Stolley JM, Garand L, Pries CM, Buckwalter KC, Hall GR: Clients with delirium, dementia, amnestic disorders, and other cognitive disorders. In Antai-Otong D, Kongable G: Psychiatric Nursing, Biological and Behavioral Concepts. Philadelphia: WB Saunders, 1995
57. Sundeen SJ: Cognitive responses and organic mental disorders. In Stuart GW, Sundeen SJ: Principles and Practice of Psychiatric Nursing, 5th ed. St. Louis: Mosby, 1995
58. Temple A, Fawdry K: King's theory of goal attainment resolving filial caregiver role strain. Journal of Gerontological Nursing 8(3):11–15, 1992
59. Trzepacz PT: The neuropathegenisis of delirium: A need to focus our research. Psychosomatis 35:374–391, 1994
60. Trzepacz PT, Brown TM, Stoudemire A: Substance-induced delirium. In Gabbard GO, editor-in chief: Treatments of Psychiatric Disorders, 2nd ed. Washington, DC: American Psychiatric Press, 1995
61. Tune L, Ross CR: Delirium: In Coffey CE, Cummings JL, Lovell MR, Pearlson GD: The American Psychiatric Press Textbook of Neuropsychiatry. Washington, DC: American Psychiatric Press, 1994
62. Whitehouse PJ, Geldmacher DS: Pharmacotherapy for Alzheimer's disease. Clinics in Geriatric Medicine 19(2):339–350, 1994
63. Wise MG, Gray KF: Delirium, dementia, and amnestic disorders. In Hales RE, Yudofsky SC, Talbott JA, eds: The American Textbook of Psychiatry, 2nd ed. Washington, DC: American Psychiatric Press, 1994
64. Wise MG: Delirium due to a general medical condition, delirium due to multiple etiologies, and delirium not otherwise specified. In Gabbard GO, editor-in chief: Treatments of Psychiatric Disorders, 2nd ed. Washington, DC: American Psychiatric Press, 1995
65. Wykle ML, Morris DL: Nursing care in Alzheimer's disease. Clinics in Geriatric Medicine 10(2):351–365, 1994

Chapter 7

1. American Psychiatric Association: DSM-IV, Diagnostic and Statistical Manual of Mental Disorders Criteria, 4th ed. Washington, DC: American Psychiatric Association, 1994
2. Anastasi JK, Sun Lee V: HIV wasting: How to stop the cycle. AJN 94(6):18–24, 1994
3. Anastasi JK, Rivera J: Understanding prophylactic therapy for HIV infections. AJN 94(2):36–41, 1994
4. Anderson BL: Psychological interventions for cancer patients to enhance the quality of life. J Consult Cl Psychology 60(4):552–568, 199
5. Fawzy FI, et al: Critical review of psychosocial interventions in cancer care. Arch Gen Psychiatry 52(2):100–113, 1995
6. Kalichman SC, et al: Use of a brief behavioral skills interventions to prevent HIV infection among chronic mentally ill adults. Psychiatric Services 46(3):275–280, 1995
7. Kaplan HI, Sadock BJ, eds: Comprehensive Textbook of Psychiatry, Vol. 1, 6th ed. Baltimore: Williams & Wilkins, 1995
8. Kelly PJ, Holman S: The new face of AIDS. AJN 93(3):26–34, 1993
9. Kim MJ, McFarland G, McLane AM (eds): Pocket Guide to Nursing Diagnoses, 6th ed. St. Louis: Mosby, 1995

10. Levenson JL: Psychiatric aspects of medical practice. In Stoudemire A (ed): Clinical Psychiatry for Medical Students, 2nd ed. Philadelphia: JB Lippincott, 1994
11. Perkins DO, et al: Somatic symptoms and HIV infection: Relationship to depressive symptoms and indicators of HIV disease. Am J Psychiatry 152(12):1776–1780, 1995
12. Price N: The role of the consultation-liaison nurse: Caring for patients with AIDS dementia complex. J Psychosoc Nurs Ment Health Serv 33(12):31–34, 1995
13. Stoudemire A (ed): Clinical Psychiatry for Medical Students, 2nd ed. Philadelphia: JB Lippincott, 1994
14. Tomb DA: Psychiatry, 5th ed. Baltimore: Williams & Wilkins, 1995
15. Whipple B, Scura KW: The overlooked epidemic: HIV in older adults. AJN 96(2):22–29, 1996

Chapter 8

1. American Psychiatric Association: Diagnostical and Statistical Manual of Mental Disorders: DSM-IV, 4th ed. Washington, DC: American Psychiatric Association, 1994
2. American Psychiatric Association: Practice guideline for the treatment of patients with substance use disorders: Alcohol, cocaine, opioids. Am J Psychiatry (Supplement) 152:11, 1995
3. Atkinson RM, Ganzini L: Substance abuse. In Coffey CE, Cummings JL, Lovell MR, Pearlson GD, eds and assoc eds: The American Psychiatric Press Textbook of Geriatric Neuropsychiatry. Washington, DC: American Psychiatric Press, 1994
4. Beck A et al: An inventory for measuring depression. Arch Gen Psychiatry 4:561–571, 1961
5. Bohn MJ: Alcoholism. Psychiatr Clin North Am 16(4):679–692, 1993
6. Brogdon KE: Improving outcomes for patients experiencing alcohol withdrawal. J Nurs Care Qual 7(3):61–70, 1993
7. Brust JCM: Neurological Aspects of Substance Abuse. Boston: Butterworth-Heinemann, 1993
8. Bukstein OG: Substance abuse. In Hersen M, Ammerman RT, Sisson LA, eds: Handbook of Aggressive and Destructive Behavior in Psychiatric Patients. New York: Plenum Press, 1994
9. Burns CM: Early detection and intervention for the hidden alcoholic: Assessment guideline for the clinical nurse specialist. Clin Nurse Spec 8(6):296–303, 1994
10. Clement JA, Williams EB, Waters C: The client with substance abuse/mental illness: Mandate for collaboration. Archives Psychiatr Nursing VII(4): 189–196, 1993
11. Cornish JW, McNicholas LF, O'Brien CP: Treatment of substance-related disorders. In Schatzberg AF, Nemeroff CB, eds: The American Psychiatric Press Textbook of Psychopharmacology. Washington, DC: American Psychiatric Press, 1995
12. Crabtree BL, Richardson D: Substance use disorders. In DiPiro JT, et al, eds: Pharmacotherapy: A Pathophysiologic Approach, 2nd ed. Norwalk, CT: Appleton & Lange, 1993

13. Dodge VH: Relaxation training: A nursing intervention for substance abusers. Arch Psychiatr Nurs V(2):99–104, 1991

14. Emrick CD: Alcoholics anonymous and other 12-step groups. In: Galanter M, Kleber HD, eds: The American Psychiatric Press Textbook of Substance Abuse Treatment. Washington, DC: American Psychiatric Press, 1994

15. Ewing J: Detecting alcoholism: The CAGE questionnaire. J Amer Medical Assoc 252(14):1905–1907, 1984

16. Foulks EF, Pena JM: Ethnicity and psychotherapy: A component in the treatment of cocaine addiction in African Americans. Psychiatric Clin North Amer 18(3):607–620, 1995

17. Frances RJ, Franklin JE: Alcohol and other psychoactive substance use disorders. In Hales RE, Yudofsky SC, Talbott JA, eds: The American Psychiatric Press Textbook of Psychiatry, 2nd ed. Washington, DC: American Psychiatric Press, 1994

18. Frances RJ, Franklin JE, Borg L: Psychodynamics. In Galanter M, Kleber HD, eds: The American Psychiatric Press Textbook of Substance Abuse Treatment. Washington, DC: American Psychiatric Press, 1994

19. Friedemann AL, Musgrove JA: Perceptions of inner city substance abusers about their families. Archives Psychiatr Nurs VIII(2):115–123, 1994

20. Friedrich RM, Kus RJ: Cognitive impairments in early sobriety: Nursing interventions. Arch Psychiatr Nurs V(2):105–112, 1991

21. Gallant D: Alcohol. In Galanter M, Kleber HD, eds: The American Psychiatric Press Textbook of Substance Abuse Treatment. Washington, DC: American Psychiatric Press, 1994

22. Gallant D: Alcoholism. In Gabbard GO, ed: Treatments of Psychiatric Disorders, Vol 1. Washington, DC: American Psychiatric Press, 1994

23. Gerety EK, McFarland GK: Impaired adjustment. In Kim MJ, McFarland GK, McLane AL: Pocket Guide to Nursing Diagnoses, 6th ed. St. Louis: Mosby, 1995

24. Gerety EK: Impaired adjustment. In Thompson JM, McFarland GK, Hirsch JE, Tucker SM: Mosby's Clinical Nursing, 3rd ed. St. Louis: Mosby Year Book, 1993

25. Gerstein DR: Outcome research: Drug abuse. In Galanter M, Kleber HD, eds: The American Psychiatric Press Textbook of Substance Abuse Treatment. Washington, DC: American Psychiatric Press, 1994

26. Gray M: Relapse prevention. In Straussner SLA, ed: Clinical Work With Substance-Abusing Clients. New York: Guilford Press, 1993

27. Halikas JA: Treatment of drug abuse syndromes. Psychiatr Clin North Amer 16(4):693–702, 1993

28. Hester RK: Outcome research: Alcoholism. In Galanter M, Kleber HD, eds: The American Psychiatric Press Textbook of Substance Abuse Treatment. Washington, DC: American Psychiatric Press, 1994

29. Inclan J, Hernandez M: Cross-cultural perspectives and codependence: The case of poor Hispanics. Am J Orthopsychiatry 62(2):245–255, 1992

30. James SL: Alcoholism in homeless veterans: A historical overview. Clin Nurse Spec 8(5):241–24, 1994

31. Janssen E: A self psychological approach to treating the mentally ill, chemical abusing and addicted (MICAA) patient. Arch Psychiatr Nurs VII(6):381–389, 1994

32. Karch AM: 1996 Lippincott's Nursing Drug Guide. Philadelphia: JB Lippincott, 1996

33. Kashka MS, Tweed SH: Substance-related disorders. In Hogstel MO, ed: Geropsychiatric Nursing, 2nd ed. St. Louis: Mosby, 1995

34. Kauffman E, Dore MM, Nelson-Zlupko L: The role of women's therapy groups in the treatment of chemical dependence. Am J Orthopsychiatry 65(3):355–363, 1993

35. Kaufman E: Psychotherapy of Addicted Persons. New York: Guilford Press, 1994

36. Lindeman M, Hawks JHH, Bartek JK: The alcoholic family: A nursing diagnosis validation study. Nurs Diagnosis 5(2):65–73, 1994

37. Lindstrom L: Managing Alcoholism: Matching Clients to Treatments. New York: Oxford University Press, 1992

38. Markowitz R: Dynamics and treatment issues with children of drug and alcohol abusers. In Straussner SLA: Clinical Work With Substance-Abusing Clients. New York: Guilford Press, 1993

39. Meyer RE: Biology of psychoactive substance dependence disorders: Opiates, cocaine, and ethanol. In Schatzberg AF, Nemeroff CB, eds: The American Psychiatric Press Textbook of Psychopharmacology. Washington, DC: American Psychiatric Press, 1995

40. Minicucci DS: The challenge of change: Rethinking alcohol abuse. Arch Psychiatr Nurs VIII(6):373–380, 1994

41. Montgomery P, Johnson B: The stress of marriage to an alcoholic. J Psychosoc Nurs Ment Health Serv 30(10):12–16, 1992

42. Morofka V: Mental health. In Thompson JM, McFarland GK, Hirsch JE, Tucker SM: Mosby's Clinical Nursing, 3rd ed. St. Louis: Mosby Year Book, 1993

43. Moss HB, Salloum IM, Fisher B: Psychoactive substance abuse. In Hersen M, Ammerman RT, Sisson LA, eds: Handbook of Aggressive and Destructive Behavior in Psychiatric Patients. New York: Plenum Press, 1994

44. Murphy G: Suicide in alcoholism. New York: Oxford University Press, 1992

45. Murphy SA: Validation of addictions nursing diagnoses in a sample of alcohol abstainers 1 year posttreatment. Arch Psychiatr Nurs VI(6):340–346, 1992

46. North American Nursing Diagnosis Association: NANDA Nursing Diagnoses: Definitions and Classification, 1995–1996. Philadelphia: NANDA, 1994

47. Ockene JK, Kristeller JL: Tobacco. In Galanter M, Kleber HD eds: The American Psychiatric Press Textbook of Substance Abuse Treatment. Washington, DC: American Psychiatric Press, 1994

48. Ockert DM, Baier AR: Assessment and treatment of clients dependent on cocaine and other stimulants. In Straussner SLA: Clinical Work With Substance-Abusing Clients. New York: Guilford Press, 1993

49. Orlin L, Davis J: Assessment and interventions with drug and alcohol abusers in psychiatric settings. In Straussner SLA: Clinical Work With Substance-Abusing Clients. New York: Guilford Press, 1993

50. Pape PA: Issues in assessment and intervention with alcohol-and drug-abusing women. In Straussner SLA: Clinical Work With Substance-Abusing Clients. New York: Guilford Press, 1993

51. Riggen OZ: The client who is addicted to alcohol. In Lego S, ed: Psychiatric Nursing: A Comprehensive Reference, 2nd ed. Philadelphia: JB Lippincott, 1996

52. Riggen OZ: The client who is abusing substances other than alcohol. In Lego S, ed: Psychiatric Nursing: A Comprehensive Reference, 2nd ed. Philadelphia: JB Lippincott, 1996

53. Schottenfeld RS: Assessment of the patient. In Galanter M, Kleber HD, eds: The American Psychiatric Press Textbook of Substance Abuse Treatment. Washington, DC: American Psychiatric Press, 1994

54. Schuckit MA: Goals of Treatment. In Galanter M, Kleber HD, eds: The American Psychiatric Press Textbook of Substance Abuse Treatment. Washington, DC: American Psychiatric Press, 1994

55. Selzer ML, Vinokur A, Rooijen EL: A self-administration short Michigan Alcoholism Screening Test (SMAST). J Studies Alcohol 36(1):117–126, 1975

56. Spiegel BR: 12-Step programs as a treatment modality. In Straussner SLA: Clinical Work With Substance-Abusing Clients. New York: Guilford Press, 1993

57. Straussner SLA: Assessment and treatment of clients with alcohol and other drug abuse problems: An overview. In Straussner SLA: Clinical Work With Substance-Abusing Clients. New York: Guilford Press, 1993

58. Swift RM: Alcohol and drug abuse in the medical setting. In Stoudemire A, Fogel BS, eds: Psychiatric Care of the Medical Patient. New York: Oxford University Press, 1993

59. Szwabo PA: Substance abuse in older women. Clin Geriatr Med 9(1):197–208, 1993

60. Westermeyer J: Cultural aspects of substance abuse and alcoholism: Assessment and management. Psychiatric Clin North Amer 18(3):589–605, 1995

61. Whipple EE, Fitzgerald HE, Zucker RA: Parent–child interactions in alcoholic and nonalcoholic families. Am J Orthopsychiatry 65(1):153–159, 1995

62. Wing DM, Hammer-Higgins P: Determinants of denial: A study of alcoholics. J Psychosoc Nurs Ment Health Serv 31(2):13–17, 1993

63. Wing DM: Applying the "Model of Recovering Alcoholics' Behavior Stages and Goal Setting" to nursing practice. Arch Psychiatr Nurs VII(4):197–202, 1993

64. Zahourek RP: The client with dual diagnosis. In Lego S, ed: Psychiatric Nursing: A Comprehensive Reference, 2nd ed. Philadelphia: JB Lippincott, 1996

Chapter 9

1. Asarnow RF, Asarnow JR: Childhood-onset schizophrenia: Editors' introduction. Schizophr Bull 20(4):591–597, 1994

2. American Psychiatric Association: DSM-IV, Diagnosis and Statistical Manual of Mental Disorders Criteria, 4th Ed. Washington, DC: American Psychiatric Association, 1994

3. Barteis SJ, Drake RE, Wallach MA: Long-term course of substance use disorders among patients with severe mental illness. Psychiatric Serv 46(3):248–251, 1995

4. Bellack AS, Meser KT: Psychosocial treatment for schizophrenia. Schizophr Bull 19(2):317–336, 1993

5. Bradshaw WH: Coping-skills training verus a problem-solving approach with schizophrenic patients. Hosp Community Psychiatry 44(11): 1102–1104, 1993

6. Bromet EJ, Dew MA, Eaton W: Epidemiology in psychosis with special reference to schizophrenia. In Tsuang MT, Tohen M, Zahner GEP, eds. Textbook in Psychiatric Epidemiology. New York: John Wiley, 1995

7. Buchsbaum MS: Charting the circuits. Nature 378: 128–129, 1995

8. Burcheri R: Auditory hallucinations in schizophrenia: Group experience in examining symptom management and individual strategies. J Psychosoc Nurs Ment Health Serv 34(2):12–25, 1996

9. Chen A: Noncompliance in community psychiatry: A review of clinical interventions. Hosp Comm Psychiatry 42(3):282–287, 1991

10. Corrigan PW, Green MF: Schizophrenic patients' sensitivity to social clues: The role of abstraction. Am J Psychiatry 150(4):589–594, 1993

11. Corrigan PS, Storzbach DM: Behavioral interventions for alleviating psychotic symptoms. Hosp Community Psychiatry 44(4):341–347, 1993

12. Corrigan PW, Toomey R: Interpersonal problem solving and information processing in schizophrenia. Schizophr Bull 21(3):345–403, 1995

13. Coursey RD, Keller, AB, Farrell EW: Individual psychotherapy and persons with serious mental illness: The client's perspective. Schizophr Bull 21(2):283–301, 1995

14. Cravener B: Establishing therapeutic alliance across cultural barriers. J Psychosoc Ment Health Nurs 30(12):10–14, 1992

15. Dassori AM, Miller AL, Saldana D: Schizophrenia among Hispanics: Epidemiology, phenomenology, course and outcome. Schizophr Bull 21(2):303–312, 1995

16. Dixon LB, et al: Modifying the PACT model to serve homeless persons with severe mental illness. Psychiatric Services 46(7):684–688, 1995

17. Eaton W W, et al: Structure and course of positive and negative symptoms in schizophrenia. Arch Gen Psychiatry 52(2):127-134, 1995

18. Eckman TA, et al: Technique for training schizophrenic patients in illness self-managment: A controlled trial. Am J Psychiatry 149(11):1549–1555, 1992

19. Forman L: Medication: Reasons & interventions for noncompliance. J Psychosoc Nurs Ment Health Serv 31(10):23–25, 1993

20. Frederick J, Cotanch P: Self-help techniques for auditory hallucinations in schizophrenia. Issues Ment Health Nurs 16(3):213–224, 1995

21. Gamble C, Midence K: Schizophrenia family work: Mental health nurses delivering an innovative service. J Psychosoc Nurs Ment Health Serv 32(10):13–16, 1994

22. Hans SL, et al: Interpersonal behavior of children at risk for schizophrenia. Psychiatry 55(4):314–335, 1992

23. Harris D, Morrison EF: Managing violence without coercion. Arch Psychiatric Nurs 9(4):203–210, 1995

24. Hatfield AB, Lefley HP: Surviving Mental Illness: Stress, Coping and Adaptation. New York: Guilford Press, 1993

25. Hegarty JD, et al: One hundred years of schizophrenia: A meta-analysis of the outcome literature. Am J Psychiatry 151(10):1409–1416, 1994

26. Hogarty GE, et al: Personal therapy: A disorder-relevant psychotherapy for schizophrenia. Schizophr Bull 21(3:379–393, 1995

27. Hogarty GE: Prevention of relapse in chronic schizophrenic patients. J Clin Psychiatry 54(3):18–23, 1993

28. Junginer J: Command hallucinations and the prediction of dangerousness. Psychiatric Services 46(9):911–914, 1995

29. Kagiaebi A: First person account: Living in a nightmare. Schizophr Bull 21(1):155–159, 1994

30. Kaplan HI, Saddock BJ: Comprehensive Textbook of Psychiatry, Vol. 1, 6th ed. Baltimore: Williams & Wilkins, 1995

31. Kaplan HI, Saddock BJ, Grebb JA, eds: Synopsis of Psychiatry, 7th ed. Baltimore: Williams & Wilkins, 1994

32. Kavanagh DJ: Schizophrenia. In Wilson PH, ed: Principles and Practice of Relapse Prevention. New York: Guilford Press, 1992
33. Keefe RSE, Harvey PD: Understanding Schizophrenia: A Guide to the New Research on Course and Treatment. New York: Free Press, 1994
34. Keith SJ: Understanding the experience of schizophrenia. Am J Psychiatry 150(11):1616–1617, 1993
35. Kim MJ, McFarland GK, McLane AM, eds: Pocket Guide to Nursing Diagnoses, 6th ed. St. Louis: Mosby, 1995
36. Kingdon DG, Turkington D: Cognitive-Behavioral Therapy of Schizophrenia. New York: Guilford Press, 1994
37. Kirkpatrick H, et al: Hope and schizophrenia: Clinicians identify hope-instilling strategies. J Psychosoc Nurs Ment Health Serv 33(6)15–19, 1995
38. Knisely JE, Northhouse L: The relationship between social support, help-seeking behavior, and psychological distress in psychiatric clients. Arch Psychatric Nurs 8(6):357–365, 1994
39. Lapierre ER, Kosiorowski B: Nonpharmacological approaches to acute symptom management. In Malone JA, ed: Schizophrenia: Handbook for Clinical Care. Thorofare, NJ: Slack, 1994
40. Leadbetter RA, et al: Multidisciplinary approach to psychosis, intermittent, hyponatremia, and polydipsia. Schizophr Bull 20(2):375–385, 1994
41. Liberman RP: Psychosocial treatment for schizophrenia. Psychiatry 57(2):104–114, 1994
42. Liberman RP, et al: Innovations in skill training for the seriously mentally ill: The UCLA social and independent living skills modules. Innovations and Research 2:43–59, 1993
43. Littrell KH: Maximizing psychosocial interventions. J Am Psychiatr Nurses Assoc 1(6):214–218, 1995
44. Lysaker P, et al: Insight and psychosocial treatment compliance in schizophrenia. Psychiatry 57(4):307–315, 1994
45. McCloskey JC, Bulechek GM, eds: Nursing Interventions Classification, 2nd ed. St. Louis: Mosby, 1995
46. McKenna PJ: Schizophrenia and Related Syndromes. Oxford: Oxford University Press, 1994
47. Miklowitz DJ: Family risk indicaators in schizophrenia. Schziophr Bull 20 (2):137–149, 1994
48. Mirsky AF, et al: Overview and summary: Twenty-five-year follow-up of high-risk children. Schizophr Bull 21(2):227–239, 1995
49. Murphy MF, Moller MD: Relapse management in neurobiological disorders: The Moller-Murphy Symptom Management Assessment Tool. Archiv Psychiatric Nurs 7(4):226–235, 1993
50. Mueser K, Bellack A, Blanchard J: Comorbidity of schizophrenia and substance abuse: Implications for treatment. J Consulting Cl Psychiatry 60(6):845–856, 1992
51. Neuzil GG, Baber VL: Acute crisis management. In Malone JA, ed: Schizophrenia: Handbook for Clinical Care. New Jersey: Slack, 1992
52. O'Connor FW: A vulnerability-stress framework for evaluating clinical interventions in schizophrenia. Image: Journal of Nursing Scholarship 26(3):231–236, 1994
53. Santos AB, et al: Research on field-based services: Models for reform in the delivery of mental health care to populations with complex clinical problems. Am J Psychiatry 152(8):1111–1123, 1995
54. Schepp KG: A symptom management program for adolescents with psychotic illnesses: Theoretical basis. JCPN 5(4):7–12, 1992

55. Schepp KG: A symptom management program for psychiatrically ill adolescents and their families: Preliminary clinical outcomes. JCNP 5(4):13–17, 1992

56. Schiller L: The Quiet Room. New York: Warner Books, 1994

57. Solomon P, Draine J: Adaptive coping among family members of persons with serious mental illness. Psychiatric Serv 46(11):1156–1160, 1995

58. Spitzer VM: Biological aspects of schizophrenia. J Am Psychiatr Nurses Assoc 1(6):204–207, 1995

59. Stoudemire A, ed: Clinical Psychiatry for Medical Students, 2nd ed. Philadelphia: JB Lippincott, 1994

60. Sullivan G, Lukoff D: Sexual side effects of antipsychotic medication: Evaluation and interventions. Hosp Community Psychiatry 41(11): 1238–1241, 1990

61. Tandon R: Neurobiological substrate of dimensions of schizophrenic illness. J Psychiat Res 29(4):255–260, 1995

62. Tesar GE: The agitated patient, Part I: Evaluation and behavioral managment. Hosp Community Psychiatry 44(4):329–331, 1993

63. Tesar GE: The agitated patient, Part II: Pharmacologic treatment. Hosp Community Psychiatry 44(7):627–629, 1993

64. Thompson JW, et al: Trends in the inpatient care of persons with schizophrenia. Schizophr Bull 21(1):75–85, 1995

65. Tollett JH, Thomas SP: A theory-based nursing intervention to instill hope in homeless veterans. Adv Nurs Sci 18(2):76–90,1995

66. Tomb DA: Psychiatry, 5th ed. Baltimore: Williams & Wilkins, 1995

67. Trappler B, Greenberg S, Friedman S: Treatment of Hasidic Jewish patients in a general hospital medical-psychiatric unit. Psychiatric Services 46(8):833–835, 1995

68. Tugrul KC: Pharmacologic treatment of schizophrenia: A review. J Am Psychiatr Nurses Assoc 1(6):208–213, 1995

69. Villenga BA, Christenson J: Persistent and severely mentally ill clients' perception of their mental illness. Issues Ment Health Nurs 15(4):359–371, 1994

70. Walkup J: A clinically based rule of thumb for classifying delusions. Schizophr Bull 21(2):223–231, 1995

71. Warner R: Time trends in schizophrenia: Changes in obstetric risk factors with industrialization. Schizophr Bull 21(3):483–501, 1995

72. Wasylenki DA: Psychotherapy of schizophrenia revisited. Hosp Community Psychiatry 43(2):123–127, 1992

73. Watzlawick P: Interpersonal aspects of schizophrenia: Some epitemological and practical conclusions. In Benedetti G, Furlan PM, eds: The Psychotherapy of Schizophrenia. Effective Clinical Approaches: Controversies, Critiques and Recommendations. Seattle: Hagrefe and Huber, 1993

74. Weiden P, Hevens L: Psychotherapeutic management techniques in the treatment of outpatients with schizophrenia. Hosp Community Psychiatry 45(6):549–555, 1994

75. Wer J, Moller M: Family-identified health educational needs regarding schizophrenia. In Malone JA, ed. Schizophrenia: Handbook for Clinical Care. Thorofare, NJ: Slack, 1992

76. Westermeyer JF, Harrow M, Marengo JT: Risk for suicide in schizophrenia and other psychotic and nonpsychotic disorders. J Nerv Ment Dis 179(5):179–259, 1991

77. Winefield HR, Harvey EJ: Needs of family caregivers in chronic schizophrenia. Schizophr Bull 20(3):557–566, 1994

78. Wynne LC: Changing approaches to schizophrenic patient and their families: 1954-1988. In Benedetti G, Furlow PM, eds: The Psychotherapy of Schizophenia: Effective Clinical Approaches, Controversies, Critiques and Recommendations. Seattle: Hogrefe and Huber, 1993

Chapter 10

1. Agency for Health Care Policy and Research, PHS, USDHHS: Depression in primary care: Detection, diagnosis, and treatment. Journal of Psychosocial Nursing and Mental Health Services 31(6):19–28, 1993
2. American Psychiatric Association: Diagnostic and Statistical Manual of Mental Disorders, DSM-IV, 4th ED. Washington, DC: American Psychiatric Association, 1994
3. Andreasen NC, Black NW: Introductory Textbook of Psychiatry, 2nd ed. Washington, DC: American Psychiatric Press, 1995
4. Badger TA: Living with depression. Family members' experiences and treatment needs. Journal of Psychosocial Nursing and Mental Health Services 34(1):21–29, 1996
5. Badger TA, Cardea JM, Biocca LJ, Mishel MH: Assessment and management of depression; An imperative for community-based practice. Archives of Psychiatric Nursing IV (4):235–241, 1990
6. Bernstein JG: Handbook of Drug Therapy in Psychiatry, 3rd ed. St. Louis: Mosby, 1995
7. Betrus PA, Elmore SK: Seasonal affective disorder, Part I: A review of the neural mechanisms for psychosocial nurses. Archives of Psychiatric Nursing V(6):357–364, 1991
8. Blixen CE, Wilkinson LK, Schuring L: Depression in an elderly clinic population: Findings from an ambulatory care setting. Journal of Psychosocial Nursing and Mental Health Services 32(6):43–49, 1994
9. Brage DG: Adolescent Depression: A review of the literature. Archives of Psychiatric Nursing IX (1):45-55, 1995
10. Burns CM, Stuart GW: Nursing care in electroconvulsive therapy. Psychiatric Clinics of North America 14(4):971–988, 1991
11. Campbell JM: Treating Depression in well older adults: Use of diaries in cognitive therapy. Issues in Mental Health Nursing 13:19–29, 1992
12. Cardell R, Horton-Deutsch SH: A model for assessment of inpatient suicide potential. Archives of Psychiatric Nursing VIII(6):366–372, 1994
13. Cataldo JK: Hardiness and death attitudes: Predictors of depression in the institutionalized elderly. Archives of Psychiatric Nursing VIII(5):326–332, 1994
14. Clark W, Vorst VR: Group therapy with chronically depressed geriatric patients. Journal of Psychosocial Nursing and Mental Health Services 32(5):9–13, 1994
15. Cummings JL: Depression in neurologic diseases. Psychiatric Annals 24(10):525–534, 1994
16. Depression Guideline Panel: Depression in Primary Care; Detection and Diagnosis, Volume 1, Clinical Practice Guideline, Number 5. Rockville, MD: USPHS, PHS, Agency for Health Care Policy and Research, 1993
17. Depression Guideline Panel: Depression in Primary Care: Treatment of Major Depression, Volume 2, Clinical Practice Guideline, Number 5. Rockville, MD: UHPHS, PHS, Agency for Health Care Policy and Research, 1993

18. Devanand DP, Sackheim HA, Prudic J: Electroconvulsive therapy in the treatment-resistant patient. Psychiatric Clinics of North America 14(4):905–923, 1991

19. Fava M, Kaji J: Continuation and maintenance treatments of major depressive disorder. Psychiatric Annals 24(6):281–290, 1994

20. Frances A, First MB, Pincus HA: DSM-IV Guidebook. Washington, DC: American Psychiatric Press, 1995

21. Gadde GM, Krishnan KR: Endocrine factors in depression. Psychiatric Annals 24(10):521–524, 1994

22. Ganzini L, Millar SB, Walsh JR: Drug-induced mania in the elderly. Drugs and Aging 3(5):428–435, 1993

23. Ganzini L, Walsh JR, Millar SB: Drug-induced depression in the elderly. Drugs and Aging 3(2):147–158, 1993

24. George MS, Ketter TA, Post RM: Activation studies in mood disorders. Psychiatric Annals 24(12):648–652, 1994

25. George MS: Introduction: The emerging neuroanatomy of depression. Psychiatric Annals 24(12):635–636, 1994

26. Gomez GE, Gomez EA: The use of antidepressants with elderly patients. Journal of Psychosocial Nursing and Mental Health Services 30(11):21–26, 1992

27. Gordon V, Matwychuk A, Sachs C, Canedy B: A three-year followup of a cognitive behavioral therapy intervention. Archives of Psychiatric Nursing 2:218–226, 1988

28. Harnett DS: Psychopharmacologic treatment of depression in the medical setting. Psychiatric Annals 24(10):545–552, 1994

29. Herr KA, Mobily PR: Geriatric mental health: Chronic pain and depression. Journal of Psychosocial Nursing and Mental Health Services 30(9):7–12, 1992

30. Himmelhoch JM: On the failure to recognize lithium failure. Psychiatric Annals 24(5):241–250, 1994

31. Hirschfeld RMA, Goodwin FK: Mood disorders. In Talbott JA, Hales RE, Yudofsky SC, eds: The American Psychiatric Press Textbook of Psychiatry. Washington, DC: American Psychiatric Press, 1988

32. Hopkin K: Will better methods yield a gene for manic depression? Journal of NIH Research 7:30–32, 1995

33. Horing-Rohan M, Amsterdam JD: Clinical and biological correlates of treatment—resistant depression: An overview. Psychiatric Annals 24(5):220–227, 1994

34. Jarrett RB, Rush AJ: Short-term psychotherapy of depressive disorders: Current status and future directions. Psychiatry 57(2):115–132, 1994

35. Jefferson JW, Greist JH: Mood disorders. In Hales RE, Yudofsky SC, Talbott JA, eds: The American Psychiatric Press Textbook of Psychiatry, 2nd ed. Washington, DC: American Psychiatric Press, 1994

36. Johnston HF, Fruehling JJ: Using antidepressant medication in depressed children: An algorithm. Psychiatric Annals 24(7):348–356, 1994

37. Kaplan HI, Sadock BJ, Grebb JA: Kaplan and Sadock's Synopsis of Psychiatry, 7th ed. Baltimore: Williams and Wilkins, 1994

38. Karch AM: Lippincott's Nursing Drug Guide 1996. Philadelphia: Lippincott-Raven, 1996

39. Kennedy GJ: The geriatric syndrome of late-life depression. Psychiatric Services 46(1):43–48, 1995

40. Ketter TA, George MS, Ring HA, Pazzaglia P, Marangell L, Kimbrell TA, Post RM: Primary mood disorders: Structural and resting functional studies. Psychiatric Annals 24(12):637–642, 1994

41. Kim E, Rovner BW: Depression in dementia. Psychiatric Annals 24(4):173–177, 1994

42. Kim MJ, McFarland GK, McLane AM: Pocket Guide to Nursing Diagnoses, 6th ed. St. Louis: Mosby, 1995

43. Kim S, Rew L: Ethnic identity, role integration, quality of life, and depression in Korean-American women. Archives of Psychiatric Nursing VIII(6):348–356, 1994

44. Kurlowicz LH: Depression in hospitalized medically ill elders: Evolution of the concept. Archives of Psychiatric Nursing VIII(2):124–136, 1994

45. Larson L: High risk for violence; self-directed. In McFarland GK, McFarlane EA: Nursing Diagnosis and Intervention: Planning for Patient Care, 2nd ed. St. Louis: Mosby, 1993

46. Maynard C: Psychoeducational approach to depression in women. Journal of Psychosocial Nursing and Mental Health Services 31(12):9–14, 1993

47. Maynard CK: Comparison of effectiveness of group interventions for depression in women. Archives of Psychiatric Nursing VII(5):277–283, 1993

48. McEnany GW: Psychobiological indices of bipolar mood disorder: Future trends in nursing care. Archives of Psychiatric Nursing IV(1):29–38, 1990

49. McFarland GK, McFarlane EA: Nursing Diagnosis and Intervention: Planning for Patient Care, 2nd ed. St. Louis: Mosby, 1993

50. McFarland GK, Wasli EL, Gerety EK: Nursing Diagnoses and Process in Psychiatric Mental Health Nursing, 2nd ed. Philadelphia: JB Lippincott, 1992

51. Metzger E, Friedman RS: Treatment-related depression. Psychiatric Annals 24(10):540–544, 1994

52. Morin GD: Seasonal affective disorder, the depression of winter: A literature review and description from a nursing perspective. Archives of Psychiatric Nursing IV(3):182–187, 1990

53. Nierenberg AA: Treatment-resistant depression in the age of serotonin. Psychiatric Annals 24(5):217–219, 1994

54. NIH Consensus Development Panel on Depression in Late Life: Diagnosis and treatment of depression in late life. JAMA 268(8):1018–1024, 1992

55. North American Nursing Diagnosis Association: Nursing Diagnoses: Definitions and Classification—1995–1996. Philadelphia: NANDA, 1994

56. Pies RW: Medical "mimics" of depression. Psychiatric Annals 24(10):519–520, 1994

57. Pollack LE: How do inpatients with bipolar disorder evaluate diagnostically homogenous groups? Journal of Psychosocial Nursing and Mental Health Services 31(10):26–32, 1993

58. Pollack LE: Improving relationships, groups for inpatients with bipolar disorder. Journal of Psychosocial Nursing and Mental Health Services 28(5):17–22, 1990

59. Pollack LE: Striving for stability with bipolar disorder despite barriers. Archives of Psychiatric Nursing IX(3):122–129, 1995

60. Pollack LE: Treatment of inpatients with bipolar disorders: A role for self-management groups. Journal of Psychosocial Nursing and Mental Health Services 33(1):11–16, 1995

61. Professional Care Guide: Psychiatric Disorders. Springhouse, PA: Springhouse Corp, 1995

62. Prudic JM, Sackeim HA, Rifas S: Medication resistance, response to ECT, and prevention of relapse. Psychiatric Annals 24(5):228–231, 1994

63. Rathus SA, Nevid JS: Abnormal Psychology. Englewood Cliffs, NJ: Prentice Hall, 1991

64. Reus V: Mood Disorders. In Goldman H: Review of General Psychiatry, 4th ed. East Norwalk, CT: Appleton & Lange, 1995

65. Rossen EK, Buschmann MBT: Mental illness in late life: The neurobiology of depression. Archives of Psychiatric Nursing IX(3):130–136, 1995

66. Rubin E, Sackeim HA, Nobler MS, Moeller JR: Brain imaging studies of antidepressant treatments. Psychiatric Annals 24(12):653–658, 1994

67. Schatzberg AF, Nemeroff CB: The American Psychiatric Press Textbook of Psychopharmacology. Washington, DC: American Psychiatric Press, 1995

68. Schwartz MF: High risk for violence: Self-directed. In Thompson JM, McFarland GK, Hirsch JE, Tucker SM: Mosby's Clinical Nursing, 3rd ed. St. Louis: Mosby, 1993

69. Simmons-Alling S: Genetic implications for major affective disorders. Archives of Psychiatric Nursing IV(1)67–71, 1990

70. Small JG: Electroconvulsive therapy for mania. Psychiatric Clinics of North America 14(4):887–903, 1991

71. Spillers GM: Suicide potential. In McFarland GK, Thomas MD: Psychiatric Mental Health Nursing: Application of the Nursing Process. Philadelphia, JB Lippincott, 1991

72. Stewart NJ, McMufllen LM, Rubin LD: Movement therapy with depressed inpatients: A randomized multiple single case design. Archives of Psychiatric Nursing VIII(1):22–29, 1994

73. Stimmel GL: How to counsel patients about depression and its treatment. Pharmacotherapy 15(6 Pt 2):100S–104S, 1995

74. Stuart GW: Detection and Treatment of Depression: The Nursing Perspective. Washington, DC: American Nurses Association, 1994

75. Tabora B, Flaskerud JH: Depression among Chinese Americans: A review of the literature. Issues in Mental Health Nursing 15:569–584, 1994

76. Thase ME, Howland RH: Refractory depression: Relevance of psychosocial factors and therapies. Psychiatric Annals 24(5):232–240, 1994

77. Ugarriza DN: Postpartum affective disorders: Incidence and treatment. Journal of Psychosocial Nursing and Mental Health Services 30(5):29–32, 1992

78. Valente SM: Electroconvulsive therapy. Archives of Psychiatric Nursing V(4):223–228, 1991

79. Valente SM: Recognizing depression in elderly patients. AJN 94(12):19–24, 1994

80. Warren BJ: Depression in African-American women. Journal of Psychosocial Nursing and Mental Health Services 32(3):29–33, 1994

81. Zauszniewski JA: Health seeking resources and adaptive functioning in depressed and nondepressed adults. Archives of Psychiatric Nursing VIII(3):159–168, 1994

82. Zauszniewski JA: Potential sequelae of family history of depression. Journal of Psychosocial Nursing and Mental Health Services 32(9):15–21, 1994

83. Zerhusen JD, Boyle K, Wilson W: Out of the darkness: Group cognitive therapy for depressed elderly. Journal of Psychosocial Nursing and Mental Health Services 29(9):16–21, 1991

Chapter 11

1. Allen SN, Bloom SL: Group and family treatment of Post-Traumatic Stress Disorder. Psychiatric Clinics of North America 17(2):425–437, 1994
2. American Psychiatric Association. Diagnostic and Statistical Manual of Mental Disorders: DSM-IV, 4th ed. Washington, DC: American Psychiatric Association, 1994
3. Ballenger JC: Benzodiazepines. In Schatzberg AF, Nemeroff CB, eds: The American Psychiatric Press Textbook of Psychopharmacology. Washington, DC: American Psychiatric Press, 1995
4. Blank AS: Clinical detection, diagnosis and differential diagnosis of post-traumatic stress disorder. Psychiatric Clinics of North America 17(2):351–383, 1994
5. Boyarsky BK, Perone LA, Lee NC, Goodman WK: Current treatment approaches to Obsessive-Compulsive Disorder. Archives Psychiatric Nursing V(5):299–306, 1991
6. Brook DW: Group psychotherapy with anxiety and mood disorders. In Kaplan HI, Sadock BJ: Comprehensive Group Psychotherapy, 3rd ed. Baltimore: Williams & Wilkins, 1993
7. Brom D, Witztum E: Recent trauma in psychiatric outpatients. Amer J Orthopsychiat 62(4):545–551, 1992
8. Brown TA, Barlow DH, Liebowitz MR: The empirical basis of Generalized Anxiety Disorder. Am J Psychiatry.151:1272–1280, 1994
9. Carroll EM, Foy D: Assessment and treatment of combat-related Post-Traumatic Stress Disorder in a medical center setting. In Foy DW, ed: Treating PTSD: Cognitive-Behavioral Strategies. New York: Guilford Press, 1992
10. Cole JO, Yonkers KA: Nonbenzodiazepine anxiolytics. In Schatzberg AF, Nemeroff CB, eds: The American Psychiatric Press Textbook of Psychopharmacology. Washington, DC: American Psychiatric Press, 1995
11. Davis GC, Breslau N: Post-traumatic Stress Disorder in victims of civilian trauma and criminal violence. Psychiatric Clinics of North America 17(2):289–299, 1994
12. deBeurs E, van Balkom AJLM, Lange A, Koele P, van Dyck R: Treatment of Panic Disorder with Agoraphobia: Comparison of fluvoxamine, placebo, and psychological panic management combined with exposure and of exposure in vivo alone. Am J Psychiatry (152)5:683–691, 1995
13. Friedman MJ, Schnurr PP, McDonagh-Coyle A: Post-Traumatic Stress Disorder in the military veteran. Psychiatric Clinics of North America 17(2):265–277, 1994
14. Goisman R, Goldenberg I, Vasile RG, Keller MB: Comorbidity of anxiety disorders in a multicenter anxiety study. Comprehensive Psychiatry 36(4):303–311, 1995
15. Goldberg RJ, Posner D. Anxiety in the medically ill. In Stoudemire A, Fogel BS, eds: The Psychiatric Care of the Medical Patient. New York: Oxford University Press, 1993
16. Hollander E, Simeon D, Gorman JM: Anxiety disorders. In Hales RE, Yudofsky SC, Talbott JA, eds: The American Psychiatric Press Textbook of Psychiatry, 2nd ed. Washington, DC: American Psychiatric Press, 1994
17. Insel TR, Winslow JT: Neurobiology of obsessive compulsive disorder. Psychiatric Clinics of North America 15(4):813–824, 1992
18. Kaplan HI, Sadock BJ, Grebb JA: Kaplan and Sadock's Synopsis of Psychiatry, 7th ed. Baltimore: Williams & Wilkins, 1994

19. Karch AM: 1996 Lippincott's Nursing Drug Guide. Philadelphia: JB Lippincott, 1996

20. Keltner NL, Folks DG: Psychotropic Drugs. St. Louis: Mosby–Year Book, 1993

21. Kirmayer LJ, Young A, Hayton BC: The cultural context of anxiety disorders. Psychiatric Clinics of North America 18(3):503–521, 1995

22. Krishnan KRR: Monoamine oxidase inhibitors. In Schatzberg AF, Nemeroff CB, eds: The American Psychiatric Press Textbook of Psychopharmacology. Washington, DC: American Psychiatric Press, 1995

23. Laraia MT: Biological correlates of Panic Disorder with Agoraphobia: Practice perspectives for nurses. Archives Psychiatric Nursing V(6):373–381, 1991

24. Levine R, Gaw AC: Culture-bound syndromes. Psychiatric Clinics of North America 18(3):523–536,1995

25. McCloskey JC, Bulechek GM, eds: Nursing Interventions Classification (NIC), 2nd ed. St. Louis: Mosby, 1996

26. McDougle CJ, Goodman WK, Leckman JF, Price LH: The psychopharmacology of obsessive compulsive disorder: implications for treatment and pathogenesis. Psychiatric Clinics of North America 16(4):749–766, 1993

27. North American Nursing Diagnosis Association: NANDA Nursing Diagnoses: Definitions & Classification 1995–1996. St Louis: NANDA 1994

28. Noyes R, Holt CS: Anxiety disorders. In Winokur G, Clayton PJ: The Medical Basis of Psychiatry, 2nd ed. Philadelphia: WB Saunders, 1994

29. Oquendo MA. Differential diagnosis of ataque de nervios. Amer J Orthopsychiat 65(1):60–65, 1994

30. Potter WZ, Manji HK, Rudorfer MV: Tricyclics and tetracyclics. In Schatzberg AF, Nemeroff CB, eds: The American Psychiatric Press Textbook of Psychopharmacology. Washington, DC: American Psychiatric Press, 1995

31. Rosenbaum JF, Pollack MH: Anxiety. In Cassem NH. Massachusetts General Handbook of General Hospital Psychiatry, 3rd ed. St. Louis: Mosby–Year Book, 1991

32. Roy-Byrne P, Wingerson D, Cowley D, Dager S: Psychopharmacologic treatment of panic, generalized anxiety disorder, and social phobia. Psychiatric Clinics of North America 16(4):719–735, 1993

33. Schweitzer PB, et al: Outcomes of group cognitive behavioral training in the treatment of panic disorder and agoraphobia. J American Psychiatric Nurses Assoc 1(3):83–91, 1995

34. Sheikh JI: Anxiety disorders. In Coffecy CE, Cummings JL, Lovell MR, Pearlson GD: Textbook of Geriatric Neuropsychiatry. Washington, DC: American Psychiatric Press, 1994

35. Sheikh JI: Anxiety disorders and their treatment. Clinics in Geriatric Medicine 8(2):411–426, 1992

36. Sipprelle RC: A vet center experience: Multievent trauma, delayed treatment type. In Foy, DW, ed: Treating PTSD: Cognitive-Behavioral Strategies. NY: Guilford Press, 1992

37. Southwick SM, Bremner D, Krystal JH, Charner DS: Psychobiologic research in post-traumatic stress disorder. Psychiatric Clinics of North America 17(20):251–264, 1994

38. Stein MB, Uhde TW: Biology of anxiety disorders. In Schatzberg AF, Nemeroff CB, eds: The American Psychiatric Press Textbook of Psychopharmacology. Washington, DC: American Psychiatric Press, 1995

39. Stemberger, RT et al: Social Phobia: an analysis of possible developmental factors. J Abnormal Psychology 104(3):526–531, 1995
40. Sutherland S, Davidson JRT: Pharmacotherapy for Post-Traumatic Stress Disorder. Psychiatric Clinics of North Amer 17(2):409–423, 1994
41. Tanaka K: Post-trauma response. In McFarland GK, Thomas MD: Psychiatric Mental Health Nursing. Philadelphia: JB Lippincott, 1991
42. Tanaka K: Development of a tool for assessing Posttrauma Response. Archives Psychiatric Nursing II(6):350–356, 1988
43. Taylor CB: Treatment of anxiety disorders. In Schatzberg AF, Nemeroff CB, eds: The American Psychiatric Press Textbook of Psychopharmacology. Washington, DC: American Psychiatric Press, 1995
44. Tomb DA. The phenomenology of post-traumatic stress disorder. Psychiatric Clinics of North America 17(2):237–250, 1994
45. Tollefson GD: Selective serotonin reuptake inhibitors.In Schatzberg AF, Nemeroff CB, eds: The American Psychiatric Press Textbook of Psychopharmacology. Washington, DC: American Psychiatric Press, 1995
46. Turner DM: Panic disorder: A personal and nursing perspective. Journal of Psychosocial Nursing and Mental Health Services 33(4):5–8, 1995
47. van der Kolk BA: Group psychotherapy with Posttraumatic Stress Disorder. In Kaplan HI, Sadock BJ: Comprehensive Group Psychotherapy, 3rd ed. Baltimore: Williams & Wilkins, 1993
48. Wells BG, Hayes PE: Obsessive-Compulsive Disorder. In DiPiro JT, Talbert RL, Hayes PE, Yee GC, Matzke GR, Posey LM, eds: Pharmacotherapy: A Pathophysiologic Approach, 2nd ed. Norwalk, CT: Appleton & Lange, 1993
49. Whitley G: Expert validation and differentiation of the nursing diagnoses anxiety and fear. Nurs Diagn 5:143–150, 1994
50. Whitley G: Anxiety (Mild, Moderate, Severe, Extreme/Panic). In McFarland GK, Thomas MD: Psychiatric Mental Health Nursing. Philadelphia: JB Lippincott, 1991
51. Whitley G: Ritualistic Behavior. In McFarland GK, Thomas MD: Psychiatric Mental Health Nursing. Philadelphia: JB Lippincott, 1991

Chapter 12

1. American Psychiatric Association: DSM-IV, Diagnostic and Statistical Manual of Mental Disorders Criteria, 4th ed. Washington, DC: American Psychiatric Association, 1994
2. Barsky AJ: Hypochondriasis and obsessive compulsive disorder. Psychiatr Clin North Am 15(4):791–801, 1992
3. Barsky AJ: Hypochondriasis: Clinical management and psychiatric treatment. Psychosomatics 37(1):48–56, 1996
4. Barsky AJ, Coeytaux RR, Sarnie MK, Cleary PD: Hypochondriacal patients' beliefs about good health. Am J Psychiatry 150(7): 1085–1089, 1993
5. Campo JV, Fritsch SI: Somatization in children and adolescents. J Am Acad Child Adolesc Psychiatry 33(9):223–1235, 1994
6. Chapman S: Outpatient chronic pain management programs. In Tollison CD, Satterthwaite JR, Tollison JW, eds: Handbook of Pain Management, 2nd ed. Baltimore: Williams & Wilkins, 1994
7. Escobar JI: Transcultural aspects of dissociative and somatoform disorder. Psychiatric Clin North Am 18(3):550–559, 1995

8. Escobar JI, et al.: Somatic symptoms after a natural disaster: A prospective study. Am J Psychiatry 149(7):965–967, 1992

9. Gabbard GO, ed: Treatments of Psychiatric Disorders, 2nd ed. Vol. 2. Washington, DC: American Psychiatric Press, 1995

10. Goodman B: When the Body Speaks Its Mind: A Psychiatrist Probes the Mysteries of Hypochondria Munchausen's Syndrome. New York: GP Putnam's Sons, 1994

11. Gothe C, Odont, CM, Nilsson CG: The environmental somatization syndrome. Psychosomatics 36(l):1–11, 1995

12. Guarnaccia PJ, Good BJ, Kleinman A: Epidemiologic studies of Puerto Rican mental health. In Mezzich JE, Jorge MR, Salloum IM, eds: Psychiatric Epidemiology: Assessment Concepts and Methods. Baltimore: John Hopkins University Press, 1994

13. Kaplan HI, Sadock BJ, Grebb JA, eds: Synopsis of Psychiatry, 7th ed. Baltimore: Williams & Wilkins, 1994

14. Keefe FJ: Behavior and cognitive-behavioral approaches to chronic pain: Recent advances and future directions. J Consult Clin Psychol 60(4):528–536, 1992

15. Kim MJ, McFarland GK, McLane AM, eds: Pocket Guide to Nursing Diagnoses, 6th ed. St. Louis: Mosby, 1995

16. Kimerling R, Calhoun KS: Somatic symptoms, social support, and treatment seeking among sexual assault victims. J Consult Clin Psychol 62(2):333–340, 1994

17. King SA, Stoudemire A: Pain disorders. In Gabbard GO, ed: Treatment of Psychiatric Disorders, 2nd ed. Washington, DC: American Psychiatric Press, 1995

18. King SA, Strain JJ: Pain disorders. In Hales RE, Yudofsky SC, eds: American Psychiatric Press Textbook of Psychiatry, 2nd ed. Washington, DC: American Psychiatric Press, 1994

19. Kirmayer LJ, Robbins JM, Dworkind M, Yaffe MJ: Somatization and the recognition of depression and anxiety in primary care. Am J Psychiatry 150(5):734–741, 1993

20. Lipsitt DR: Hypochondriasis and body dysmorphic disorder. In Gabbard GO, ed: Treatment of Psychiatric Disorders, 2nd ed. Washington, DC: American Psychiatric Press, 1995

21. Lloyd GC: Psychiatry in general medicine. In Kendell RE, Zealley AK, eds. Companion to Psychiatric Studies, 5th ed. Edinburgh: Churchill Livingstone, 1993

22. Maxmen JS: Essential Psychopathology and Its Treatment, 2nd ed, rev. for DSM-IV. New York: WW Norton, 1994

23. McCloskey JC, Bulechek GM, ed: Nursing Interventions Classification (NIC) , 2nd ed. St. Louis: Mosby, 1995

24. Pavalonis D, DeCarr M, Shultz MS: Nursing roles for chronic pain management in the seriously mentally ill. J Am Psychiatr Nurs Assoc 1(4):107–111, 1995.

25. Phillips KA: Body dysmorphic disorder: The distress of imagined ugliness. Am J Psychiatry 148(9):1138–1149, 1991

26. Pliskin KL: Dysphoria and somatization in Iranian culture. West J Med 157(3):295–300, 1992

27. Roberts SJ: Somatization in primary care. The common presentation of psychosocial problems through physical complaints. Nurs Pract 19(5):47, 50–56, 1994

28. Rogler LH, Cortes DE, Malgady RG: The mental health relevance of idioms of distress. Anger and perceptions of injustice among New York Puerto Ricans. J Nerv Ment Dis 182(6):327–330, 1994

29. Rosen JC, Reiter J, Orosan P: Cognitive-behavioral body image therapy for body dysmorphic disorder. J Consult Cl Psychol 63(2):263–269, 1995

30. Ryan CM, Morrow LA: Dysfunctional buildings or dysfunctional people: An examination of the sick building syndrome and allied disorders. J Consult Clin Psychol 60(2):220–224, 1992

31. Saxe GN, et al: Somatization in patients with dissociative disorders. Am J Psychiatry 151(9):1329–1334, 1994

32. Simon GE, VonKorff M: Somatization and psychiatric disorder in the NIMH Epidemiologic Catchment Area study. Am J Psychiatry 148(11):1494–1500, 1991

33. Smith GR: The course of somatization and its effects on utilization of health care resources. Psychosomatics 35(3):263–267, 1994

34. Stern R, Fernandez M: Group cognitive and behavioral treatment for hypochondriasis. BMJ 303(6812):1229–1231, 1991

35. Stoudemire A, ed: Clinical Psychiatry for Medical Students, 2nd ed. Philadelphia: JB Lippincott, 1994

36. Tomb DA: Psychiatry, 5th ed. Baltimore: Williams & Wilkins, 1995

Chapter 13

1. American Psychiatric Association: Diagnostic and Statistical Manual of Mental Disorders: DSM-IV, 4th ed. Washington, DC: American Psychiatric Association, 1994

2. Eisendrath SJ: Factitious physical disorders: Treatment without confrontation. Psychosomatics 30(4):383–387, 1989

3. Folks DG: Munchausen's Syndrome and other factitious disorders. Neurologic Clinics 13(2):267–281,1995

4. Gerety EK, McFarland GK: Personal identity disturbance. In Thompson JM, McFarland GK, Hirsch JE, Tucker SM: Mosby's Clinical Nursing, 3rd ed. St. Louis: Mosby–Year Book, 1993

5. Guziec J, Lazarus A, Harding JJ: Case of a 29-year-old nurse with factitious disorder: The utility of psychiatric intervention on a general medical floor. Gen Hosp Psychiatry 16:47–43, 1994

6. Kaplan HI, Sadock BJ, Gregg JA: Factitious disorders. In Kaplan and Sadock's Synopsis of Psychiatry: Behavioral Sciences, Clinical Psychiatry, 7th ed. Baltimore: Williams & Wilkins, 1994

7. Kass FC: Identification of persons with Munchausen's syndrome: Ethical problems, Gen Hosp Psychiatry 7:195–200, 1985

8. Nickoloff SE, Neppe VM, Ries RK: Factitious AIDS. Psychosomatics 30(3):342–345, 1989

9. Meadow R. The history of Munchausen by Proxy. In Levin AV, Sheridan MS. Munchausen Syndrome by Proxy: Issues in Diagnosis and Treatment. New York: Lexington, 1995.

10. Pankratz L, Jackson J: Habitually wandering patients. New England J Medicine 331:1752–1755(December 29), 1994

11. Pankratz L: Continued appearance of factitious posttraumatic stress disorder [letter]. Amer J Psychiatry 147:811–812, 1990

12. Pankratz L, Lezak M: Cerebral dysfunction in the Munchausen syndrome. Hillside J Clin Psychiatry 9:195–206, 1987
13. Parker PE: A case report of Munchausen Syndrome with mixed psychological features. Psychosomatics 34(4):360–364, 1993
14. Plassmann R: Munchausen syndromes and factitious diseases. Psychother Psychosom 62:7–26, 1994
15. Plewes JM, Fagan JG: Factitious disorders and malingering. In Hales RE, Yudofsky SC, Talbott JA, eds: The American Psychiatric Press Textbook of Psychiatry, 2nd ed. Washington, DC: American Psychiatric Press, 1994
16. Reich P, Gottfried LA: Factitious disorders in a teaching hospital. Annals Internal Medicine, 99:240–247, 1983
17. Rosenberg DA: Web of deceit: A literature review of Munchausen Syndrome by Proxy. Child Abuse & Neglect 11:547–563, 1987
18. Seigal M, Altmark D: Adult victims. In Levin AV, Sheridan MS. Munchausen Syndrome by Proxy: Issues in Diagnosis and Treatment. New York: Lexington, 1995
19. Schwarz K, Harding R, Harrington D, Farr B: Hospital management of a patient with intractable factitious disorder. Psychosomatics 34(3):265–267, 1993
20. Sheridan, Levin AV. Summary. In Levin AV, Sheridan MS: Munchausen Syndrome by Proxy: Issues in Diagnosis and Treatment. New York: Lexington, 1995
21. Smith NJ, Ardern MH: "More in sickness than in health": A case study of Munchausen by Proxy in the elderly. J Family Therapy 11:321–334, 1989
22. Snowden J, Solomons R, Druce H: Feigned bereavement: Twelve cases. Br J Psychiat 133:15–19, 1978
23. Sparr L, Pankratz L: Factitious posttraumatic stress disorder. Amer J Psychiatry 140:8:1016–1019, 1983
24. Spivak H, Rodin G, Sutherland A: The psychology of factitious disorders: A reconsideration. Psychosomatics 35(1):25–34, 1994
25. Yorker BC, Kahan BB: Munchausen's Syndrome by Proxy as a form of child abuse. Archives of Psychiatric Nursing IV(5):313–318, 1990

Chapter 14

1. American Psychiatric Association: Diagnostic Criteria From DSM-IV. Washington, DC: American Psychiatric Association, 1994
2. Halm MA: The impact of technology on patients and families. Nurs Clin North Am 28(21):443–457, 1993
3. Hornstein NL, Putnam FW: Clinical phenomenology and adolescent dissociation disorders. J Am Acad Child Adolesc Psychiatry 31(6): 1077–1085, 1992
4. Hulse JR: Humor: A nursing intervention for the elderly. Geriatr Nurs 15(2):88–90, 1994
5. Kaplan HI, Sadock BJ, Grebb JA, eds: Synopsis of Psychiatry, 7th ed. Baltimore: Williams and Wilkins, 1994
6. Kim MJ, McFarland GK, McLane AM, eds: Pocket Guide to Nursing Diagnoses, 6th ed. St. Louis: Mosby, 1995
7. Living and working with MPD. J Psychosoc Nurs Ment Health Serv 32(8):17–22, 1994

8. McCloskey JC, Bulechek GM, ed: Nursing Interventions Classification (NIC), 2nd ed. St. Louis: Mosby, 1996

9. Nevid JS, Rathus SA, Green B: Abnormal Psychology in a Changing World, 2nd ed. Englewood Cliffs, NJ: Prentice Hall, 1994

10. Pinegar C: Screening for dissociative disorders in children and adolescents. JCAPN 8(1)5–16, 1995

11. Riley E: "I am what I am": Inpatient treatment for people with dissociative identity disorder. Capsules and Comments in Psychiatric Nursing 2(2):94–103, 1995

12. Spiegel D: Dissociation: Culture, Mind, and Body. Washington, DC: American Psychiatric Press, 1994

13. Stafford LL: Dissociation and multiple personality disorder; A challenge for psychosocial nursing. J Psychosoc Nus Ment Health Serv 31(1):15–20, 1993.

14. Stoudemire A, ed: Clinical Psychiatry for Medical Students, 2nd ed. Philadelphia: JB Lippincott, 1994

15. Tomb DA: Psychiatry, 5th ed. Baltimore: Williams and Wilkins, 1995

Chapter 15

1. Abel GG, Osborn CA: Pedophilia. In Gabbard GO, ed: Treatments of Psychiatric Disorders, Vol. II, 2nd ed. Washington, DC: American Psychiatric Press, 1995

2. Abel GG, Rouleau JL: Sexual abuses. In Levine SB, ed: Clinical sexuality. Psychiatric Clinics of North America 18(1), 1995

3. American Psychiatric Association: DSM-IV, Diagnostic and Statistical Manual of Mental Disorders Criteria, 4th ed. Washington, DC: American Psychiatric Association, 1994

4. Carney NG: Suicidal ideation and child abusers: Three case studies. Jo Psychosoc Nurs Ment Health Serv 32(11):34–46, 1994

5. Elliott DM, Smiljanich K: Sex offending among juveniles: Development and response. J Pediatr Health Care 8(3):101–105, 1994

6. George WH, Marlatt GA: Introduction. In Laws RD, ed: Relapse Prevention with Sex Offenders. New York: Guilford Press, 1989

7. Kaplan HI, Sadock BJ, Grebb JA, eds: Synopsis of Psychiatry, 7th ed. Baltimore: Williams & Wilkins, 1994

8. Kaplan HS: Sexual desire disorders (hypoactive sexual desire and sexual aversion). In Gabbard GO, ed: Treatments of Psychiatric Disorders, Vol. 2, 2nd ed. Washington, DC: American Psychiatric Press, 1995

9. Kim MJ, McFarland GK, McLane AM, eds: Pocket Guide to Nursing Diagnoses, 6th ed. St. Louis: Mosby, 1995

10. Larson NR: Female sex offenders: Can we treat them? Treatment Today 7(4):26–27, 1996

11. Lego S: Masochism: Implications for psychiatric nursing. Arch Psychiatr Nurs 6(4):224–229, 1992

12. Levine SB: Sexual Life: A Clinician's Guide. New York: Plenum Press, 1992

13. Marshall WL, Hudson SM, Ward T: Sexual deviance. In Wilson PH, ed: Principles and Practice of Relapse Prevention. New York: Guilford Press, 1992

14. Maxmen JS: Essential Psychopathology and Its Treatment, 2nd ed. New York: WW Norton, 1994

15. McCloskey JC, Bulechek GM, ed: Nursing Interventions Classification (NIC), 2nd ed. St. Louis: Mosby, 1995
16. Mena M, Binik YM: Painful coitus: A review of female dyspareunia. J Nervous Ment Dis 182(5):264–272, 1994
17. Risen CB: A guide to taking a sexual history. In Levine SB, ed: Clinical sexuality. Psychiatric Clinics of North America 18(1), 1995
18. Rosen RC, Leiblum SR: Hypoactive sexual desire. In Levine SB, ed: Clinical sexuality. Psychiatric Clinics of North America 18(1), 1995
19. Rosenbaum M: Female sexual arousal disorder and female orgasmic disorder. In Gabbard GO, ed: Treatments of Psychiatric Disorders, Vol II, 2nd ed. Washington, DC: American Psychiatric Press, 1995
20. Schiavi RC: Male erectile disorder. In Gabbard GO, ed: Treatments of Psychiatric Disorders, Vol II, 2nd ed. Washington, DC: American Psychiatric Press, 1995
21. Stoudemire A, ed: Clinical Psychiatry for Medical Students, 2nd ed. Philadelphia: JB Lippincott, 1994
22. Tomb DA: Psychiatry, 5th ed. Baltimore: Williams & Wilkins, 1995
23. Travin S, Protter B: Sexual Perversion: Integrative Treatment Approaches for the Clinician. New York: Plenum, 1993
24. Wincze JP: Sexual Dysfunction: A Guide for Assessment and Treatment. New York: Guilford Press, 1991

Chapter 16

1. American Psychiatric Association: Diagnostic and Statistical Manual of Mental Disorders: DSM-IV, 4th ed. Washington, DC: American Psychiatric Association, 1994
2. American Psychiatric Association: Practice Guideline for Eating Disorders. Washington, DC: American Psychiatric Association, 1993
3. Cahill C: Implementing an inpatient eating disorders program. Perspectives in Psychiatric Care 30(3):26–30, 1994
4. Childs-Clarke A: Nursing care of bulimia with cognitive behavioural therapy. Nursing Times 90(40):40–42, 1994
5. Conrad N, Sloan S, Jedwabny J: Resolving the control struggle on an eating disorders unit. Perspectives in Psychiatric Care 28(3):13–18, 1992
6. de Zwaan M, Mitchell JE: Medical complications of anorexia nervosa and bulimia nervosa. In Kaplan AS, Garfinkle PE, eds: Medical Issues and the Eating Disorders: The Interface (Eating Disorders Monograph Series No. 7). New York: Brunner/Mazel, 1993
7. Fontaine KL: The conspiracy of culture: Women's issues in body size. Nursing Clin North Amer 26(3):669–676, 1991
8. Garner DM, Rosen LW: Eating disorders. In Hersen M, Ammerman RT, Sisson LA, eds: Handbook of Aggressive and Destructive Behavior in Psychiatric Patients. New York: Plenum Press, 1994
9. Gerety EK, McFarland GK: Body image disturbance. In Thompson JM, McFarland GK, Hirsch JE, Tucker SM: Mosby's Clinical Nursing, 3rd ed. St. Louis: Mosby, 1993
10. Gold E: Nursing. In Piran N, Kaplan AS, eds: A Day Hospital Group Treatment Program for Anorexia Nervosa and Bulimia Nervosa (Eating Disorders Monograph Series No. 3). New York: Brunner/Mazel, 1990

11. Halmi KA: Eating disorders: Anorexia nervosa, bulimia nervosa, and obesity. In Hales RE, Yudofsky SC, Talbott JA, eds: American Psychiatric Textbook of Psychiatry. Washington, DC: American Psychiatric Press, 1994

12. Hock HW et al: Impact of urbanization on detection rates of eating disorders. Am J Psychiatry 152(9):1272–1278, 1995

13. Hoffman L, Halmi K: Psychopharmacology in the treatment of anorexia nervosa and bulimia nervosa. Psychiatric Clin North Am 16(4):767–778, 1993

14. Hofland SL, Dardis PO: Bulimia nervosa: Associated physical problems. J Psychosoc Nurs Ment Health Serv 30(2):23–27, 1992

15. Horne RL, Van Vactor JC, Emerson S: Disturbed body image in patients with eating disorders. Am J Psychiatry 148(2):211–215, 1991

16. Jensen H: Bulimia Nervosa: Predictor of recovery and treatment intervention. J Health Education 25(6):338–341, 1994

17. Kaplan AS: Medical and nutritional assessment. In Kaplan AS, Garfinkle PE, eds: Medical Issues and the Eating Disorders: The Interface (Brunner/Mazel Eating Disorders Monograph Series No. 7). New York: Brunner/Mazel, 1993

18. Karch AM: 1996 Lippincott's Nursing Drug Guide. Philadelphia: JB Lippincott, 1996

19. Kennedy SH, Shapiro C: Medical management of the hospitalized patient. In Kaplan AS, Garfinkle PE, eds: Medical Issues and the Eating Disorders: The Interface (Eating Disorders Monograph Series No. 7). New York: Brunner/Mazel, 1993

20. Kerr AG, Piran N: Comprehensive group treatment program. In Piran N, Kaplan AS, eds: A Day Hospital Group Treatment Program for Anorexia Nervosa and Bulimia Nervosa (Eating Disorders Monograph Series No. 3). New York: Brunner/Mazel, 1990

21. Leach AM: The psychopharmacotherapy of eating disorders. Psychiatric Annals 25(10):628–633, 1995

22. Love CC, Seaton H: Eating disorders: Highlights of nursing assessment and therapeutics. Nursing Clin North Am 26(3):677–697, 1991

23. Meades S: Suggested community psychiatric nursing interventions with clients suffering from anorexia nervosa and bulimia nervosa. J Advanced Nurs 18(3):364–370, 1993

24. Michielli DW, Dunbar CC, Kalinski MI: Is exercise indicated for the patient diagnosed as anorectic? J Psychosoc Nurs Ment Health Serv 32(8):33–35, 48–49, 1994

25. Miller DAF, McCluskey-Fawcett K, Irving LM: Correlates of bulimia nervosa: Early family mealtime experiences. Adolescence 28(111):621–635, 1993

26. Miller KD: Body-image therapy. Nurs Clin North Am 26(3):727–736, 1991

27. Morofka V: Mental health. In Thompson JM, McFarland GK, Hirsch JE, Tucker SM: Mosby's Clinical Nursing, 3rd ed. St. Louis: Mosby Year Book, 1993

28. Myer SA, O'Brien A: Multisystem complications of bulimia: A critical care case. DCCN 12(4):194–203, 1993

29. North American Nursing Diagnosis Association: NANDA Nursing Diagnoses: Definitions & Classification, 1995–1996. Philadelphia: NANDA, 1994

30. Olivardia R et al: Eating disorders in college men. Am J Psychiatry 152(9):1279–1285, 1995

31. Piran N: Treatment model and program overview. In Piran N, Daplan AS, eds: A Day Hospital Group Treatment Program for Anorexia Nervosa and Bulimia Nervosa (Eating Disorders Monograph Series No. 3). New York: Brunner/Mazel, 1990

32. Riley ER: Eating disorders as addictive behavior: Integrating 12-step programs into treatment planning. Nurs Clin North Am 26(3):715–726, 1991

33. Stein KF: The self-schema model: A theoretical approach to the self-concept in eating disorders. Arch Psychiatr Nurs X(2):96–109, 1996

34. Weiss MG: Eating disorders and disordered eating in different cultures. Psychiatric Clin North Am 18(3):537–553, 1995

35. Weltzin TE, Fernstrom MH, Fermstrom JD: Acute tryptophan depletion and increased food intake and irritability in bulimia nervosa. Am J Psychiatry 152(11):1668–1671, 1995

36. White JH: Women and eating disorders. AWHONNS Clinical Issues Perinatal Women's Health Nurs 4(2):227–235, 1993

37. Woodside DB: Genetic contributions to eating disorders. In Kaplan AS, Garfinkle PE, eds: Medical Issues and the Eating Disorders: The Interface (Eating Disorders Monograph Series No. 7). New York: Brunner/Mazel, 1993

Chapter 17

1. Alward RR: Part 4, Sleep as a circadian rhythm: The impact of shiftwork. American Nurse 27(2):20–21, 1995

2. American Psychiatric Association: Diagnostic and Statistical Manual of Mental Disorders, DSM-IV, 4th ed. Washington, DC: American Psychiatric Association, 1994

3. Andreasen NC, Black DW: Introductory Textbook of Psychiatry, 2nd ed. Washington, DC: American Psychiatric Press, 1995

4. Bliwise DL, Hughes M, McMahon PM, Kutner N: Observed sleep/wakefulness and severity of dementia in an Alzheimer's Disease Special Care Unit. Journal of Gerontology 50A(6):303–306, 1995

5. Cannard G: On the scent of a good night's sleep. Nursing Standard 9(34):21, 1995

6. Chokroverty S: An approach to a patient with sleep complaints. In Chokroverty S: Sleep Disorders Medicine: Basic Science, Technical Considerations and Clinical Aspects. Boston: Butterworth-Heinemann, 1994

7. Dowling G: Part 5. Sleep problems in older adults. American Nurse 27(3):24–25, 1995

8. Dudas S. Kim MJ: Sleep pattern disturbance. In Kim MJ, McFarland GK, McLane AM: Pocket Guide to Nursing Diagnoses, 6th ed. St. Louis: Mosby, 1995

9. Duxbury J: Avoiding disturbed sleep in hospitals. Nursing Standard 9(10):31–34, 1994

10. Fitzsimmons L. Verderber A, Shively M: Enhancing sleep following coronary artery bypass graft surgery. J Cardiovasc Nurs 7(2):86–89, 1993

11. Floyd JA: Another look at napping in order adults. Geriatric Nursing 16(3):136–138, 1995

12. Floyd JA: The use of across-method triangulation in the study of sleep concerns in healthy older adults. Adv Nurs Sci 16(2):70–80, 1993

13. Foreman MD, Wykle M: Nursing standard-of-practice protocol: Sleep disturbances in elderly patients. Geriatric Nursing 16(5):238–243, 1995

14. Frances A, First MB, Pincus HA: DSM-IV Guidebook. Washington, DC: American Psychiatric Press, 1995
15. Jensen DP, Herr KA: Sleeplessness. Advances in Clinical Nursing Research 28(2):385–405, 1993
16. Johnson AH, Wise MS, Jimmerson KR: The nurse practitioner's role in a pediatric sleep clinic. Journal of Pediatric Health Care 9(4):162–166, 1995
17. Kim MJ, McFarland GK, McLane AM: Pocket Guide to Nursing Diagnoses, 6th ed. St. Louis: Mosby, 1995
18. Knapp M: Night shift: The restorative sleep specialists. J Gerontological Nursing 19(5):38–42, 1993
19. Kryger MH, Roth T, Dement WC, eds: Principles and Practice of Sleep Medicine, 2nd ed. Philadelphia: WB Saunders, 1994
20. Kupfer DJ, Buysse DJ, Nofzinger EA, Reynolds CF: Sleep disorders. In Widiger TA, Frances AJ, Pincus HA, First MB, Ross R, Davis W: DSM-IV Sourcebook, Vol. 1. Washington, DC: American Psychiatric Association, 1994
21. Lee KA: Part 6. Sleep in infants, young children and adolescents. American Nurse 27(3):26–27, 1995
22. Lynch S, Priest R: Treating insomnia: Fitting the therapy to the cause. Prescriber March 5:37–52, 1992
23. McCall WV: Management of primary sleep disorders among elderly persons. Psychiatric Services 46(1):49–54, 1995
24. Mirka T, Rukholm E: Understanding postoperative psychosis ad sleep deprivation: A case approach. Canadian Journal of Cardiovascular Nursing. 3(4):3–5, 1993
25. Morin CM: Insomnia: Psychological Assessment and Management. New York: Guilford Press, 1993
26. North American Nursing Diagnosis Association: Nursing Diagnoses: Definitions and Classification 1995–1996. Philadelphia: NANDA, 1994
27. Neylan TC, Reynolds CF, Kupfer DJ: Sleep disorders. In Hales RE, Yudofsky SC, Talbott JA, eds: The American Psychiatric Press Textbook of Psychiatry, 2nd ed. Washington, DC: American Psychiatric Press, 1994
28. Othmer E, Othmer SC: The Clinical Interview Using DSM-IV. Volume 1: Fundamentals. Washington, DC: American Psychiatric Press, 1994
29. Prinz P, Vitiello M, et al: Geriatrics: sleep disorders and aging. N Engl J Med 323:520–526, 1990
30. Pulling C: Sleep: A reality or dream for the hospitalized adult? Canadian Journal of Cardiovascular Nursing 3(4):7–12, 1993
31. Reynolds CF, Kupfer DJ, Buysse DJ. Coble PA, Fasiczka A: Subtyping DSM-III-R Primary Insomnia. In Widiger TA, Frances AJ, Pincus HA, First MB, Ross R, Davis W: DSM-IV Sourcebook, Vol. 1. Washington, DC: American Psychiatric Association, 1994
32. Satlin A: Sleep disorders in dementia. Psychiatric Annals 24:186–191, 1994
33. Shaver JLF, Landis CA: Part 1, Understanding the behavior of sleep. American Nurse October 1994
34. Shaver JLF, Landis CA: Part 3, Helping people manage primary insomnia. American Nurse 27(1):22–23, 1995
35. Shaver JLF, Rodgers AE: Part 2, Screening for sleep-related disorders: Sleep apnea and narcolepsy. American Nurse November/December, 1994
36. Southwell MT: Sleep in hospitals at night: Are patients' needs being met? Journal of Advanced Nursing 21(6):1101–1109, 1995
37. Spenceley SM: Sleep inquiry: A look with fresh eyes. IMAGE: Journal of Nursing Scholarship 25(3):249–256, 1993

38. Wieseke A, Twibell R, et al: A content validation study of the nursing diagnoses by critical care nurses. Heart and Lung 23(4):345–351, 1994

39. Wood AM: A review of literature relating to sleep in hospital with emphasis on the sleep of the ICU patient. Intensive and Critical Care Nursing 9(2):129–136, 1993

40. Wooten V: Sleep disorders in geriatric patients. Clinics in Geriatric Medicine 8(2):427–439, 1992

41. Yarcheski A, Mahon NE: A study of sleep during adolescence. Journal of Pediatric Nursing 9(6):357–366, 1994

Chapter 18

1. American Psychiatric Association: DSM-IV Diagnostic and Statistical Manual of Mental Disorders Criteria, 4th ed. Washington, DC: American Psychiatric Association, 1994

2. Corrigan PW, Yudofsky SC, Silver JM: Pharmacological and behavioral treatments for aggressive psychiatric inpatients. Hosp Community Psychiatry 44(2): 125–133, 1993

3. Gold KL: Pyromania. Treatment Today 7(4):14–15, 1996

4. Goldman MJ: Kleptomania: Making sense of the nonsensical. Am J Psychiatry 148(8):986–996, 1991.

5. Kaplan HI, Sadock BJ, Grebb JA, eds: Synopsis of Psychiatry, 7th ed. Baltimore: Williams & Wilkins, 1994

6. Kim MJ, McFarland GK, McLane AM, eds: Pocket Guide to Nursing Diagnoses, 6th ed. St. Louis: Mosby, 1995

7. Lancee WJ, et al: The relationship between nurses' limit-setting styles and anger in psychiatric inpatients. Psychiatric Services 46(6) 609–613, 1995

8. Lion JR, Scheinberg AW: Disorders of impulse control. In Gabbard GO, ed: Treatments of Psychiatric Disorders. Washington, DC: American Psychiatric Press, 1995

9. McCloskey JC, Bulechik GM, ed: Nursing Interventions Classification (NIC), 2nd ed. St. Louis: Mosby, 1995

10. McCown W, VandenBos GR: Treating the impulsive patient. Hosp Community Psychiatry 45(11):1075–1077, 1994

11. Maxmen JS: Essential Psychopathology and Its Treatment, 2nd ed. New York: WW Norton, 1994

12. Selzer J: Borderline omnipotence in pathological gambling. Arch Psychiatric Nurs 6(4):215–218, 1992

13. Wise MG, Tierney JG: Impulse control disorders not elsewhere classified. In Hales RE, Yudolsky SC, Talbott JA, eds: The American Psychiatric Press Textbook of Psychiatry, 2nd ed. Washington, DC: American Psychiatric Press, 1994

Chapter 19

1. American Psychiatric Association: Diagnostic and Statistical Manual of Mental Disorders, DSM-IV, 4th ed. Washington, DC: American Psychiatric Association, 1994

2. Andreasen NC, Black DW: Introductory Textbook of Psychiatry, 2nd ed. Washington, DC: American Psychiatric Press, 1995

3. Antai-Otong D, Kongable G: Psychiatric Nursing: Biological and Behavioral Concepts. Philadelphia: WB Saunders, 1995
4. Asnis GM, Friedman TA, Sanderson WC, Kaplan ML: Suicidal behaviors in adult psychiatric outpatients, I: Description and prevalence. Am J Psychiatry 150(1):108–112, 1993
5. Carroll R: Mourning: A concern for medical-surgical nurses. Medsurg Nurs 2(4):301–303, 1993
6. Copeland JRM, Abou-Saleh MT, Blazer DG, eds: Principles and Practice of Geriatric Psychiatry. New York: John Wiley & Sons, 1994
7. Costello J: Helping relatives cope with grieving process. Prof Nurse 11(2):89–92, 1995
8. Drench ME: Changes in body image secondary to disease and injury. Rehabil Nurs 19(1):31–36, 1994
9. Dunner DL: Current Psychiatric Therapy. Philadelphia: WB Saunders, 1993
10. Engel G: Grief and grieving. AJN 64(9):93–98, 1964
11. Fortinash KM, Holoday-Worret PA: Psychiatric Nursing Care Plans, 2nd ed. St. Louis: Mosby, 1995
12. Frances A, First MB, Pincus HA: DSM-IV Guidebook. Washington, DC: American Psychiatric Press, 1995
13. Gabbard GO, ed: Treatments of Psychiatric Disorders, Vol 2. Washington, DC: American Psychiatric Press, 1995
14. Gamlin R, Kinghorn S: Using hope to cope with loss and grief. Nurs Stand 9(48):33–35, 1995
15. Gerety EK, McFarland GK: Anticipatory grieving, dysfunctional grieving. In McFarland GK, McFarlane EA: Nursing Diagnosis and Intervention: Planning for Patient Care. St. Louis: CV Mosby, 1994
16. Gerety EK: Grieving, anticipatory grieving, dysfunctional grieving. In McFarland GK, Thomas MC: Psychiatric Mental Health Nursing. Philadelphia: JB Lippincott, 1991
17. Glaser B, Strauss A: Awareness of Dying. Chicago: Aldine Publishing, 1968
18. Glaser B, Strauss A: Time for Dying. Chicago: Aldine Publishing, 1968
19. Greenberg WM, Rosenfeld DN, Ortega EA: Adjustment disorder as an admission diagnosis. An J Psychiatry 152(3):459–461, 1995
20. Heiney SP, Dunaway NC, Webster J: Good grieving: An intervention program for grieving children. Oncol Nurs Forum 22(4):649–655, 1995
21. Holahan CJ, Moos RH: Life stressors and mental health: advances in conceptualizing stress resistance. In Avison WR, Gotlib IH: Stress and Mental Health: Contemporary Issues and Prospects for the Future. New York: Plenum Press, 1994
22. Jacob SR: An analysis of the concept of grief. J Adv Nurs 18(11):1787–1794, 1993
23. Kim MJ, McFarland GK, McLane AM: Pocket Guide to Nursing Diagnoses, 6th ed. St. Louis: Mosby, 1995
24. Kovacs M, Ho V, Pollock MH: Criterion and predictive validity of the diagnosis of adjustment disorder: A prospective study of youths with new-onset insulin-dependent diabetes mellitus. Am J Psychiatry 152(4):523–528, 1995
25. Kübler-Ross E: On Death and Dying. New York: Macmillan, 1969
26. Leinhaas MA, Hedstrom NJ: Low vision: How to assess and treat its emotional impact. Geriatrics 49(5):53–56, 1994

27. Lindemann E: Symptomatology and management of acute grief. Am J Psychiatry 101(2):141–148, 1944

28. Lloyd-Williams M: Bereavement referrals to a psychiatric service: An audit. Eur J Cancer Care 4(1):17–19, 1995

29. McFarland GK, Gerety EK: Dysfunctional grieving. In Thompson JM, McFarland GK, Hirsch JE, Tucker SM: Mosby's Clinical Nursing, 3rd ed. St. Louis: Mosby, 1993

30. McFarland GK, Wasli EL, Gerety EK: Nursing Diagnoses and Process in Psychiatric Mental Health Nursing, 2nd ed. Philadelphia: JB Lippincott, 1992

31. McLean DE, Link BG: Unraveling complexity. In Avison WR, Goitlib IH: Stress and Mental Health: Comtemporary Issues and Prospects for the Future. New York: Plenum Press, 1994

32. Mulcahey AL, Young MA: A bereavement support group for children fostering communication about grief and healing. Cancer Proct 3(3):150–156, 1995

33. North American Nursing Diagnosis Association: Nursing Diagnoses: Definitions and Classification 1995–1996. Philadelphia: NANDA, 1994

34. Noshpitz JD: Treatment for stress-related disorders. In Noshpitz JD, Coddington RD: Stressors and the Adjustment Disorders. New York: John Wiley & Sons, 1990

35. Noshpitz JD, Coddington RD: Stressors and the Adjustment Disorders. New York: John Wiley & Sons, 1990

36. Oltmanns TF, Emery RE: Abnormal Psychology. Englewood Cliffs, NJ: Prentice-Hall, 1995

37. Othmer E, Othmer SC: The Clinical Interview Using DSM-IV, Volume 2: The Difficult patient. Washington, DC: American Psychiatric Press, 1994

38. Othmer E, Otmer SC: The Clinical Interview Using DSM-IV, Volume I: Fundamentals. Washington, DC: American Psychiatric Press, 1994

39. Oxman TE, Barrett JE, Freeman DH, Manheimer E: Frequency and correlates of adjustment disorder related to cardiac surgery in older patients. Psychosomatics 35(6):557–568, 1994

40. Pies RW: Clinical Manual of Psychiatric Diagnosis and Treatment: A Biopsychosocial Approach. Washington, DC: American Psychiatric Press, 1994

41. Pilkington FB: The lived experience of grieving the loss of an important other. Nurs Sci Q 6(3):130–139, 1993

42. Razavi D, Stiefel F: Common psychiatric disorders in cancer patients. I. Adjustment disorders and depressive disorders. Support Care Cancer 2(4):223–232, 1994

43. Shives LR: Basic Concepts of Psychiatric-Mental Health Nursing, 3rd ed. Philadelphia: JB Lippincott, 1994

44. Skodol AE, Dohrenwend BP, Link BG, Shrout PE: The nature of stress: Problems of measurement. In Noshpitz JD, Coddington RD, eds: Stressors and the Adjustment Disorders. New York: John Wiley & Sons, 1990

45. Steeves RH, Kahn DL, Wise CT, Baldwin AS, Edlich RF: Tasks of bereavement for burn center staffs. J Burn Care Rehabil 14(3):386–397, 1993

46. Stolberg AL, Mahler J: Enhancing treatment gains in a school-based intervention for children of divorce through skill training, parental involvement, and transfer procedures. J Consult Clin Psychol 62(1):147–156, 1994

47. Strain JJ, Newcorn J, Wolf D, Fulop G: Adjustment disorder. In Hales RE, Yudofsky SC, Tablott JA, eds: The American Psychiatric Press Textbook of Psychiatry, 2nd ed. Washington. DC: American Psychiatric Press, 1994

48. Strain JJ: Adjustment disorders. In Gabbard GO. ed: Treatment of Psychiatric Disorders, 2nd ed. Washington, DC: American Psychiatric Press, 1995

49. Townsend MC: Psychiatric/Mental Health Nursing: Concepts of Care. Philadelphia: FA Davis, 1993

Chapter 20

1. American Psychiatric Association: DSM-IV, Diagnostic and Statistical Manual of Mental Disorders Criteria, 4th ed. Washington, DC: American Psychiatric Association, 1994

2. Black DW, Baumgard CH, Bell SE: A 16- to 45-year follow-up of 71 men with antisocial personality disorder. Comprehensive Psychiatry 36(2):130–140, 1995

3. Bornstein RF: The Dependent Personality. New York: Guilford Press, 1993

4. Dresser J & Doyne JL: Borderline personality disorders: Strategies for interrupting self-mutilation. Paper presented at Psychiatric Nursing `95, Gerontological Nursing `95, May 17–19, 1995 Philadelphia, PA.

5. Gabbard GO: Psychodynamic Psychiatry in Clinical Practice, DSM-IV Edition. Washington, DC: American Psychiatric Press, 1994

6. Gabbard GO, Wilkinson SM: Management of Countertransference with Borderline Patients. Washington, DC: American Psychiatric Press, 1994

7. Gallop R: Self-destructive and impulsive behavior in the patient with a borderline personality disorder: Rethinking hospital treatment and management. Arch Psychiatr Nurs 6(3):178–182, 1992

8. Greene H, Ugarriza DN: The "stably unstable" borderline personality disorder: History, theory, and nursing intervention. J Psychosoc Nurs Mental Health Serv 33(12):26–30, 1995

9. Groopman LC, Cooper AM: Narcissistic personality disorder. In Gabbard GO, ed: Treatments of Psychiatric Disorders, Vol II, 2nd ed. Washington, DC: American Psychiatric Press, 1995

10. Gunderson JG & Links P: Borderline personality disorder. In Gabbard GO, ed: Treatments of Psychiatric Disorders, Vol II, 2nd ed. Washington, DC: American Psychiatric Press, 1995

11. Horowitz MJ: Histrionic personality disorder. In Gabbard GO, ed: Treatment of Psychiatric Disorders, Vol II, 2nd ed. Washington, DC: American Psychiatric Press, 1995

12. Kantor M: Distancing. A Guide to Avoidance and Avoidant Personality Disorder. Westport, CT: Praeger, 1993

13. Kaplan HI, Sadock BJ, Grebb JA, eds: Synopsis of Psychiatry, 7th ed. Baltimore: Williams & Wilkins, 1994

14. Kim MJ, McFarland GK, McLane AM, eds: Pocket Guide to Nursing Diagnoses, 6th ed. St. Louis: Mosby, 1995

15. Lewis CE: Neurochemical mechanism of chronic antisocial behavior (psychopathy): A literature review. J Nerv and Ment Dis 179(2):720–727, 1991

16. Linehan MM: Skills Training for Treating Borderline Personality Disorders. New York: Guilford Press, 1993

17. Linehan MM, et al: Interpersonal outcome of cognitive behavioral treatment for chronically suicidal borderline patients. Am J Psychiatry 151(12):1771–1776, 1994

18. Lyons MJ: Epidemiology of personality disorders. In Tsuang MT, Tohen M, Zahner GEP, eds: Textbook in Psychiatric Epidemiology. New York: John Wiley, 1995

19. Marziak E, Munroe-Blum H: Interpersonal Group Psychotherapy for Borderline Personality Disorder. New York: Basic Books, 1994

20. Masterson JF, Klein R, eds: Disorders of the Self, New Therapeutic Horizons. The Masterson Approach. New York: Brunner/Mazel, 1995

21. Maxmen JS: Essential Psychopathology and Its Treatment, 2nd ed. New York: W.W. Norton, 1994

22. McCloskey JC, Bulechek GM, ed: Nursing Interventions Classification, 2nd ed. St. Louis: Mosby, 1994

23. Meissner WW: Paranoid personality disorder. In Gabbard GO, ed: Treatments in Psychiatric Disorders, Vol. II, 2nd ed. Washington, DC: American Psychiatric Press, 1995

24. Meloy JR: Antisocial personality disorder. In Gabbard GO, ed: Treatments in Psychiatric Disorders, Vol. II, 2nd ed. Washington, DC: American Psychiatric Press, 1995

25. McCullough PK, Maltsberger JT: Obsessive-compulsive personality disorder. In Gabbard GO, ed: Treatments of Psychiatric Disorders, Vol. II, 2nd ed. Washington, DC: American Psychiatric Press, 1995

26. Miller SG: Borderline personality disorder from the patient's perspective. Hosp Community Psychiatry 45(12):1215–1219, 1994

27. Millon T: An Integrative Theory of Personality and Psychopathology. Personality and Psychopathology: Building a Science. Selected Papers of Theodore Millon. New York: John Wiley, 1996

28. Nehls N: Group therapy for people with borderline personality disorder: Interventions associated with positive outcomes. Issues Ment Health Nurs 13(3):255–269, 1992

29. Nehls N: Brief hospital treatment plans: Innovations in practice and research. Issues Ment Health Nurs 15(1):1–11, 1994

30. Norris J: Nursing interventions for self-esteem disturbances. Nursing Diagnosis 3(2):48–53, 1992

31. Perry JC: Dependent personality disorder. In Gabbard GO, ed: Treatments of Psychiatric Disorders, Vol. II, 2nd ed. Washington, DC: American Psychiatric Press, 1995

32. Shearin E, Linehan MM: Cognitive behavioral therapy for borderline personality disorders. In Paris J, ed: Borderline Personality Disorder: Etiology and Treatment. Washington, DC: American Psychiatric Press, 1993

33. Siever LJ, Davis KL: A psychobiological perspective on the personality disorders. Am J Psychiatry 148 (12):1647–1658, 1991

34. Soloff PH, et al: Self-mutilation and suicidal behavior in borderline personality disorder. J Pers Disord 8:257–267, 1994

35. Stein KF: Affect instability in adults with a borderline personality disorder. Arch Psychiatr Nurs 10(1):32–40, 1996

36. Stevenson J, Mears R: An outcome study of psychotherapy for patients with borderline personality disorder. Am J Psychiatry 149(3):358–363, 1992

37. Stone M: Schizoid and schizotypal personality disorders. In Gabbard GO, ed: Treatments in Psychiatric Disorders, Vol. II, 2nd ed. Washington, DC: American Psychiatric Press, 1995

38. Stoudemire A, ed: Clinical Psychiatry for Medical Students, 2nd ed. Philadelphia: JB Lippincott, 1994
39. Sutherland SM, Frances A: Avoidant personality disorder. In Gabbard GO, ed: Treatments of Psychiatric Disorders, Vol. II, 2nd ed. Washington, DC:. American Psychiatric Press, 1995
40. Tomb DA: Psychiatry, 5th ed. Baltimore: Williams & Wilkins, 1995
41. Waldinger RJ: The role of psychodynamic concepts in the diagnosis of borderline personality disorder. Harvard Rev Psychiatry 1:158–167, 1993

Index

Page numbers followed by *f* indicate figures; those followed by *t* indicate tables.